Mi

About the Author

Ryan M. Niemiec, PsyD, (pronounced "knee-mick") is Education Director of the VIA Institute on Character, the global, nonprofit positive psychology organization that educates people about the latest science and practice of character strengths. He is a licensed psychologist, certified coach, international workshop leader, and is Adjunct Professor at Xavier University in Cincinnati, Ohio. He is co-author of *Positive Psychology at the Movies* (2014) and *Movies and Mental Illness* (2010). In 2011, Ryan received the Distinguished Early Career Award from the American Psychological Association (Division 46).

Ryan has led several hundred mindfulness meditation groups for clinical and nonclinical populations over the last decade, and has delivered mindfulness retreats, seminars, and workshops to a variety of groups, including physicians, counselors, religious leaders, and the general public.

Ryan created Mindfulness-Based Strengths Practice (MBSP) out of his ongoing passion for the two topics. MBSP marks the first, structured character strengths program and one of the first mindfulness programs to explicitly focus on what is best in people. He has enjoyed training the early pioneers in this approach.

He is a member of the mindfulness community Being Peace Sangha just outside of Cincinnati. His dharma name, in the Thich Nhat Hanh lineage, is Fullest Breath of the Heart.

Ryan's invited workshops and presentations span a number of universities and organizations, including the United States Air Force Academy, Harvard University, the University of Pennsylvania, Washington University, Universidad Iberoamericana, International Positive Psychology Association, American Psychological Association, and European Positive Psychology Association. He blogs for Psychology Today and PsychCentral, and his work has been featured by a variety of sources including Dr. Oz, USA Today, the Huffington Post, Positive Psychology News Daily, and Greater Good.

Ryan's signature strengths are hope, curiosity, love, appreciation of beauty, fairness, perspective, and gratitude. He enjoys spending time with family, playing sports, watching positive psychology movies, traveling, teaching, and collecting Pez dispensers.

Mindfulness and Character Strengths

A Practical Guide to Flourishing

Ryan M. Niemiec

VIA Institute on Character
Cincinnati, OH

Library of Congress Cataloging-in-Publication Data
is available via the Library of Congress Marc Database under the
LC Control Number 2013937860

National Library of Canada Cataloguing in Publication Data

Niemiec, Ryan M, author
    Mindfulness and character strengths : a practical guide to flourishing / Ryan Niemiec, VIA
Institute on Character, Cincinnati, OH.

Accompanied by audio CD.
Includes bibliographical references and index.
Issued in print and electronic formats.
ISBN 978-0-88937-376-1 (pbk.).--ISBN 978-1-61676-376-3 (pdf).--ISBN 978-1-61334-376-0 (epub)

    1. Meditation. 2. Attention. 3. Character. 4. Self-actualization
(Psychology). 5. Mindfulness-based cognitive therapy. I. Title.

BF637.M4N53 2013   158.1   C2013-902560-X
                                                             C2013-903356-4

© 2014 by Hogrefe Publishing

Cover illustration by Monica Watha-Niemiec © 2013

PUBLISHING OFFICES
USA: Hogrefe Publishing, 38 Chauncy Street, Suite 1002, Boston, MA 02111
                Phone (866) 823-4726, Fax (617) 354-6875; E-mail customerservice@hogrefe-
                publishing.com
EUROPE: Hogrefe Publishing, Merkelstr. 3, 37085 Göttingen, Germany
                Phone +49 551 99950-0, Fax +49 551 99950-425, E-mail publishing@hogrefe.com

SALES & DISTRIBUTION
USA: Hogrefe Publishing, Customer Services Department,
                30 Amberwood Parkway, Ashland, OH 44805
                Phone (800) 228-3749, Fax (419) 281-6883, E-mail customerservice@hogrefe.com
EUROPE: Hogrefe Publishing, Merkelstr. 3, 37085 Göttingen, Germany
                Phone +49 551 99950-0, Fax +49 551 99950-425, E-mail publishing@hogrefe.com

OTHER OFFICES
CANADA: Hogrefe Publishing, 660 Eglinton Ave. East, Suite 119 - 514, Toronto,
                Ontario M4G 2K2
SWITZERLAND: Hogrefe Publishing, Länggass-Strasse 76, CH-3000 Bern 9

Hogrefe Publishing
Incorporated and registered in the Commonwealth of Massachusetts, USA, and in Göttingen, Lower
Saxony, Germany

Printed and bound in the USA
ISBN 978-0-88937-376-1

Praise for the Book

In this remarkable book, Ryan Niemiec brings alive the synergy between the rich body of mindfulness teachings and a pioneering model for understanding character strengths. By demonstrating how mindful attention can be directed in a systematic and precise way to awaken our full potential, this guidebook makes a unique contribution to the field of transformation and spiritual awakening.

Tara Brach, PhD, author of Radical Acceptance *and* True Refuge

Mindfulness and Character Strengths is a cogent, nuanced articulation of the principles and practice of mindfulness as applied in the context of positive psychology. Ryan's rich experience as a meditation practitioner illuminates the work.

Sharon Salzberg, author of Lovingkindness, The Force of Kindness, *and* Real Happiness: The Power of Meditation, *and co-founder of the Insight Meditation Society*

By bringing together two powerful practices – mindfulness and character strengths – Ryan Niemiec has created a practical, effective, and inspiring program that can benefit individuals and organizations. Reading and applying the ideas in this book can help you fulfill your potential for happiness and success.

Tal Ben-Shahar, PhD, bestselling author of Happier *and* Being Happy

The fields of positive psychology and mindfulness have been separate for too long. This fascinating book shows how mindfulness and character strengths complement and enhance each other and describes an innovative 8-week program for anyone seeking awareness, insight, and the cultivation of the best within themselves.

Ruth A. Baer, PhD, Professor at University of Kentucky; Editor of Mindfulness-Based Treatment Approaches *and* Assessing Mindfulness and Acceptance Processes in Clients

Ryan Niemiec, with solid scholarship in both mindfulness and character strengths, has now become the first scholar to integrate these two paths of healing and growth in his book *Mindfulness and Character Strengths* to create an avenue that offers powerful healing and flourishing to many. Using his own strengths of humility, love of learning and creativity, Ryan has synthesized two relevant fields, producing a brilliant and profound mélange of ideas which gently nudge readers to observe themselves mindfully and also let their awareness not escape their innate goodness of kindness, compassion, curiosity and gratitude so they can harness their inbuilt negativity bias. Ryan's book is a unique blend of elegant ideas melded in innovative methods – all rooted in good science. It is a must read for anyone who is interested in exploring contentment – of their own and of those around them.

Tayyab Rashid, PhD, CPsych, Psychologist & Researcher, University of Toronto Scarborough, Canada

Mindfulness and Character Strengths weaves together the perennial wisdom of mindfulness with the modern scientific study of character strengths, in a beautiful tapestry that will benefit professionals across many disciplines, as well as the people whose lives they touch.

Shauna Shapiro, PhD, Associate Professor at Santa Clara University, CA and co-author of The Art and Science of Mindfulness: Integrating Mindfulness into Psychology and the Helping Professions

This book is amazing! Dr. Niemiec has both a deep understanding of mindfulness and a working expertise in the strengths-based approach of positive psychology. This book adds unique insights, and represents an important contribution to the field. The writing is both clear and detailed – I highly recommend this book.

Richard Sears, PsyD, MBA, ABPP, faculty member of the Doctor of Psychology Program at Union Institute and University and Director of the Center for Clinical Mindfulness and Meditation; lead author of Mindfulness in Clinical Practice

An excellent and very practical book that well integrates mindfulness and the development of character strengths. The book is surely to be helpful to many people from all walks of life and blends positive psychology with this important contemplative approach. Many tips and examples are well-supported with evidence-based research findings too. I'll surely recommend the book to clients, colleagues, and students, which I know will be well received and appreciated.

Thomas G. Plante, PhD, ABPP, The Augustin Cardinal Bea, S.J. University Professor and Director of Spirituality & Health Institute, Santa Clara University, CA; author of Religion, Spirituality, and Positive Psychology *and* Contemplative Practices in Action

Character strengths have been shown to be involved in a variety of positive outcomes in private and work life and their use is beneficial to adults and youth. This book goes one step further and introduces Mindfulness-Based Strengths Practice (MBSP), a program combining mindfulness and strengths that is aimed at guiding individuals and organizations to flourishing. This new book by Ryan Niemiec includes a variety of useful worksheets, exercises, homework assignments, etc. that the reader and trainee will enjoy.

Willibald Ruch, PhD, Professor of Psychology; Director of Character Strengths Lab, University of Zurich, Switzerland

For Rhys

my precious son

how might I completely express my love for you?

words alone cannot

actions alone cannot

savoring cannot

time spent cannot

mindfulness use cannot

strengths use cannot

my only hope …

is to model a life well-lived

Disclaimer Notice

The authors/editors and publisher have made every effort to ensure that the information contained in this publication is in accordance with current scientific standards and practices at the time of publication. Despite the care taken in the production and correction of the text, errors cannot be completely ruled out. The authors/editors and publisher make no representations or warranties of any kind and assume no liabilities of any kind with respect to the accuracy or completeness of the contents (procedure, therapy, amounts, doses, applications etc.) and specifically disclaim any implied warranties of merchantability or fitness of use for a particular purpose. Neither the authors/editors nor the publisher shall be held liable or responsible to any person or entity with respect to any loss or incidental or consequential damages caused, or alleged to have been caused, directly or indirectly, by the information contained herein. Trademarks and registered names are not distinguished in the text; the absence of such explicit marking does not mean that any name is not a trademarked name.

Foreword

Ryan Niemiec is one of the foremost practitioners of well-being research in the world today. I have had the good fortune of hearing him present his work on a number of occasions, both in the context of the Master of Applied Positive Psychology (MAPP) program I direct at the University of Pennsylvania and at the World Congress on Positive Psychology organized by the International Positive Psychology Association (IPPA). Our pedagogical model in the MAPP program is to include not only instruction by Martin Seligman and other faculty from the University of Pennsylvania but also to invite many of the world's leading researchers and practitioners in positive psychology and related fields to address our students directly. For several years now, we have asked Ryan to lead a module on the VIA Classification of Strengths and Virtues for our students. We have found him to be deeply informed, passionate, and compassionate in his presentations on strengths, and our students respond by giving him standing ovations.

When Ryan told me he was considering writing a book connecting strengths and mindfulness, I told him I thought it was a good idea. Now that I have had the privilege of reading the resulting book, I think it is an outstanding idea. As you will shortly see, Ryan masterfully leverages the expertise on strengths he has honed as the Education Director of the VIA Institute on Character (the nonprofit organization that funded the development of the VIA Classification) together with his extensive experience leading hundreds of mindfulness meditation groups over the last ten years. What he has accomplished as a result – and what is so beautifully illustrated on the cover – is a work of insightful integration.

Most obviously, this book integrates two evidence-based domains of well-being research and practice. Academic research tends to develop in silos, with scholars rewarded for conducting studies on a single topic or approach. Evidence-based practice all too often follows academic precedent by focusing on the delivery of a single type of in-

tervention, or by cobbling together a series of interventions. In contrast, Ryan's accomplishment here is to provide a deep practical integration of two influential lines of research. Beyond simply pointing out that both mindfulness meditation and character strengths are important for human flourishing, he argues convincingly that strengths can enhance mindfulness and that mindfulness can deepen strengths. Even more importantly, his Mindfulness-Based Strengths Practice (MBSP) program provides a detailed model for putting these insights into practice. Ryan's work constitutes an outstanding example that I hope other researchers and practitioners will follow to integrate other domains for the enhanced cultivation of human flourishing.

Less obvious, perhaps, than the integration of mindfulness and character strengths (but just as important) is the contribution Ryan's work makes toward the integration of other aspects of human flourishing that should not be separated. First is the unfortunate divide between the mind and the body. In positive psychology, many of the leading researchers come from the tradition of cognitive psychology, so it is not surprising that so many positive interventions have a cognitive emphasis. Although the body is necessary to carry out these positive interventions, it is almost always treated incidentally, with no explicit instructions on how a specific use of the body can enhance the effectiveness of the intervention. The philosopher Richard Shusterman (2012) has argued extensively that biases against the body in Western culture have constituted an obstacle to human flourishing. To counteract these biases, he founded the field of somaesthetics, which "concerns the body as a locus of sensory-aesthetic appreciation (aesthesis) and creative self-fashioning" (p. 27). One effect of Ryan's work in this present volume is to help bring the body to positive psychology practices to enhance the cultivation of human flourishing. With its great emphasis on an awareness of the body, mindfulness meditation introduces a welcome somatic dimension in work on character strengths, a dimension that is largely lacking outside of the MBSP approach.

A second general integrative contribution Ryan's work has to do with the overall orientation of psychological interventions. Kenneth Pargament (2007) has pointed out that psychology (at least in the United States) is largely a "psychology of control," since it focuses on helping people gain greater control in their lives. He contrasts this with a "psychology of acceptance," which focuses on helping people come to terms with the things in their lives they cannot control. Clearly, both of these approaches are important in the right balance. Applying this distinction to the themes of this book, it seems clear that character strengths tend to focus on helping people gain more control in their lives and mindfulness meditation tends to focus on helping people toward greater acceptance. Of course, this distinction is not absolute, since some character strengths (gratitude and spirituality, for example) seem more oriented toward acceptance, and since mindfulness relies on our ability to control our attention and may result in greater control over our behavior. By bringing strengths and mindfulness together, however, Ryan invites us to examine this distinction in greater detail and opens up possibilities for a more effective balance between control and acceptance in human life.

Finally, Ryan's work points out the value of an integration of the science of well-being and the culture of human flourishing and of the application of this integration in practice. Both the VIA Classification of strengths and virtues and mindfulness meditation demonstrate the value of a partnership between science and culture. In both these cases, advances have been made because scientists have looked to culture for an understanding of the nature of human flourishing and for ways of cultivating it. Culture has provided a wealth of wisdom and practical knowledge, and science has contributed empirical methods of inquiry that are used to document the value of this cultural treasure and to investigate the most effective ways of applying it in various contexts. These examples indicate that the quest for human flourishing must be an interdisciplinary endeavor and that it progresses best through a collaboration between science and culture, a collaboration that is moving forward in fascinating ways in a number of disciplines (Pawelski & Moores, 2013).

In sum, I believe this book is path breaking in several ways: It brings together two key elements in the quest for human flourishing; it uses an integrative approach that provides a robust model for future work in positive interventions; and it helps overcome harmful oppositions between the mind and the body, between the psychology of control and the psychology of acceptance, and between science and culture. I hope you will have an opportunity to hear Ryan present this material in person – as a part of a future MAPP class, at an upcoming IPPA World Congress on Positive Psychology, or at some other venue. In the meantime, I hope that you enjoy this book as much as I have and that you are able to put its contents to good use in your own life and in the lives of those you touch.

James O. Pawelski
April 2013

References

Pargament, K. (2007). *Spiritually integrated psychotherapy: Understanding and addressing the sacred.* New York, NY: The Guilford Press.

Pawelski, J. O., & Moores, D. J. (Eds.). (2013). *The eudaimonic turn: Well-being in literary studies.* Madison, NJ: Fairleigh Dickinson University Press.

Shusterman, R. (2012). *Thinking through the body: Essays in somaesthetics.* Cambridge, UK: Cambridge University Press.

Table of Contents

Section IV: Resources

Audio CD Tracks

Track 1   Introduction
Track 2   Body-Mindfulness Meditation
Track 3   You at Your Best and Strength-Spotting
Track 4   Character Strengths Breathing Space
Track 5   Strengths Gatha
Track 6   Loving-Kindness Meditation
Track 7   Strength-Exploration Meditation
Track 8   Fresh-Look Meditation
Track 9   Signature Strengths Breathing Space
Track 10   Best Possible Self

Preface

The faculty of bringing back a wandering attention, over and over again, is the very root of judgment, character, and will...an education which should improve this faculty would be <u>the</u> education par excellence.

William James

It's an honor to write this book.

I am on the same journey of awareness and growth as each person reading these sentences, and it is humbling to describe my observations, experiences, and understanding of the sciences and practices relating to these topics.

These topics are extraordinary ones. To merge mindfulness and character strengths is to bring a deep awareness to our best qualities and to use these qualities to improve our awareness. Mindfulness and character strengths deepen one another. Mindfulness offers *the how* for the practice of character strengths. In other words, to practice using strengths with mindfulness is to be intentional and conscious about noticing and deploying your best qualities. Character strengths draw upon mindfulness itself (e.g., curiosity, self-regulation), providing *the fuel* to help you make mindfulness an ongoing part of your daily life. Truly, this integration is a uniting of our mind and heart.

Beginnings

My formal connection and practice with mindfulness began in the 1990s when I was introduced to the work of Thich Nhat Hanh, a humble and prolific Buddhist monk. I began to read and practice the principles contained in several of his books, especially *The Miracle of Mindfulness*, *Being Peace*, and *Peace is Every Step*. His observations on tuning into the present moment struck a deep chord in me. I was astonished at how the words and the practices were simultaneously simple and deep. They were simple in that they were immediately understandable and could

be quickly applied in daily life in a meaningful way, and his words were deep in that upon reflection it was clear that they offered solid wisdom about how to live a fulfilling life. This naturally led me to the work of other popular mindfulness teachers. One of these was Jon Kabat-Zinn who wrote *Full Catastrophe Living*, a book that documents the rationale, research, and practice of the most popular mindfulness program on the planet (Mindfulness-Based Stress Reduction).

I attended mindfulness retreats and conferences and seriously studied mindfulness as espoused by both secular and nonsecular teachers (including both Buddhists and Christians), and more important, applied mindfulness in my daily life – practicing meditation, engaging in mindful walking, applying mindfulness to mundane tasks such as washing the dishes, and using mindfulness when stressed or anxious. As a psychologist, I found that mindfulness connected well with my holistic conceptualization of people, fit neatly with the emerging trend toward mind-body therapies, and offered a powerful path that could help clients who were suffering. I began to lead meditation experiences for a wide range of clients, helping professionals, and the general public, and I used these workshops to teach participants how to integrate Eastern and Western philosophies and practices. Soon, I was being invited to lead day-long mindfulness training programs for practitioners and weekend mindfulness retreats for the general public. At this time, interest in mindfulness was spreading; however, it was in its infancy stage compared to its popularity in today's world.

One day, in 2002, the late Dr. Bob Wilke, the director of the Psychology and Religion Program at Saint Louis Behavioral Medicine Institute, called me into his office. He was pleased with the success of the mindfulness groups I'd been leading for priests, nuns, friars, and other ministers. Bob pointed to a green book on his desk titled *Mindfulness-Based Cognitive Therapy for Depression,* and he said, "Ryan, I want you to *do* this in our program." Being a fairly agreeable person, trusting the director's judgment, and intrigued by the book's title, I responded, "Sure." I soon came to understand that the research and practice in this book was both solid and significant, as well as cutting-edge psychology. I studied the approach, attended workshops on the topic, continued my personal mindfulness practice, and weaved MBCT into my work.

A hybrid model was emerging in my practice – one that merged the wisdom and mindful living qualities of Thich Nhat Hanh, the structured, scientific-based approach of MBCT, and the widely applied scientific work of Jon Kabat-Zinn. I was privileged to bring mindfulness to groups and individuals, to those suffering with medical and mental illness, addictions, and everyday problems and stressors. This involved leading hundreds of groups in clinical and nonclinical settings. I was inspired by the immediate joy people often experienced, the "healing" that came about, and the excitement that was generated when someone began to grow and change as a result of implementing these new behaviors and practices.

Many years later I was hired by a nonprofit organization, the VIA Institute on Character, where I currently educate both clinicians and nonclinicians about the latest science and best practices in working with character strengths. This position allowed me to spend most of my time exploring the research on working with strengths in general as well as the latest specific research on each of the 24 character strengths, connecting with leading scientists and practitioners in the field, practicing from a strengths-based approach, and teaching practitioners around the world how to improve their work with strengths.

While conducting trainings, the topic of mindfulness as a mechanism for working with strengths repeatedly came up. In addition, the two main models for working with character strengths aware-explore-apply (Niemiec, 2013) and aware-align-appreciate (VIA Institute) each happen to begin with mindfulness. Research was documenting more and more that mindfulness could be ap-

plied successfully to help people manage a variety of problems, disorders, and struggles, and, at the same time, bring about greater balance, coping, and resources. So why not bring mindfulness explicitly to what is best in individuals? An important synergy was developing.

Despite widespread popularity, there were no programs focused exclusively on training individuals and groups on the VIA character strengths. I saw a natural opportunity and began to experiment with integrating these topics. I presented on the integration in several countries, had conversations with practitioners in each field, and developed several iterations of what eventually became Mindfulness-Based Strengths Practice (MBSP). Early versions of the program were tested by me and a handful of expert practitioners from several countries and the original data were positive (see Chapter 6). Both practitioners and clients were enthusiastic about this new approach.

MBSP is described in detail in Section III of this book.

Humble About Our Limitations

About a decade ago I was asked to be part of a mindfulness colloquium that involved professors, educators, and meditators from different disciplines along with a special presentation by a Bhikkhu. A Bhikkhu is an ordained Buddhist monastic and this particular Bhikkhu was a well-known scholar who was widely revered. The "star" of the show, the Bhikkhu, opened his candid presentation with humor and humanity. He wished to show the audience that he was a human being with normal emotions and playfulness just like everyone else. And, knowing that I, "the psychologist," was to be presenting after him, he decided to offer a joke at my expense. He commented about the limitations of the profession of psychology and added, "Psychology has been around for over 100 years and look at how much progress society has made," he quipped. The audience roared with laughter.

While I realize my profession is an easy target (just watch any movie that portrays a psychologist or psychiatrist), I wasn't happy that the monk had made no effort to clarify or explain what psychology has accomplished. Instead, he sat down, leaving the comment for further audience interpretation and potential perpetation of stereotypes.

Later, when it was my turn to present, I stood up and arranged my PowerPoint presentation to the opening slide with my credentials thus revealing my vulnerability to the Bhikkhu's earlier comment – my topic was the integration of mindfulness in psychotherapy. I turned to the audience of a few-hundred people, with my PowerPoint slide looming large over my head, and said, bowing deeply, "With all due respect to the Bhikkhu, Buddhism has been around for not 100 but 2,500 years, and look at how much progress society has made."

Perhaps my statement was not exemplary from the perspective of forgiveness and letting go but there is a message of humility in this story. We need to be humble about what has been accomplished and what remains. Mindfulness, when practiced well, beckons us to humility … to let go of a focus on ourselves and to be present to our true nature, our connectedness with others.

My comment, similar to the Bhikkhu's, was merely good-natured teasing. Indeed, both Buddhism and psychology have accomplished much over the decades (in the case of Buddhism, over the centuries). Of course, a core lesson of Buddhism is that suffering will always be present, but there are also numerous examples of successes, achievements, and goodness that can and should be celebrated.

It is important for me to express humility in regard to the topics in this book and their integration. Both science and practice have taught humanity about these areas; however, there is a substantial amount of work that still needs to be done. New research and practices are emerging and being developed each month that will continue to inform, update, and improve the integration of mindfulness and character strengths.

We All Need Support

One week I was running late for my sangha gathering (a "sangha" is a meditation community in which members support one another in their meditation practice). My sangha is a mindfulness community called Being Peace Sangha, near Cincinnati, Ohio; this particular sangha practices in the tradition of Thich Nhat Hanh.

While making a quick turn onto one of the side roads, I safely but abruptly cut off another car. As I continued to drive along, I found myself hoping the person I cut off would turn down a side-street. Instead, they continued on behind me. They were not chasing me; they were simply the car behind me on a divided road.

When I made the turn down the long quarter-mile driveway toward the sangha building, the other car turned as well. My embarrassment elevated. This was a road that dead-ended right at my destination and I would soon be face-to-face with the individual I had cut off. We got out of our cars at the same time. I recognized the man from our weekly gatherings. I initially hoped he didn't realize that I was the person who had cut him off. He smiled at me in a way that demonstrated that he sensed my embarrassment. His expression was soft, friendly, and forgiving.

I turned to him and apologized, noting: "Now you understand why I need to come to sangha?"

As mindfulness teacher, Jon Kabat-Zinn has commented, "There are not too many people I know who cannot benefit from a higher dose of awareness." This is true for me now, and I am convinced will remain true for the rest of my life.

A Harmony We Can All Hear

The topics in this book are new and old at the same time. Mindfulness has a deep, wide, and rich history, as does the study of virtues and strengths and the other positive qualities that reveal our humanness. At the same time, the scientific study of mindfulness and of character strengths are both quite young; each has a smattering of studies and important articles that date back a few decades. However, it has only been in the last decade that each has flourished, especially mindfulness.

As is common with new psychological domains that promise to help others, practice often jumps out ahead of science. This is particularly true of the science of character, which has moved along nicely for a new field; however, not nearly as rapid as the explosion of studies, programs, and practices involving mindfulness meditation.

Interestingly, almost nothing has been written on the formal integration of these two fascinating areas. Apart from an unpublished study, a blog or two, and a couple of recent publications[1], there's not much one can find on how mindfulness informs character strengths and how character strengths inform mindfulness practice. This book fills this gap.

To be sure, the history of Buddhism – the original home of mindfulness – has much to say about certain strengths such as compassion and wisdom. Over the centuries, works by Buddhist scholars and spiritual leaders generally limit their attention to one or two strengths but certainly have not made an effort to systematically go through the entire panoply of positive traits (e.g., the 24 character strengths within the VIA Classification).

formal training program of character strengths. This chapter offers important details for running MBSP, including the internal structure of sessions, details about various elements in the sessions (e.g., the virtue circle, journaling vs. tracking), tips for leading mindfulness exercises, core processes woven into sessions, and managing challenges. This chapter also includes pilot data on MBSP. Chapters 7 through 14 describe each session of MBSP and include outlines, handouts, scripts, exercises, debriefing strategies, case examples, and practices. Chapter 15 details a number of ways MBSP can be adjusted to fit certain populations and settings.

While I use hundreds of references to support the approach, research, and practices, every practitioner should use appropriate caution in implementing MBSP. Additional research will be needed before MBSP can be identified as an empirically-validated program.

The Approach at Hand

I'll begin with chapters that offer primers on mindfulness (Chapter 1) and on character strengths (Chapter 2). These treat each area as a separate topic, examining the core concepts, related ideas, research, and practices. Chapter 3 offers a theoretical rationale for the integration of mindfulness and character strengths, and summarizes the existing research on correlations and consequences of mindfulness and each of the 24 character strengths. Chapters 4 and 5 look closely at the two main ways to integrate these areas – bringing character strengths to mindfulness (referred to as strong mindfulness) and bringing mindfulness to character strengths (referred to as mindful strengths use). Chapter 6 marks the third section of the book – Mindfulness-Based Strengths Practice (MBSP) – a program designed to foster strong mindfulness and mindful strengths use. MBSP is the first

The Audience for This Book

This book is written for the practitioner, whatever his or her profession. There are many professions that help people, and therefore many professionals who can put the ideas in this book to good use. A few examples include:

- Counselors, psychologists, and social workers
- Coaches, mentors, medical professionals, and other helping professionals
- Educators and teachers working with children, youth, and university students
- Business professionals, such as managers, executives, consultants, executive coaches, and various leaders in organizations
- Researchers, who will find a programmatic template that can be studied empirically

This is intentionally a wide net. The benefits of mindfulness and character strengths extend far beyond such categories. These are universal concepts that help people become stronger. For the astute layperson, this book offers introductory, intermediate, and advanced concepts in learning about mindfulness and character strengths practices that can help the individual deepen his or

---

[1] I have recently published two articles appearing in peer-review journals on the integration of mindfulness and character strengths, and mindfulness scholars Ruth Baer and Emily Lykins wrote a chapter on the linkage for a positive psychology textbook (see Baer & Lykins, 2011; Niemiec, 2012; Niemiec, Rashid, & Spinella, 2012).

her mindfulness practice and/or enhance well-being. The book includes numerous practical tips for enhancing these ideas in daily life.

I encourage practitioners and researchers to study the program, and I welcome your comments and questions. Feel free to contact me by e-mail and peruse the denoted websites for articles, sample meditations, and other MBSP resources and updates.

With gratitude for your inherent goodness, and with the hope that it be expressed widely and mindfully.

Ryan M. Niemiec
rmjn@sbcglobal.net
www.viacharacter.org/mindfulness
www.ryanniemiec.com
Cincinnati, Ohio
April 2013

Acknowledgments

The most cherished section of any book I write is this one (in addition to the dedication). This is because I can highlight and express my strength of gratitude to the wonderful people who have inspired me and contributed to the words on these pages.

There are giants in the area of character strengths, but no greater than the under-recognized thought leader, Neal Mayerson, who has taught me far more about the topic than any other person. Indeed, it is not possible to quantify the number of lives that have been touched because of Neal's pioneering work as chairman and founder of the VIA Institute but also his philanthropic work and nonprofit business developments. His is a legacy for the ages.

In the character strengths world, the best models are often the humble ones who are also using a seemingly larger capacity of wisdom and kindness than the rest of us. One such example is Donna Mayerson. She personifies mindful strengths use.

In addition to Neal and Donna, I'm fortunate to have several cherished colleagues onsite at the VIA Institute, namely Kelly Aluise, Breta Cooper, and Chris Jenkins, all of whom are the type of individuals who will drop whatever they are doing – at seemingly any moment – to offer constructive and helpful support and counsel. I'm also very grateful that VIA has several formal consultants – Tayyab Rashid, Mark Linkins, Michelle McQuaid, and Bob McGrath – each of whom carries an international reputation because of their brilliance in their particular specialty relating to character strengths.

The world is full of many inspiring teachers of mindfulness, those who directly teach it and those who indirectly model it. My favorites are those who do both well; those who happened to have had the most profound effect on my life over the last couple decades are, without a doubt, Thich Nhat Hanh, and Jon Kabat-Zinn. Zindel Segal has also been an important model. It should be no surprise that traces of their work can be seen sprinkled throughout Mindfulness-Based Strengths Practice.

I've appreciated the encouragement of many scholars at the intersection of mindfulness, positive psychology, and character strengths, who directly or indirectly pushed me forward in this work, namely Emily Lykins, Tayyab Rashid, Marcello Spinella, Chris Perrier, Jean Kristeller, Todd Kashdan, Ricardo Arguis Rey, Aaron Jarden, and Ruth Baer. Other practitioners in the area who offered strong encouragement included Richard Sears, Michael Bready, Geraldine Dougherty, Amanda Horne, Nina Ekman, Sille Lundquist, and Dev Curtis.

Thanks also to the late Chris Peterson who led the groundbreaking creation of the VIA Classification, as well as the support of Kelley McCabe (from e-Mindful), David Black (of mindfulexperience.org), Mads Bab, Jeremy Clyman, Dan Tomasulo, and my "Aristotelian friend" James Pawelski, whose insights and Socratic questioning helped me push through the early challenges of writing this book.

A special thanks goes to Emily Lykins and Judy Lissing, both MBSP practitioners, who went out of their way to read early drafts of various chapters and offer instrumental feedback and counsel.

My brave and intelligent publisher, Rob Dimbleby, continues to take risks in the service of producing meaningful material for the world. He is a joy to work with. I also wish to thank the talented staff at Hogrefe for their hard work on the design and layout, namely the creatively talented Lisa Bennett, whom I look forward to giving a big hug of gratitude to someday for her work on this book.

My early mindfulness supporters – Sr. Marilyn Wussler, the late Fr. Dave Kraus, Br. Bill Johnson (B.J.), the late Fr. Bob Aaron, Judy Highfill, Marsha Hatfield-Baker, Charles Burbridge, Lynn Rossy, Paul Duckro, Ron Margolis, and my inimitable, beloved mentor/colleague Danny Wedding. Each of these incredible human beings provided me unique opportunities to share mindfulness with others, before it was "en vogue" to do so. Not only did they move against the popular grain in psychology but they provided me confidence, collaboration, and strategies along the way.

The support from workshop participants across four continents has been striking, especially those attending workshops in the US, UK, Denmark, Canada, Hong Kong, Singapore, and Australia. These particular individuals attended 1–2-day workshops and decided to spend additional, optional time at gatherings on the integration of mindfulness and character strengths. They offered support, interest, feedback, and reinforcement for this work.

A special note of gratitude and dedication goes to the late Bob Wilke – supervisor, mentor, colleague, and friend – who despite driving me to emotional extremes, was ultimately a beloved wisdom catalyst. He was a man of authenticity and goodness, whose example inspired me to pursue new avenues of mindfulness at a pivotal moment in my career. Bob's legacy lives on in the pages of this book.

The MBSP Program

To the first-ever group of MBSP participants: your participation and efforts will not be forgotten. Thank you Paul, Hugh, Twyla, Erica, Edie, Ginger, Mimi, and Marilyn!

To the first five MBSP pilot leaders, Anne-Sophie Dubanton (Portugal), Kay Bruce (France), Catriona Rogers (Hong Kong), Gitte Elkaer (Denmark), and Judy Lissing (Australia). You are the early pioneers of MBSP. You took risks, you worked hard, and you innovated. Your advice, feedback and encouragement helped strengthen the MBSP program. In the future, I hope that many people will take MBSP under your compassionate and competent leadership.

Another deep bow of gratitude goes to Donna Fossier, Barry Scott Myers, Phuong Nguyen, Camille Fengolio, Julie Rowbotham, Anne Hartmann, and Donna Burns. In addition, to all those at Good Shepherd Parish, especially the socially intelligent, kind-hearted Jack Peltz, the dynamic duo of Art and Laurie Ftacink, and several delightful beings including Marti, Mary C., Judy, Mary H., Bob, Ann, Chris, Mary Lynne, Martha, and Lonetta.

I'm grateful to Tayyab Rashid, who might not know it, but indirectly led me to change the name of the program to Mindfulness-Based Strengths Practice (MBSP).

Appreciation goes out to the many people in the VIA online courses who offered insights and personal examples in regard to integrating mindfulness and character strengths; as this is a diverse international audience, it provides additional validity to this approach. Many thanks to my friend, the humble and wise leader of Being Peace Sangha, Paul Davis, OI (Order of Interbeing), who has experienced MBSP, led portions of it, and encouraged me implicitly.

Family

Writing books and simultaneously maintaining a consistent and strong connection with family presents a variety of challenges. It would not occur without – to paraphrase St. Francis de Sales – a cup of understanding, a barrel of love, and an ocean of patience on the part of my family.

I wish to thank my entire family for their ongoing encouragement of me to express who I am through writing. Specifically, I'd like to point out my parents, Sue Popson and Joe Niemiec who never put boundaries or contingencies on who I was or who I might become; they never pigeonholed me into a particular profession or line of work but instead allowed me to make my choices and then championed me along the way.

Special thanks goes to my kind and talented sister-in-law, Monica Watha Niemiec (go to www.monicawatha.com), whose artwork is featured on the cover, created just for this book. She displayed exemplary perseverance, creativity, understanding, flexibility, and compassion with this project. I am so grateful that she was able to paint the image that had been residing in my head.

I also wish to thank my aunt and uncle, Gwen and Don Juszczyk, who came into my life only recently, but in doing so made an already good life even better.

As I worked through much of this book, my wife, Rachelle, and son, Rhys, waited for me to finish. Your support and presence sustained me and allowed me to rally perseverance. Rhys climbed on top of me, stomped on my computer, and in one instance, the 21-month-old tapped on my keys and deleted the entire book (which thankfully was backed up). My gratitude to you both, my dear ones, as you watched me work harder and longer than I had anticipated, and too often I struggled in futility to mindfully multi-task my attention to you and the book. I'm finished now, so I'm all yours … let's go play!

Section I: Primers

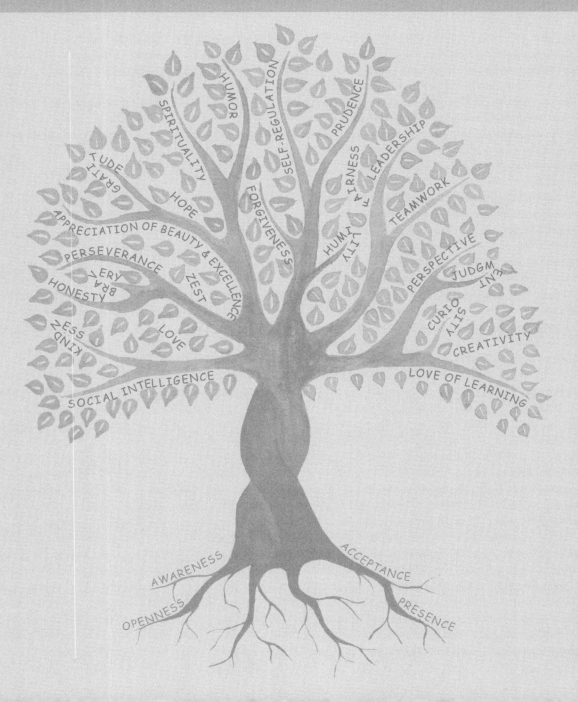

Chapter 1
A Primer on Mindfulness

My experience is what I agree to attend to.

William James

 Chapter Snapshot

Mindfulness has become a widely popular topic in the social sciences, in both research and practice. This chapter offers a primer on mindfulness, reviewing some general concepts and ideas such as scientific and practical definitions, misconceptions, the nature of autopilot, and the mindfulness continuum. Important background and historical information on mindfulness are discussed, followed by the presentation of research on a variety of mindfulness programs, underlying mindfulness mechanisms, and mindfulness in everyday life. Mindfulness practices are then discussed and practice tips are reviewed throughout the chapter.

 Opening Story

During weeklong retreats with renowned mindfulness teacher Thich Nhat Hanh (referred to as "Thay," which is Vietnamese for "teacher"), there is an opportunity for participants to pose a question to the venerable teacher to respond to. On one retreat, I recall Thay's sharing about an instance with a nuclear physicist who came up to the front of the retreat hall to ask a question in front of nearly one thousand retreatants. The physicist shared that as he began to deepen his mindfulness practice and see his life more clearly, he was coming to realize that his work seemed to be contributing to the advancement of potential danger and destruction rather than helping or creating a better world. He explained the suffering he began to feel because of this and his emerging thoughts of quitting his job. "What should I do?" he asked Thay. After a few deep breaths and careful reflection, Thay turned to the man and encouraged him to continue practicing mindfulness at his job; he explained that with a position of that level of seriousness, it's better to have someone practicing mindfulness giving deep thought and reflection to each action and potential action rather than to have someone functioning mindlessly and carelessly.

A core theme of mindfulness emerges from this story: whatever you are doing, do it mindfully. As the story indicates, rather than trying to take away the bad, avoid the negative, change who you are, or make a series of life changes, often the best response is to bring greater mindfulness to the current task.

Mindfulness Background/History

Mindfulness is an ancient practice that has come into focus in recent years. Psychologists, neuroscientists and a variety of clinical professionals are investigating and/or applying mindfulness in their work. Mindfulness originates in ancient Buddhist practices from over 2,500 years ago and has been brought to Western countries by teachers who have emigrated and Westerners who have travelled to Asia in order to study and practice it before it became known in the West. Many people in research and clinical mental health fields have become mindfulness practitioners (and vice versa), so it was probably only a matter of time before Western culture started to examine mindfulness in a thorough and serious way, moving beyond regarding it as an Eastern curiosity or esoteric practice.

In the Buddhist framework, mindfulness is one of several qualities of mind that is exercised in order to ultimately achieve "awakening" or "enlightenment," a state in which one experiences physical and emotional pain without suffering. This involves an experience of self-transcendence and is accompanied by a great sense of well-being, compassion, and altruistic motivation. Mindfulness is mentioned in the earliest known Buddhist texts of Theravada Buddhism (the Pali Canon), but as a core essential of Buddhist principles it has remained a central part of Buddhism as it spread across cultures and time, including Mahayana (e.g., Zen) and Vajrayana (e.g., Tibetan) schools. Formal Buddhist meditations are sometimes simplified into two basic practices: samatha or samadhi (concentration, one-pointed meditation) and vipassana (insight meditation). The former refers to the development of calm and concentration while the latter refers to looking deeply and developing insight. Indeed, many Western mindfulness practitioners integrate both concentration practice and insight meditation into the framework of mindfulness groups and programs. In Buddhism, negativity emerges from misperceptions and misunderstandings about others and the universe, and the fundamental life motivation is viewed as the quest for happiness (Wallace & Hodel, 2008).

One could argue that mindfulness came to the awareness of Westerners through Buddhism because Buddhism places such a central emphasis on mindfulness and has developed a wide variety of practices to develop it among practitioners. Buddhist psychology is also explicitly aimed at the reduction of suffering and promotion of well-being, which makes it easily applicable to Western research and clinical fields. Further, Buddhism places a great deal of emphasis on empirical observation over faith, and as such does not require any particular "beliefs" that cannot be verified through observation. The effectiveness of mindfulness techniques does not require subscribing to any particular religious beliefs.

While Buddhism is the tradition that is most responsible for articulating and introducing mindfulness to Western cultures, mindfulness is arguably present to a considerable degree in all of the major world religions. Elements of mindfulness are most evident in the "mystical" or contemplative branches of religions emphasizing introspection, humility, and patience, including Christianity (e.g., the Desert Fathers of the third century Egypt, Carrigan, 2001, and numerous mystics such as St. Teresa of Avila and St. John of the Cross), Sufi Islam, Jewish Kabbalah, Taoism, and Hinduism (e.g., Advaita Vedanta). For example, there are equivalent terms for the attentional aspect of mindfulness developed in contemplative traditions: *recollection* in Christianity, *zikr* in Islam, *kavanah* in Judaism, and *samadhi* in Buddhism and Hinduism. Anthony de Mello, a renowned and widely published Jesuit scholar from India, integrated Buddhist and Hindu prayer forms into Christian spirituality. His first book *Sadhana* (de Mello, 1978) offers a number of practices on beginner's mind, gratitude, perspective, spirituality, appreciation of beauty, and mindfulness of body, breath, and sounds. The book's title is an Indian word with many meanings – discipline, technique, spiritual exercises, and approach to God. In more recent history, Christian scholars have examined mindfulness and framed it as "finding God in all things" (Rehg, 2002).

Mindfulness is also addressed in several secular philosophies. For example, Pyrrho of Elis and other Skeptic philosophers trained themselves to regard thoughts and experiences with a suspension of belief, leading to a sense of tranquility, i.e., ataraxia (Kuzminski, 2007). This is essentially the "decentering" aspect of mindfulness discussed later in the chapter. The 18th century Scottish economist, Adam Smith, suggested adopting the perspective of an "impartial spectator" of one's experience to overcome difficult emotions and act in an empathic and ethical manner.

More contemporary views include Herbert Benson, a Harvard physician who emphasized the concentration aspect of mindfulness and who stated that, regardless of a person's religious or nonreligious practice, the following four elements are present:

1. A quiet environment
2. A mental device (a constant stimulus)
3. A passive attitude (redirecting attention)
4. A comfortable position (a posture sustained for at least 20 minutes, e.g., sitting, kneeling, swaying)

He called the experience that is triggered by these four elements the relaxation response (Benson, 1975). Benson added additional advice that is consistent with mindfulness practice: to not cling to a single posture or technique, to not force the practice onto oneself, and to not expect particular results.

Jon Kabat-Zinn is one of the individuals most responsible for popularizing mindfulness in the West. He created Mindfulness-Based Stress Reduction (MBSR), which is the original, structured mindfulness program that has led to numerous other such programs that serve a variety of populations around the world. Kabat-Zinn and his work were unique in the late 1970s in that he was one of the few figures studying the effects of mindfulness and he was doing the work at a prominent medical institution – the University of Massachusetts Medical School.

Thich Nhat Hanh, a Zen Buddhist monk, has also had a profound influence on mindfulness practices around the world. He has authored over 100 books on peace and mindfulness, was nominated for the Nobel Peace Prize in 1979, and continues to travel the world widely leading mindfulness retreats for practitioners and laypeople, averaging around 1,000 attendees at each retreat.

Of course, there are a number of other mindfulness teachers from Eastern and Western backgrounds that have served as catalysts for the popularity of mindfulness in the world, especially in the West. There are far too many to list here but some include Tara Bennett-Goleman (2001), Tara

Brach (2003), Pema Chodron (1997), Joseph Goldstein (1976), Jack Kornfield (1993), Lama Surya Das (1999), and Sharon Salzberg (1995).

The widespread accessibility and applicability of mindfulness makes it very amenable to study and implement in Western contexts, outside of any particular cultural or religious belief system. Despite the heavy Buddhist influence on the development of mindfulness practices in the West, and the ongoing dialog between Buddhist teachers and Western scientists, it is clear that mindfulness seems to be a universal human phenomenon that does not belong to any one religion, and it even cuts across religious/secular distinctions. This is not an attempt to divest mindfulness of any spiritual significance for those who practice it in that context. To the contrary, it reinforces the relevance and importance of the practice and application.

Mindfulness – General Concepts

Mindfulness: The 2-Part Definition

Mindfulness is a universal quality with wide relevance to the lives of humans.

> … mindfulness, precisely because it is not formulaic, and because it has to do with the quality of our experience as human beings and the degree to which we can pay attention in our lives, is truly universal in scope, and therefore relevant in virtually all circumstances (Kabat-Zinn & Kabat-Zinn, 1997, p. 35).

In a word, mindfulness is awareness. However, this does not fully capture the essence or fullness of mindfulness. Even better, consider one of the most quoted definitions of mindfulness which states that mindfulness means to pay attention in a particular way – on purpose, in the present moment, and nonjudgmentally (Kabat-Zinn, 1994). Thus, mindfulness involves deliberately focusing on what's happening in our moment-to-moment experience in a way that is noncritical and nonjudging. One concern with this definition is the third part – if mindfulness is nonjudging, then what is it? This presents an interesting conundrum that scientists have investigated.

Mindfulness has become a robust area of scientific inquiry and hence a number of definitions and conceptualizations of mindfulness have emerged. In an attempt to consolidate this thinking and to offer direction for the future study of mindfulness, a diverse team of mindfulness scholars and researchers gathered to review the previous work on mindfulness and create and propose a consensual, operational definition of mindfulness. A two-part definition emerged from this work; they described mindfulness as the *self-regulation* of attention with the use of an attitude of *curiosity*, openness, and acceptance (Bishop et al., 2004). It is interesting to highlight that within this conceptualization, there is strong emphasis on two character strengths: self-regulation and curiosity. These two components are common to nearly every definition of mindfulness and may represent a maximally parsimonious definition for it (Coffey, Hartman, & Fredrickson, 2010).

This definition should not be taken lightly as mindfulness has been a challenging construct to pin down. In part, this is because there are many qualities that are developed alongside mindfulness practice as well as some constructs that are natural outcomes of mindfulness practice (e.g., patience, wisdom, compassion).

Mindfulness practice involves sustaining and shifting attention (e.g., focusing and refocusing on the present experience when the mind wanders). This requires the letting go of one's entrenchment in automatic and ruminative thinking. Core to this discussion is metacognition (thinking about our thinking). Teasdale (1999) distinguished between *metacognitive knowledge*, i.e., knowing that one's thoughts may not always be accurate, and *metacognitive insight*, a direct experiential realization that one's thoughts are not a direct representation of reality, but rather mental events, or cognitive activity in the field of one's awareness. As metacognition grows, one is more easily able to step back and discard vicious circles of negativity that are part of one's subjective experiences. Segal, Williams, and Teasdale (2002) discuss this aspect of mindfulness as *decentering*, where thoughts and other psychological phenomena are viewed as temporary, mental events passing through awareness.

Acceptance has long been recognized as a beneficial characteristic in Western and Eastern religious and philosophical sources and literary works (Williams & Lynn, 2010–2011). Acceptance involves what many mindfulness scholars refer to as a deliberate attitude of *allowing*, rather than resistance, toward current thoughts, feelings, and sensations (Hayes, Strosahl, & Wilson, 1999; Kabat-Zinn, 1990; Segal, Williams, & Teasdale, 2002). This is similar to *equanimity*, a concept in Buddhist psychology which refers to an attitude of impartiality toward pleasant, unpleasant, or neutral present moment experiences.

In short, when we are being mindful we are taking control of what we focus on – we are controlling our attention (self-regulation). Research has found that mindfulness is more than the mere absence of mindlessness (Ritchie & Bryant, 2012); rather, there is a level of activity with our attention. As we attend to our present moment – whether this be to an emotion, a thought, a belief, an impulse, a sensation, or to something in our surrounding environment – we approach it with an open and accepting attitude (curiosity).

Another definition for mindfulness that can be applied here is Thich Nhat Hanh's (1979) view that mindfulness means to keep one's attention alive in the present reality. This "aliveness" captures both the self-regulation of attention and the approach of curiosity. When our mind is alive it is awake, tuned in, and ready, and concepts like openness and curiosity can readily be applied. This "aliveness" quality also offers a counterpoint to our tendencies toward autopilot, which are discussed later in the chapter.

Mindfulness, ultimately, is about shifting in the way we relate to ourselves. It's about seeing and experiencing ourselves in a different way. While cognitive-behavior therapy has made strides in helping individuals find ways to think differently by changing the content of thoughts, challenging the negative patterns in our thoughts, thinking differently about our emotions, and using our thinking to enact behavior changes, mindfulness does something different. Mindfulness helps us not to change our thoughts but to relate to thoughts (and ourselves) in a different way – a way that is balanced and nonjudgmental, curious, and accepting.

Misconceptions

Most people do not view mindfulness meditation in the ways just described. Instead, the words mindfulness meditation conjure up immediate images of people sitting on cushions, placing their thumbs and forefingers together, closing their eyes, repeating certain syllables or words, and being isolated and quiet for long periods of time. While some mindfulness experiences involve these qualities, many others do not. Since mindfulness means to cultivate awareness, curiosity, and acceptance, any aspect of life can become part of the practice of mindfulness.

Alongside these aforementioned images are common misconceptions and beliefs strongly implanted in people's minds such as "meditation is too difficult," "I can't do it," "I don't have time," and "I don't see the point." Such beliefs lead people to avoid mindfulness.

It is easy to see why so many individuals believe meditation is too difficult. Consider the following pressures or self-imposed expectations:

- One must sit still on a cushion for a prolonged period of time.
- Something wonderful, often mystical, is supposed to happen, such as profound relaxation, an experience of oneness, or an immediate transformation. One will achieve these outcomes if one does the meditation "correctly."
- Meditation will offer a quick relief of my symptoms or problems.

There are kernels of truth in these points; however, each is more misleading than accurate. One useful distinction made by some mindfulness teachers is to explain that mindfulness is a *horizontal process*, where the intent is greater awareness, whereas other types of meditation (e.g., transcendental meditation, mantra meditation, and similar forms) can be viewed as a *vertical process* where the intent is relaxation or inner peace. This book places emphasis on mindfulness as a horizontal process.

Mindfulness is a type of meditation that can be cultivated not just by sitting on a cushion or chair, but also by getting in touch with the present moment. One can therefore practice this during any activity in life. The purpose of mindfulness is NOT relaxation, inner oneness, or symptom relief, although these are all possible "side effects" of mindfulness practice. Individuals completing mindfulness trainings or programs may say to their friends, "I used to have depression but now I have mindfulness instead" or "I just meditate to get rid of my stress." These statements can eas-

ily relegate mindfulness to be a type of curative agent. When such statements are coupled with the vast amount of positive studies now supporting mindfulness and the attention mindfulness is receiving in today's culture, it is no wonder some may see mindfulness as a panacea!

However, mindfulness is best viewed and practiced as a way of being, or as an approach to daily life. To see mindfulness as simply a technique or a tool to overcome a stressor is quite limiting. The purpose of mindfulness is to build greater *awareness* of the "here and now" – a greater awareness of the changing moment-to-moment experience of our minds and bodies. Mindfulness therefore becomes more about letting go than about getting more.

What Is the Present Moment?

If we are asked this question, the typical practitioner might say something similar to "It's the here and now" or "It's being aware of our experience as it unfolds." While useful on a practical or conceptual level, this is insufficient from the perspective of the anatomy of our consciousness. Technically speaking, a present moment is:

> The span of time in which psychological processes group together very small units of perception into the smallest global unit (a gestalt) that has a sense of meaning in the context of a relationship. Objectively, present moments last from 1 to 10 seconds with an average around 3 to 4 seconds. Subjectively, they are what we experience as an uninterrupted *now*. The present moment is structured as a micro-lived story with a minimal plot and a line of dramatic tension made up of vitality affects. It is thus temporally dynamic. It is a conscious phenomenon, but need not be reflectively conscious, verbalized, or narrated. It is viewed as the basic building block of relationship experiences. (Stern, 2004, p. 245).

This description comes from Daniel Stern (2004) who offers a phenomenological perspective of the present moment. He adds that there are several features of present moments. Here are a few examples of these features that Stern notes:

- *Awareness or consciousness is a necessary condition for a present moment.* Here, Stern explains that present moments are felt experiences of what occurs during a period of consciousness.

- *The present moment is not the verbal account of an experience*. Instead, he explains that the present moment *is* the lived experience.
- *The felt experience of the present moment is whatever is in awareness now, during the moment being lived*. Stern notes that present moments are simply that which is on our mental stage.
- *Present moments are of short duration*. Stern explains these moments last for usually a few seconds, however, exceptions can be found when individuals achieve certain meditation states.
- *The present moment has a psychological function*. These moments are typically around events that break through ordinary living.
- *Present moments are holistic happenings*. They are a gestalt or organized grouping of smaller units such as thoughts, feelings, actions, and sensations.

William James, sometimes referred to as the "grandfather of positive psychology," compared the human stream of consciousness to the life of a bird that contains flights and perchings. The perchings are the present moments and the flights are the spaces between periods of consciousness that are not accessible (discussed in Stern, 2004).

So what does all of this mean? The present moment is highly transient and at the same time it's vitally important. There is always a brief opportunity to make the most of something – to engage in the now. And, at the same time, when one realizes the moment is gone, one is in another moment to cherish, to use consciously, or to simply be connected with.

The Habitual Mind

As noted, present moments are relatively brief and transient. We spend far more time unaware of present moments than aware of them. The mindfulness literature refers to the tendency of the human mind to wander off as going into automatic pilot (Segal et al., 2002).

There is much our mind can get distracted with. Research has shown that our minds can process about seven items (sounds, odors, images, emotions) at once and it has been estimated it takes just 1/18 of a second to process each item. The result is 126 pieces of information every second (half a million per hour) (Csikszentmihalyi, 1997). That's a lot of "options" we can potentially bring our attention to! There is far more that is *not* attended to by our mindful awareness than attended to. Csikszentmihalyi adds that the majority of our thoughts are the same as yesterday. Thus, our habitual mind is simply recycling old thoughts, difficult interactions, painful memories, or mundane and trivial experiences.

Mindfulness is contrasted with automaticity, a state of unawareness that occupies a significant portion of our daily living, in which we are going through the motions of an activity, not tuned in or aware of our internal experience. Meditation teachers often refer to our mind's ability to hop around from thought to thought as "monkey mind," because at these times our mind is like a group of monkeys in trees, chattering about as they randomly hop around from branch to branch and from tree to tree. One purpose of mindfulness is to "wake up" from monkey mind and habitual living and to become present and attend closely to what is happening internally and externally in the present moment.

Practice Tip: Catch AP-ASAP

This abbreviation stands for a key principle in mindfulness practice: Catch auto-pilot as soon as possible. The mind can wander off in the blink of an eye and sometimes it is gone for quite awhile, having jumped to several topics, elicited different feeling reactions, and even tapped into core beliefs we have about ourselves and the world. This occurs right behind our nose, outside of our awareness. However, the sooner we catch where our mind has headed off, the quicker we can make the decision to bring it back to the present moment, allow it to continue wandering, or make some other decision.

When leading mindfulness groups or individual sessions, I write this principle on a board or a sheet of paper to highlight its importance. I emphasize how this can be viewed as one of the first steps in establishing greater mindfulness in oneself and in one's environment. Humility and appreciation of beauty

& excellence can be used to respond to our autopilot in a balanced way. We can sit back in awe and wonder about how our minds are able to head into autopilot so often; and we can be humbled by the ability of our mind to control so much of our lives. We can thus offer a metaphoric bow of respect to ourselves and to our minds.

There are countless examples of autopilot. The most prevalent, concrete examples occur during our daily routines, such as while driving, working, reading, walking, and eating. When driving, we go off into autopilot and perhaps miss our exit or suddenly realize we are a lot further along on the drive than we thought; yet our body-mind was still driving the car safely and successfully. Our mind was off in autopilot. When eating, we often lose focus and forget to savor the food; the taste and texture of the food vanishes as our mind wanders elsewhere. When talking with others we might mindlessly nod our heads as if we're listening closely but our mind is thinking about something else entirely. While reading, we can lose track of the story or the content of the book for a period of time and then suddenly realize that we are no longer comprehending the words. We then turn back a page or two and ask ourselves something like "Ok, where was I last mindful?"

All of this is occurring yet we continue to function throughout our day, often because of autopilot. Part of the reason for this is our mind functions quite well on autopilot. Similar to the airline pilot placing the airplane on autopilot, our mind flies us from activity to activity, from multi-tasking to single-tasking, often only requiring minimal attention on our part. Therefore, the habitual mind should not be viewed as something bad or negative. We should not denigrate our autopilot nature, we should be humbled by it, attempt to be acutely aware of it, and even *praise* it. We are able to operate heavy machinery, figure out complex tasks, perform many tasks at once, persevere on projects, and accomplish many things in our daily life because of our autopilot. Indeed, it's hard to imagine our lives without it.

Each individual's habit energy is different and can present unexpected twists and turns. I recall the first time I led a mindful eating exercise. It was with a psychotherapy client who was chronically depressed and experiencing a lot of suffering. I explained to him that we would be practicing with a particular exercise and I handed him one raisin. As soon as the raisin touched the palm of the man's hand, he had popped it in his mouth and swallowed it. A couple of seconds later, the man realized his automated response, and expressed embarrassment. Sometimes our autopilot is so strong that it impacts our behavior, despite the novelty of the situation; even though this man had mental and physical fatigue and slowed responses, his autopilot was unabated (perhaps even stronger than if he were not depressed). Several-hundred clients and students later, I've never experienced someone repeat that behavior with the raisin exercise.

Mindfulness is a challenge, even for those well-practiced. While no one is a mindful listener all the time, in some situations the exhibition of mindlessness is more striking. One example was a long-time meditator who was in my mindfulness community (sangha) many years ago. I had previously spoken with this middle-aged man briefly on three or four occasions. This was the first time we began to ask more personal questions. I asked him a couple questions about his work to which he shared; I then began to share about my work. The conversation was flowing nicely, off to a good start. I was four or five sentences into explaining my work and the man suddenly looked over to the side at someone who caught his attention and then simply turned his body away from mine and walked away calmly to the other person. He did not say a word about this abrupt transition. I stood there stunned in mid-sentence. The conversation was suddenly over. It was a bit mystifying as the man had seemed quite engaged in the conversation and we appeared to be connecting with one another.

Interestingly, this example of a fairly dramatic shift from one present moment activity (conversation) to another (walking away to engage in another conversation) mirrors what happens in meditation practice and in daily activities. A well-intentioned meditator gives full attention to the breath in the present moment until an intriguing thought arises and the meditator unknowingly shifts their focus completely to this thought. While this thought did emerge in the present moment, the meditator is no longer aware that they have been carried away from the focus on the breath in the present moment. Similar experiences occur while savoring the delights of the first few bites of dinner until the sixth or seventh bites arrive and one's attention is far away thinking about plans for after dinner.

Mind wandering is difficult to control, hard to recognize, and difficult to prevent (Mrazek, Smallwood, & Schooler, 2012), therefore it can become so pervasive and frequent that it might seem as though we are barely living our life. For some it will appear as if they've been living life as an automaton or zombie, shifting from unconsciously existing to mindlessly consuming. This can also be referred to as living a "substitute life" (Bayda, 2002), in which we fabricate a maze of thoughts and strategies to avoid being present to life as it is, and then we believe and act from the fabrications and beliefs.

Mind wandering is not without risk as it can compromise a number of cognitive skills, interfering with one's ability to integrate present moment experience into a general context which may lead to additional problems (Smallwood, Mrazek, & Schooler, 2011). Other drawbacks of mindlessness have been noted by Killingsworth and Gilbert (2010) who developed an iPhone application to contact participants at random moments during their typical day and ask them about their happiness level, their activity, and whether or not their mind was wandering. Mind wandering occurred in about 47% of the samples and the researchers estimated that this frequency was higher than what is typically seen in scientific labs. They concluded that "a human mind is a wandering mind, and a wandering mind is an unhappy mind. The ability to think about what is not happening is a cognitive achievement that comes at an emotional cost" (p. 932).

Ellen Langer, a Harvard scientist who has studied mindfulness and mindlessness processes for decades, explains that much of the time humans are mindless and too unaware to even make note that they are not there! The human tendency to be unaware of one's own unawareness is indeed an ironic phenomenon. Langer (2009) explains that mindlessness occurs either through repetition (e.g., going into autopilot when driving) or a single exposure to information. She notes that when information appears irrelevant, is presented as an absolute, or is given by an au-

thority figure, then it usually does not occur to humans to question it. This means the individual has locked him-/herself into a limited mindset and thereby inhibits his/her own learning.

When we are "mindless" and lost in our thinking, we lose touch with our internal and external environment. Two things often result: (1) We miss the details (in many instances, the positives) of life. (2) We miss opportunities to grow or challenge ourselves. The good news is there are ways to break this mindlessness. By jumping back into mindfulness in any of these moments, we are opening a door of opportunity to these potentials. Research has found that mindful breathing, even simply eight minutes, can decrease mind wandering, compared with other tasks including relaxation (Mrazek et al., 2012).

Mindlessness and mindfulness are opposing constructs (Mrazek et al., 2012). Consider Figure 1.1 which offers a teaching tool for understanding mindfulness and mindlessness as a continuum of awareness, along with related concepts. Being a continuum, there is no endpoint for a perfect, complete mindfulness or for total mindlessness.

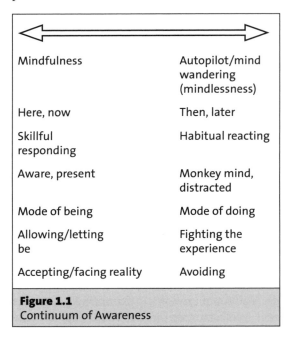

Mindfulness	Autopilot/mind wandering (mindlessness)
Here, now	Then, later
Skillful responding	Habitual reacting
Aware, present	Monkey mind, distracted
Mode of being	Mode of doing
Allowing/letting be	Fighting the experience
Accepting/facing reality	Avoiding

Figure 1.1
Continuum of Awareness

This diagram contains a variety of examples that partially characterize the mindfulness experience and the autopilot experience. It is not intended to indicate that the left side is completely good and that the right side completely bad. Also, while reviewing this diagram, one should not assume that each point on each side is highly correlated with the other points; for example, one might be in a "mode of doing" and not be mindless and distracted. Instead, view this figure as a heuristic for reviewing important processes relating to mindfulness.

Figure 1.2 is an excerpt from *The Dhammapada*, a classic work that has been described by meditation teacher Jack Kornfield (2005) as "the most beloved of all Buddhist texts, both poetic and profound" (p. ix). This excerpt captures the complexity of the habitual mind and the fruits of mindfulness in bringing self-regulation to mind wandering.

Practice Tip: Discover Mindfulness During the Extremes

This can be a useful exploration exercise for those who are new to the practice of mindfulness and struggling to understand it.

We've had many moments in our lives when we were jolted to awareness. There is a natural heightening of awareness during periods where we experience extremes – the highs, lows, and intensities of life. These "human" experiences present an opportunity for us to increase our mindfulness throughout the rest of our day.

- Funerals, weddings, transitions, rites of passage
- Natural disasters or other tragedies – the aftereffects and impact on others
- Early on with love/sexual relationships
- The experience of physical or emotional pain
- Mystical experiences, feeling "moved" or a sense of "oneness"
- Fear experiences – shock
- Compassion for others, e.g., a woman struggling on the side of road with four kids after a car accident

Reflect on one or more of the above experiences from your life. Did the experience lead to greater clarity and self-awareness? What did you learn about mindfulness from this experience? When you experience one of these situations in the future, take notice of the intensity of the mindfulness generated in the moment and throughout the hours and days that follow.

"The Mind"[1]

The restless, agitated mind,
Hard to protect, hard to control,
The sage makes straight,
As a fletcher the shaft of an arrow.

Like a fish out of water,
Thrown on dry ground,
This mind thrashes about,
Trying to escape Mara's[2] command.

The mind, hard to control,
Flighty – alighting where it wishes –
One does well to tame.
The disciplined mind brings happiness.

The mind, hard to see,
Subtle – alighting where it wishes –
The sage protects.
The watched mind brings happiness

Far-ranging, solitary,
Incorporeal and hidden
Is the mind.
Those who restrain it
Will be freed from Mara's bonds.

For those who are unsteady of mind,
Who do not know true Dharma,
And whose serenity wavers,
Wisdom does not mature.

For one who is awake,
Whose mind isn't overflowing,
Whose heart isn't afflicted
And who has abandoned both merit and demerit,
Fear does not exist.

Knowing this body to be like a clay pot,
Establishing this mind like a fortress,
One should battle Mara with the sword of insight,
Protecting what has been won,
Clinging to nothing.

All too soon this body
Will lie on the ground,
Cast aside, deprived of consciousness,
Like a useless scrap of wood.

Whatever an enemy may do to an enemy,
Or haters, one to another,
Far worse is the harm
From one's own wrongly directed mind.

Neither mother nor father,
Nor any other relative can do
One as much good
As one's own well-directed mind.

Figure 1.2
Excerpt from The Dhammapada

[1] From *The Dhammapada*, by Gil Fronsdal, pp. 9–11, © 2005 by Gil Fronsdal. Reprinted by arrangement with Shambhala Publications Inc., Boston, MA. www.shambhala.com
[2] In Buddhist literature, Mara often represents the personification of temptation.

Mindfulness Research

Research on the study and benefits of mindfulness meditation and mindfulness-based practices has increased dramatically in recent years (Brown, Ryan, & Creswell, 2007; Sears, Tirch, & Denton, 2011). Since the year 2000, mindfulness research has increased nearly twenty-fold. See Figure 1.3 that delineates the surge in mindfulness publications. A recent meta-analysis on the psychological impact of meditation showed clear evidence that meditation has a positive effect on well-being, similar to the effect achieved by therapeutic and behavioral approaches in psychotherapy (Sedlmeier et al., 2012).

Mindfulness-related meditation has been integrated into psychological approaches to treat a variety of psychological disorders and problems, including stress, anxiety, depression, relationship problems, borderline personality disorder, substance abuse, binge eating disorder, insomnia, bipolar disorder, and psychotic symptoms (Baer, 2003; Grossman, Niemann, Schmidt, & Walach, 2004; Nyklicek, Vingerhoets, & Zeelenberg, 2010; Segal et al, 2002; Shapiro & Carlson, 2009).

Ellen Langer (1989; 1997; 2009), who emphasizes cognitive aspects of mindfulness involving novelty and thinking in alternative categories, has found that increases in mindfulness results in greater competence, health, longevity, positive affect, creativity, and charisma. There is also research that shows the benefits of mindfulness on relationship functioning (Carson, Carson, Gil, & Baucom, 2004). In addition, Shapiro, Schwartz, and Santerre (2002) discuss the impact of mindfulness on interpersonal functioning by citing Tloczynski and Tantriella (1998) who found that breath meditation for six weeks was superior to a relaxation group and a control group in significantly decreasing interpersonal problems.

Why Is Mindfulness an Effective Practice?

Because the impact of mindfulness-based approaches on psychological well-being has been well established, a natural further area of investigation is to explore *why* mindfulness is effec-

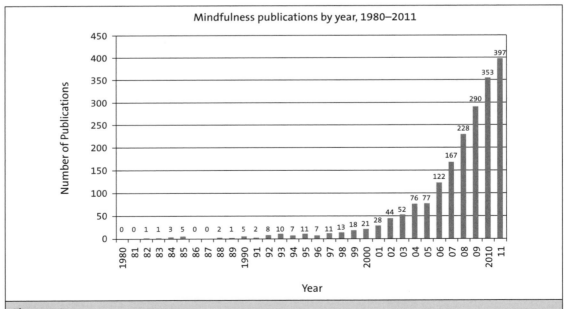

Figure 1.3
Mindfulness research over the decades
Note. Figure reprinted with permission from David S. Black. Available from Mindfulness Research Guide (see Black, 2010) at www.mindfulexperience.org

tive in helping a number of populations, ranging from those who are high in well-being to those who are suffering from physical and psychological problems. A decade ago, Ruth Baer (2003) explored the science of mindfulness from a conceptual and empirical approach. She hypothesized a number of important explanations for the effectiveness of mindfulness. These included:

- *Exposure:* being with fear to create a change opportunity; nonjudgmental observation; particularly important for anxiety conditions.
- *Cognitive change:* nonjudgmental acceptance; metacognition; particularly important in depression and eating disorders.
- *Self-management:* coping resources; self-criticism/judgment that is more general and global is replaced; focus on self-care; particularly important for depression.
- *Relaxation:* letting go; physiological relaxation; slowing down; particularly helpful for stress and worry.
- *Acceptance:* closely linked with change; understanding that one does not have to change all unpleasant symptoms.

Researchers have also looked at the connection between mindfulness and two aspects of mental health (flourishing and psychological distress) and found important contributing factors are clarity of one's inner life, managing negative emotions, nonattachment, and rumination (Coffey et al., 2010).

Further progress has been made in understanding the mechanisms of action involved in mindfulness processes (Baer, 2010; Carmody, Baer, Lykins, & Olendzki, 2009). In her edited book studying the processes of change in mindfulness interventions, Baer (2010) closely explores a number of pathways that offer a compelling picture accounting for the success of mindfulness programs and meditation in general:

- *Mindfulness:* The practice of mindfulness itself – both in groups and in home practice – is an obvious factor accounting for change. In a study of Mindfulness-Based Stress Reduction (MBSR), changes in mindfulness occurred at week 2 whereas changes in perceived stress did not occur until week 4, indicating that improvement in mindfulness skills is a critical

factor in accounting for the impact that mindfulness has on psychological well-being (Baer, Carmody, & Hunsinger, 2012).
- *Decentering:* Decentering, also described as reperceiving or defusion, refers to the observation of one's thoughts and feelings as temporary and transient events in the mind and not necessarily truths or facts. Researchers have found mindfulness and decentering to be highly overlapping constructs (Carmody et al., 2009).
- *Psychological flexibility:* This is a complex construct that refers to a wide range of human qualities, such as adapting to situational demands, shifting mindsets and behaviors, keeping balance in life domains, and being aware, open, and committed to acting from one's values (Kashdan & Rottenberg, 2010).
- *Values:* Thinking about what is most important in life and then identifying behaviors that are aligned with values is a core feature in Acceptance and Commitment Therapy (ACT) and accounts for some of this program's success (Wilson, Sandoz, Flynn, Slater, & DuFrene, 2010).
- *Emotion regulation:* This involves not trying to decrease or change emotions but increasing awareness and acceptance of emotions as well as experiencing them by decreasing emotional reactivity and promoting responsive, goal-directed behavior.
- *Self-compassion:* This involves taking a kind and friendly approach to oneself that manifests as love, understanding, and gentleness. In a study of experienced and inexperienced meditators, mindfulness and self-compassion correlated with well-being and meditation experience suggesting that these processes play an important role in the connection between psychological well-being that comes from mindfulness training (Baer, Lykins, & Peters, 2012). A study of MBSR and a waitlist control also found mindfulness and self-compassion to be key processes of change (Keng, Smoski, Robins, Ekblad, & Brantley, 2012).
- *Spirituality:* Mindfulness is a secular process, yet can be viewed as inherently linked with spirituality (depending on how one defines spirituality). Studies have shown that mind-

fulness increases spirituality and that these changes are linked with several domains of psychological functioning (Baer, 2010; Carmody, Reed, Kristeller, & Merriam, 2008).

- *Changes in the brain, attention, and working memory:* Neuroscience applied to mindfulness is a rapidly emerging field that has revealed many findings about the impact on structural changes in the brain, as well as attention and memory (Davidson & Begley, 2012).

Mindfulness in Everyday Life

The practice of mindfulness in everyday life, referred to generally as mindful living, has had less systematic research. Mindful living practices such as mindful walking, eating, and talking are typically embedded practices and homework exercises in mindfulness programs.

Research has focused far more on the study of formal meditation practice than on aspects of mindful living. However, in a study of MBSR participants, the self-reported time that was spent practicing formal mindfulness meditation predicted the tendency to be mindful in daily life; this then led to reduced stress and improved psychological functioning (Carmody & Baer, 2008).

Another exception can be found in Easterlin and Cardena (1999) who compared beginning and advanced meditators who received random daily pages in which they were to respond to particular questions relating to the present moment. The advanced meditators reported less stress and anxiety and more positive mood, greater acceptance of the present moment, and a higher capacity for metacognition (thinking about thinking). These researchers explain that metacognition emerges in everyday life because our consciousness is divided between being in a particular experience (e.g., feeling tired) and observing/witnessing the experience (e.g., noticing tiredness from moment-to-moment, observing sensations of tiredness in the body). This distinction can be applied to daily activities – we can be absorbed in the experience of washing dishes and we can observe the sensations we experience while washing the dishes.

A small qualitative review found that intentional (mindful) living was one of the key outcomes of mindfulness practice (Rothaupt & Morgan, 2007). The researchers also noted three additional outcomes – connectedness (interconnection), gratitude (and spirituality), and actively inviting others to increase their mindful living.

Researchers have also found a connection between savoring the moment and the experience of everyday positive events (referred to as "uplifts"). Participants who were lower on savoring had fewer uplifts and those higher on savoring had more uplifts (Hurley & Kwon, 2012).

Mindfulness Programs: Different Types of Launching Pads

The study of mindfulness meditation and mindfulness-based practices in the last decade or so has increased voluminously (Brown et al., 2007) and has led to a number of effective mindfulness and mindfulness-based psychological interventions (Allen, Bromley, Kuyken, & Sonnenberg, 2009; Baer, 2003). Indeed, meta-analyses of mindfulness programs have yielded positive results in terms of improving mental health and reducing distress (Fjorback, Arendt, Ornbøl, Fink, & Walach, 2011; Grossman et al., 2004; Marchand, 2012). Mindfulness training has been formalized into different structured programs used to treat a myriad of psychological and medical conditions, for example, chronic pain (Kabat-Zinn, 1990), anxiety (Hayes et al., 1999), depression (Segal et al., 2002), substance abuse (Bowen et al., 2009), binge eating (Kristeller & Wolever, 2011), and borderline personality (Linehan, 1993), to name a few. Research has found there are large differences in the way mindfulness is conceptualized and practiced in meditation interventions (Chiesa & Malinowski, 2011).

Jon Kabat-Zinn (2003) describes mindfulness programs and practices as:

> … merely launching platforms or particular kinds of scaffolding to invite cultivation and sustaining of attention in particular ways. They are the menu, so to speak, not the meal; the map, rather than the territory, the traditional admonition being not to mistake the finger pointing at the moon for the moon. (p. 147).

A number of mindfulness programs have emerged and serve as launching pads for the cultivation of a deeper, wiser attention to the present moment. The four most studied programs that heavily emphasize mindfulness are Mindfulness-Based Stress Reduction (MBSR), Mindfulness-Based Cognitive Therapy (MBCT), Dialectical Behavior Therapy (DBT), and Acceptance and Commitment Therapy (ACT) (Baer, 2010). The core of these and other mindfulness-based programs is to practice self-awareness, present moment awareness, acceptance, observation of thoughts, feelings, and sensations, and to apply mindfulness in the context of distress or problems.

MBSR

An important explanation for the dramatic increase in both the scholarship and popularity of mindfulness is the pioneering work of Kabat-Zinn and his MBSR program at the University of Massachusetts Medical School (Kabat-Zinn, 1990). In the 1970s, Kabat-Zinn masterfully took some of the best practices of Buddhism and meditation and translated them into a practically-based program to help patients who suffered from chronic illnesses. At the medical center, Kabat-Zinn worked with the most challenging patients whom physicians from various specialty areas stated there was no other conventional treatment they could offer them. These patients were individuals who had experienced multiple surgeries, debilitating pain, and serious medical conditions. A compelling video of the MBSR program depicting the work with patients over eight weeks was created by Bill Moyers (1993) a couple decades ago and is worth viewing (some mindfulness programs still show this video to clients as part of the mindfulness training).

MBSR is the original, structured, secular mindfulness program. It set forth a framework for many outgrowths of mindfulness to emerge (Kabat-Zinn, 1990). MBSR consists of 8 sessions, typically of 2.5 hours in length, along with an additional "day of mindfulness" retreat. MBSR is the most studied mindfulness program, and research has found that subjects experienced improved general health, decreases in medical symptom complaints, and decreases in psychological distress,

anxiety, and depression (Reibel, Greeson, Brainard, & Rosenzweig, 2001). An assumption of MBSR programs is that the intensive mindfulness work will enhance veridical perception (Grossman et al., 2004), a phrase which refers to perceiving things as they actually are.

Several meta-analyses have been conducted on MBSR among clinical and nonclinical clients. Those that have focused on healthy subjects have found MBSR has a strong effect on improving psychological well-being (Eberth & Sedlmeier, 2012) and significantly reduces stress, although the latter was found to be equal to standard relaxation training for stress management (Chiesa & Serretti, 2009). For clinical populations, MBSR has had a small effect on depression, anxiety, and distress among individuals with chronic medical disease (Bohlmeijer, Prenger, Taal, & Cuijpers, 2010), a positive impact on mental health – but inconclusive on physical health – for cancer patients (Ledesma & Kumano, 2009), and some positive although limited findings in managing sleep disturbance (Winbush, Gross, & Kreitzer, 2007).

MBSR has been used to treat anxiety conditions. Kabat-Zinn et al. (1992) found a significant decrease in anxiety among generalized anxiety disorder, panic disorder, and agoraphobia. Mindfulness seems to impact information processing and activate metacognitive plans that help to improve control of thinking (Roemer & Orsillo, 2002; 2009). This helps the anxious individual to disconnect their maladaptive beliefs and to strengthen a more flexible response to threats where they can detect early signs of anxiety, experience less tension overall, and learn how to detach from mental phenomena (Kabat-Zinn, 1990). Gains in anxiety reduction were maintained at 3-year follow-up (Miller, Fletcher, & Kabat-Zinn, 1995).

Favorable effects of MBSR have been found in the treatment of chronic pain. Patients being treated with MBSR experienced significant reductions in present moment pain, negative body image, inhibition of activity by pain, mood disturbance, depression, anxiety, and pain-related drug use, in addition to increases in self-esteem (Kabat-Zinn, 1982). Gains were maintained at 15 month follow-up. The rationale for the gains is that MBSR involves the teaching of self-regulation, cultivation of a detached observation of the pain experience, and separation of physical sensations from accompanying thoughts about pain (Kabat-Zinn, 1982; Kabat-Zinn, Lipworth, & Burney, 1985).

MBCT

Mindfulness-Based Cognitive Therapy (MBCT) is an 8 session program, modeled on MBSR, and was created by a team of researchers – Zindel Segal, Mark Williams, and John Teasdale (2002; 2013). Some of the core themes of MBCT include: automatic pilot, acceptance (allowing and letting be), thoughts are not facts, self-care, and relapse prevention. A video of MBCT featuring Segal was filmed as a teaching tool for students (American Psychological Association, 2004) and received favorable reviews (Niemiec, 2005).

The original studies of MBCT compared it with treatment as usual among individuals with recurrent major depression who had 3 or more depression episodes in their past. MBCT significantly reduced depression relapse, yet was not significant for those with one or two depression episodes (Segal et al., 2002; Teasdale et al., 2000). The researchers account for this noting that the first and second episodes of depression are usually triggered by major life events, however, as the frequency of episodes increases it becomes more likely that the depression episode is triggered by mood and negative rumination, which are areas that MBCT trains individuals to target with nonjudging awareness. A more recent meta-analysis noted that in addition to four studies finding effectiveness for recurrent depression, there was also benefit for reducing residual depression, anxiety disorders, and anxiety symptoms associated with bipolar disorder (Chiesa & Serretti, 2011). A subsequent, randomized controlled study found efficacy for MBCT over the control group regardless of the number of depression episodes (one or more) (Geschwind, Peeters, Huibers, van Os, & Wichers, 2012).

In MBCT, decreasing rumination is considered a key change mechanism (Kingston, Dooley, Bates, Lawlor, & Malone, 2007). Decentering, which is taught in most mindfulness-based programs, is one way to reduce rumination (Baer,

2010), and decentering along with curiosity may underlie its effectiveness (Bieling et al., 2012). This means that the success of MBCT is partly due to increases in metacognition (thinking about thinking) in that there is higher accessibility to metacognitive sets than experienced by those who are depressed (Teasdale et al., 2000). A novel aspect of MBCT (different from cognitive-behavior therapy) is that MBCT creates a change in the relationship individuals have with their negative thoughts (i.e., distinct from changing the thought content). Said another way: negative thoughts and feelings are experienced as mental events rather than as facts or truths about the self. Teasdale (1999) also explains that in MBCT participants' autobiographical memory is modified, in that more specific memories (e.g., I screwed up at my last job when I skipped 5 days of work) rather than general memories (e.g., I've been a failure in all my work) are focused on. In a qualitative study of participants' MBCT experiences, the core construct that emerged was "relating mindfully" (Bihari & Mullan, 2012). This improvement in one's relationship with oneself led to profound changes in participants' relationships with others.

DBT

DBT was developed by Marsha Linehan at the University of Washington. She studied the biographical accounts of holocaust survivors and torture victims to geain a deeper understanding of the nature of suffering and along the way learned that acceptance was a key feature of many of the survivors' experiences. She combined this learning with her interest in Zen Buddhism and incorporated concepts of mindfulness and acceptance into DBT. The DBT program involves three adjunctive modules in addition to core mindfulness training, which is repeated throughout the DBT process. The other modules involve skill-building in emotion regulation, distress tolerance, and interpersonal effectiveness. DBT has been used to treat a number of conditions; however, perhaps most striking is its success in treating challenging clientele such as individuals with severe suicidality, self-injurious behavior, trauma, and borderline personality disorder (Baer, 2010; Linehan, 1993).

ACT

ACT was developed by Steven Hayes, Kirk Strosahl, and Kelly Wilson in the late 1970s and emphasizes the importance of separating oneself from identifying with one's thoughts, accepting internal experiences, clarifying values, and committing to behaviors that are consistent with one's goals (Hayes et al., 1999). Mindfulness is a core underlying process in ACT work. ACT has been successfully applied to a large number of disorders, including depression, anxiety, anger, substance abuse, self-harm, chronic pain, and work stress (Hayes, Luoma, Bond, Masuda, & Lillis, 2006).

MBRP

Mindfulness meditation has been applied to different populations of substance abusers. The most popular structured approach is Mindfulness-Based Relapse Prevention (MBRP), developed by Alan Marlatt and colleagues. Compared to treatment as usual, MBRP led to lower substance use, greater decreases in craving, and increases in acceptance and acting with awareness (Bowen et al., 2009). Among smokers, a brief mindfulness exercise on managing urges led to fewer cigarettes smoked over a 7-day period compared to a control group (Bowen & Marlatt, 2009).

Another mindfulness program for substance abusers, called Mindfulness-Oriented Recovery Enhancement was employed with alcohol-dependent adults, and results revealed enhanced self-awareness and improved coping with emotional distress and addictive impulses (Garland, Schwarz, Kelly, Whitt, & Howard, 2012). A systematic review of mindfulness meditation for substance abuse disorders found that preliminary evidence exists for the efficacy and safety of mindfulness; however, further studies are needed with this population (Zgierska et al., 2009). Character strengths have been hypothesized and explored as accounting for some of the successes of recovery from mindfulness-based interventions to facilitate recovery from addictions (Selvam, 2012).

MB-EAT

A number of studies have found benefit in the use of mindfulness for individuals with eating disorders or related difficulties. Jean Kristeller created a formalized 8-week program for individuals with binge-eating disorder called Mindfulness-Based Eating Awareness Training (MB-EAT). This program led to various improvements in eating and mood (Kristeller & Hallett, 1999; Kristeller, Wolever, & Sheets, 2013). MB-EAT seems to work on a number of levels: increasing awareness and self-monitoring of both hunger cues and satiety cues, and reducing eating that is on autopilot, a result of negative affect or a reaction to environmental triggers (Kristeller & Hallett, 1999; Kristeller & Wolever, 2011), which all help to cultivate a different approach to eating that is characterized by mindfulness, acceptance, and self-compassion.

Other mindfulness-related programs have been successful in treating clinical disorders (e.g., anorexia and bulimia) and nonclinical problems (e.g., overeating), for example, Appetite Awareness Training (Craighead & Allen, 1995), ACT (Lillis, Hayes, Bunting, & Masuda, 2009), and DBT (Wisniewski & Kelly, 2003). Perhaps the biggest issue in weight management is the high frequency of weight regain. A recent mindfulness program involving themes of maintenance and relapse prevention is Enhancing Mindfulness for the Prevention of Weight Regain (EMPOWER). This program has led to changes in eating behavior, thinking patterns, emotional reactivity, and increased acceptance, planning and goal-accomplishment (Caldwell, Baime, & Wolever, 2012). In this program, participants learn standard mindfulness practices (e.g., body scan, sitting meditation), less common mindfulness practices (e.g., Stop-Breathe-Connect, Stop-Breathe-Bite, and 20 Breaths), and tools for healthy eating (e.g., meal planning, reading food labels, and healthy restaurant dining).

MBRE

Mindfulness-Based Relationship Enhancement (MBRE) was developed by James and Kimberly Carson and colleagues as an intervention to enrich the relationships of nondistressed couples (Carson at al., 2004). They showed MBRE compared to wait-list controls had a positive impact on relationship satisfaction, closeness, mutual acceptance and relationship distress, in addition to positive effects on individual optimism, spirituality and relaxation, with benefits at 3-month follow-up. In the follow-up study, the researchers found that the gains in MBRE could be attributed largely to partners' sense they were participating in exciting, self-expanding activities together (Carson, Carson, Gil, & Baucom, 2007).

MBRE is modeled on MBSR with interventions and meditations that are adapted to couples, for example, couples focus on one another during loving-kindness meditation, incorporate one another in yoga exercises, build mutual awareness during shared activities, and engage in mindful touch, dyadic eye-gazing, share the goodness of one another, and apply mindfulness to relationship difficulties.

Compassion Training

The formal training of compassion has surged in recent years and a large number of programs have emerged including Compassion-Focused Therapy (CFT) and Compassion Mind Training (CMT) (Gilbert, 2009; 2010), general compassion meditation programs (e.g., Pace et al., 2009), and Compassion Cultivation Training (CCT; Jazaieri et al., 2012). In general, these programs focus directly on training compassion through mindfulness, loving-kindness, self-compassion, and related practices, and reveal favorable results relating to psychological and physical well-being. The latter program found that specific domains of compassion can be targeted and successfully trained, e.g., compassion for others, receiving compassion from others, and self-compassion. Compassion programs have been tailored to specific populations such as at-risk youth. Another program, Cognitively-Based Compassion Training (CBCT), did not produce improvements in psychosocial functioning; however, the strength of hope did increase among the adolescents in the compassion group (Sheethal et al., 2013).

Contexts

These and other mindfulness programs have been applied to a number of different contexts, including medicine, psychotherapy, law, and education. The adaptation of mindfulness, namely Mindful-

ness-Based Strengths Practice (MBSP), across contexts is discussed in Chapter 15. A fairly new context in which mindfulness is being directly applied is coaching (e.g., life coaching, wellness/health coaching, executive coaching). Passmore and Marianetti (2007) discuss the use of mindfulness in coaching and relay four specific applications for coaches to consider: the use of mindfulness as preparation prior to the coaching session, to help maintain focused attention during sessions, to help remain emotionally detached in sessions, and as a practice that can be taught to coachees.

Neuroscience

It is striking how much attention mindfulness has received in the world of neuroscience. At the same time, contributing factors are easy to spot, such as neuropsychologist Richard Davidson's innovative research lab at the University of Wisconsin, as well as the Mind & Life dialogs the Dalai Lama has been having with neuroscientists and other top Western scientists for over 25 years. This has led to a number of book publications (e.g., Goleman, 1997) and has contributed to the flourishing of science in the area. One of the most salient research findings to emerge is that mindfulness has an impact on neuroplasticity. Neuroplasticity refers to the brain's ability to rewire and restructure itself through learning and experience. Lab studies of meditators has shown that repetitive mindfulness practice drives positive changes in neuroplasticity leading to greater emotional balance, compassion, happiness, and the buffering of stress and trauma, which reflect greater mental/physical well-being (Lutz, Dunne, & Davidson, 2007).

Mindfulness training seems to change individuals' emotional set-points, even among those individuals whose brains are wired more for psychological disorders such as depression and anxiety. Research on meditation has led to a number of other findings: Concentration, mindfulness, and relaxation seem to be uniquely different brain states (Dunn, Hartigan, & Mikulas, 1999); meditation experience has been linked with increased cortical thickness (Lazar et al., 2005); and mindfulness meditation training has led to significant boosts in the immune system (Davidson et al., 2003).

Mindfulness Practice

Types of Practice

Any time an individual brings his/her attention to the present moment with curiosity, openness, and/or acceptance, then they are practicing mindfulness. This can occur at "any" time, whether it is attention to how one is sitting, one's movement while walking, one's breathing while working, the road and landscape while driving, the food one is eating, or the smile on a loved one's face while talking.

Kabat-Zinn (1990) offers the practical distinction of practicing mindfulness formally and informally. Both are crucial in the development of any mindfulness practice. Here are four general categories of practice:

Formal

Some people practice mindfulness meditation for a certain amount of time each day. It is a "formal" practice when one carves out part of daily living to practice mindfulness, for example, 2 ×/ day for 15 minutes each or every morning from 9:00 AM – 9:30 AM. The most common form of mindfulness is concentrating on one's breathing while sitting.

Informal

Informal practice means to "use it when you need it." When one is stressed, anxious, depressed, overwhelmed, or helpless, informal practice suggests the individual take a moment to slow down, to pause and "just be" with the discomfort. The individual focuses on breathing and becoming aware of his or her body, thoughts, emotions, behavior, and environment in the present moment. Some guiding questions include:
- What is your body saying to you right now?
- What are you thinking about?
- What emotions are you present to right now?
- What do you need?

- What would "self-care" look like for you in this moment?

In-the-Moment

This form of practice means to purposefully thread mindfulness into daily activities (see Nhat Hanh, 1991). Some general ideas include:
- Practice returning your attention to the present moment whenever your mind wanders off.
- Whenever possible, do one thing at a time (multi-tasking can lead to mindlessness)
- Pay full attention (using all five senses, when possible) to what you are doing right now
- Practice "being" while you are eating, driving, talking, listening, working, praying, etc.

Cued

This means to set up external cues to bring oneself back to the present moment. One's autopilot mind and busy lifestyle make it easy to lose one's mindfulness. Environmental cues act as triggers to remind oneself to be open and curious to what is going on around oneself. Some people place sticky notes in their various living quarters as a cue.

Example

For example, consider Fr. Dave, a priest who was part of a mindfulness group I was leading for clergy. Fr. Dave was practicing bringing mindfulness more into his daily life but explained that his autopilot mind was becoming a significant challenge to contend with. He decided to set up cues for himself. He placed small sticky notes in places that would surprise him, such as his wallet, on the inside of his mindfulness folder, and on the milk container in his refrigerator. Whenever he spotted one of these cues, he would pause, take two slow breaths and check in with his body tension and where his mind was wandering. Fr. Dave also placed sticky notes in places that he commonly walked by, such as his bathroom door, his work desk, and his closet at church. He found that his mind quickly habituated to these locations that were "out in the open" and after a week or two his autopilot took over and he no longer noticed them. Thus, he set himself a reminder to move these particular cues in different places once every two weeks.

Practice Tip: Take a Moment to "Just Be"

Individuals new to basic meditation, such as sitting meditation or breath meditation, will inevitably benefit from some explanation of the purpose of meditation and how to practice. Of course, no amount of reading about meditation will replace the actual practice. The influential Zen teacher Ezra Bayda (2002) explains the basics in terms of three aspects of sitting: being-in-the-body, labeling and experiencing, and opening into the heart of experiencing.

1. *Being-in-the-body:* Notice your body, its posture, and your sensations. Tune into the sensations of your breath in the body.
2. *Labeling and experiencing:* As you notice thoughts and emotions occur, label them as thoughts or emotions. Meditation scholar Jack Kornfield (1993) has suggested you might say to yourself "judging mind" or "planning mind" to label thoughts of self-criticism or thoughts of the day's plans that emerge. Emotions, such as anxiety, sadness, joy, and peace can also be labeled as such and experienced in the moment as one gets stronger in the practice.
3. *Opening into the heart of experiencing:* This aspect of sitting meditation involves persevering through the struggles of sitting meditation and realizing that obstacles are simply part of the practice. Bayda encourages breathing into the space of the heart and to stick with the heart-space for "just one more breath," which in turn, builds perseverance with the practice.

With each of these, the challenge is to let go of the mind's tendency to want to "do." The mind will chatter away about your plans of the day, situations that occurred yesterday, conversations you've had recently, and the many things that you should be doing instead of sitting. The mind will be very convincing that you should not be sitting there. But, just breathe and be where you are – in the moment. Like everything with mindfulness, taking time to "just be" is a practice you can cultivate.

Where's Your Client at With Their Mindfulness Practice?

If the client is brand new to mindfulness: Recommend that the client take it slowly but steady. They should make note of the mindfulness practice that strikes them the most – mindful walking, mindful eating, mindful sitting – and practice it daily. Encourage them to set up a way to stay motivated and stick with this daily practice. It would be helpful if they joined a mindfulness meditation group in their community, or asked a relationship partner or friend to check in on their practice regimen each week. If they are having problems staying motivated, help the client set up a reinforcement system where they track their experiences each day (see the tracking forms used in MBSP in Section III).

If the client has some mindfulness knowledge and practical experience: Work with the client to first consider what is already working with their practice of mindfulness – how can they build upon the positives that they are already taking action with? Also, encourage them to consider their strengths. Introduce the character strengths to them. Which strengths might help them deepen their practice? If they're high in love of learning, perhaps they could tackle a new mindfulness book; if they're high in love or kindness, perhaps develop a loving-kindness meditation practice (listen to Track 6 of the attached CD for an example of loving-kindness meditation). If they're high in teamwork, they could consider engaging in a regular practice with a friend and discussing their experiences or weave in a practice of mindful listening/mindful speaking with a loved one.

If the client has significant experience in the practice of mindfulness: Encourage them to read this book! If they take a "beginner's mind" approach to certain chapters, such as Chapter 4 which deals with strengthening one's mindfulness practice with character strengths, there will be some new insights that are likely to positively impact on their practice. In addition, invite them to imagine what it would be like to boost their knowledge and practice of character strengths to the same level of their mindfulness practice. What benefits might emerge?

Practice Tip: Takeaway Tip-Sheet:

- *Observe your "monkey-mind":* Since our mind often chatters incessantly, rather than trying to stop it, take a stance of watching it, just as one might enjoy sitting back and watching a group of monkeys climb, jump, and swing in the trees.
- *Weave your parachute every day*: Kabat-Zinn (1990) used this metaphor to emphasize that mindfulness should be cultivated and practiced each day. Just as you wouldn't begin weaving your parachute as you're jumping out of a plane, you'd want to weave it each day so that when you need it, it might be strong enough to hold you up.
- *When possible, limit your multi-tasking:* When you are eating, just eat … when you are walking, just walk. Practice giving your full attention to whatever you are doing.
- *Set up "bells" of mindfulness:* Make a plan to return your attention to the present moment when you hear an actual bell or a cue you set up in your environment.
- *Always back to the breath*: When your mind wanders, bring it back to the breath no matter where you are and what you are doing. Repeat this over and over the rest of your life.
- *Be curious about your distractions:* If your mind repeatedly heads off to a particular topic or always seems to avoid a specific emotion, consider bringing an approach of curiosity and interest to your mind and the topic.

Chapter 2
A Primer on Character Strengths

Character is fate.

Heraclitus

Chapter Snapshot

This chapter offers a primer on character strengths. Definitions, key concepts, misconceptions, research, and a variety of character strengths interventions will be reviewed. Several general principles for conceptualizing and distinguishing character strengths are discussed. Practical tips are offered throughout the chapter and it closes with some core ideas that can be viewed as important teaching points.

Opening Story

One of the biggest transitions in my life was catalyzed by the use of a variety of my character strengths. I was living in St. Louis and recently married. Everything was going very strong with my career in clinical psychology, directing and creating new programs, leading retreats, writing books, and building a regional reputation. However, there was one problem: My wife and I were far away from family. We had many tense discussions about whether we should move. My wife didn't have a location in mind, just that she was ready to leave St. Louis which was far away from her closest connections. I was settled and comfortable, unable to fathom giving up everything I had worked so hard to develop. We had this disagreement too many times to count.

One day, while driving back to St. Louis, the same discussion emerged again. As tension began to rise, I decided a different approach was needed. Something clicked in me. "What if?" I said to myself. "What if we were to move?" For the very first time, I allowed myself to fully envision this other reality, to see things from a very new perspective. I was exercising my judgment/critical thinking – a middle-range character strength for me. This allowed me to be open to a different perspective, one that I had previously rejected in my head without genuinely listening to other views or reviewing any details. As I considered what I would be letting go, I also took notice of what I would gain (e.g., closer proximity to family, new career possibilities). My signature strengths of hope and curiosity began to bloom and a wave of excitement arose. As I began to express these thoughts to my amazed wife, the pieces began to fit into place. In that conversation, we selected with certainty that our new destination would be Cincinnati, even though I'd never visited the city before, and knew very little about it. Something seemed exactly right, even though it was not entirely rational. We began to put this enormous transition into motion and made the move within a year.

Several years later, we reflect upon this decision, catalyzed in one moment through strength use, as one of the best decisions of our lives.

Character Strengths Background/History

Philosophers, theologians, educators, ethicists, psychologists, and scholars have long been interested in virtues, ethics, strengths, and the good life. A limitation has been that there was no common language for discussing the best qualities in people. While there does exist popular classification systems for studying what is wrong with people – the *DSM-IV* (American Psychiatric Association, 1994) and the *ICD-10* (World Health Organization, 1990), there was nothing comparable for human strengths.

In the late 1990s and early 2000s, the emerging field of positive psychology sought to apply science to bring a clearer understanding to what is best in people. Positive psychology had been conceptualized as the scientific study of the conditions and processes that contribute to flourishing or optimal functioning (Gable & Haidt, 2005), as well as "nothing more than the scientific study of ordinary human strengths and virtues" (Sheldon & King, 2001, p. 216). Martin Seligman gave the field a voice while president of the American Psychological Association. His intention was not to introduce something brand new but to bring together disparate research groups around the world studying positive aspects of human nature, and to promote new research initiatives. Another driving force was the intention to bring further balance to the psychology field which had focused far more on what's wrong with people than what's right with people. One example of this gap is reflected in psychology professor David Myers' study (2000) of positive social interactions and relationships. He calculated the ratio of peer-reviewed studies of negative emotional experiences to positive emotional experiences and found a 21 : 1 disparity in studies between 1967 and 2000. Indeed, psychology had made significant progress in developing research and practices around addiction, abuse, and various psychological disorders, however, its focus had been lopsided.

Seligman (1999) offered three main pathways for scientific inquiry into the positive: positive subjective experiences (positive emotions), positive traits (character strengths), and positive institutions. One of the biggest projects in this new

field was the collaboration of 55 scientists who embarked on a three-year project led by Chris Peterson, a university professor and researcher. The scientists' mission was to review a couple-hundred works throughout time that have attempted to categorize or discuss human virtue, strength, or goodness. The literature dated back 2,500 years to Buddhism and the approach was systematic. In addition to reviewing previous attempts to classify virtue, an empirical approach was driven by two questions: Would the virtue catalogs of early thinkers converge? Would certain virtues, regardless of tradition or culture, be widely valued? (Dahlsgaard, Peterson, & Seligman, 2005; Peterson & Seligman, 2004). The researchers looked for "coherent resemblance," reflecting that "the higher order meaning behind a particular core virtue lined up better with its cross-cultural counterparts than with any other core virtue" (Dahlsgaard et al., 2005, p. 204). What emerged were six similar themes (virtues) emerging across the traditions of Athenian philosophy, Confucianism, Taoism, Buddhism, Hinduism, Christianity, Judaism, and Islam. These paralleling themes are wisdom, courage, humanity, justice, temperance, and transcendence. These became the six virtue categories in the VIA Classification.

Following historical review, other analyses were conducted, including the application of various criteria to determine the strengths that reside under the virtues. It was paramount that the strengths be both universal across cultures and measurable. Data from over 30 nations supported the ubiquity of character strengths (Peterson & Seligman, 2004), and a couple years later data was published on the universality of character strengths across 52 countries (Park, Peterson, & Seligman, 2006). Other research has replicated and expanded this work (McGrath, in press). In addition, Biswas-Diener (2006) conducted some pioneering cross-cultural research offering further support that these characteristics were more than a Western cultural phenomenon. He traveled to remote areas to speak with various cultures about the existence of these 24 strengths and whether the strengths met various criteria. For example, Biswas-Diener met with the Maasai tribal people in Kenya and the Inuit people in Northern Greenland, each selected for their representation of far-ranging differences in language, technological development, cultural and spiritual practices, geography, and history. His research team found high rates of agreement on the existence, importance, and desirability of the 24 character strengths in these cultures. The cultures also acknowledged the possibility that people of any age and gender could develop the strengths and that there are cultural institutions to foster them.

Following the establishment of the 24 character strengths, a measurement tool was then validated to assess the strengths; this is known as the *VIA Survey* or the *VIA Inventory of Strengths* (Park & Peterson, 2006c; Peterson & Seligman, 2004). The VIA Classification of 24 character strengths and six virtues is detailed in Table 2.1, and described in full in Peterson and Seligman (2004).

Table 2.1
VIA Classification of Character Strengths and Virtues

---

1. **Wisdom and Knowledge** – Cognitive strengths that entail the acquisition and use of knowledge
   - *Creativity* [originality, ingenuity]: Thinking of novel and productive ways to conceptualize and do things; includes artistic achievement but is not limited to it
   - *Curiosity* [interest, novelty-seeking, openness to experience]: Taking an interest in ongoing experience for its own sake; finding subjects and topics fascinating; exploring and discovering
   - *Judgment* [critical thinking, open-mindedness]: Thinking things through and examining them from all sides; not jumping to conclusions; being able to change one's mind in light of evidence; weighing all evidence fairly
   - *Love of Learning:* Mastering new skills, topics, and bodies of knowledge, whether on one's own or formally; related to the strength of curiosity but goes beyond it to describe the tendency to add systematically to what one knows
   - *Perspective* [wisdom]: Being able to provide wise counsel to others; having ways of looking at the world that make sense to oneself/others
2. **Courage** – Emotional strengths that involve the exercise of will to accomplish goals in the face of opposition, external or internal
   - *Bravery* [valor]: Not shrinking from threat, challenge, difficulty, or pain; speaking up for what's right even if there's opposition; acting on convictions even if unpopular; includes physical bravery but is not limited to it
   - *Perseverance* [persistence, industriousness]: Finishing what one starts; persevering in a course of action in spite of obstacles; "getting it out the door"; taking pleasure in completing tasks
   - *Honesty* [authenticity, integrity]: Speaking the truth but more broadly presenting oneself in a genuine way and acting in a sincere way; being without pretense; taking responsibility for one's feelings and actions
   - *Zest* [vitality, enthusiasm, vigor, energy]: Approaching life with excitement and energy; not doing things halfway or halfheartedly; living life as an adventure; feeling alive and activated
3. **Humanity** – Interpersonal strengths that involve tending and befriending others
   - *Love* (capacity to love and be loved): Valuing close relations with others, in particular those in which sharing and caring are reciprocated; being close to people
   - *Kindness* [generosity, nurturance, care, compassion, altruistic love, "niceness"]: Doing favors and good deeds for others; helping them; taking care of them
   - *Social Intelligence* [emotional intelligence, personal intelligence]: Being aware of the motives/ feelings of others and oneself; knowing what to do to fit into different social situations; knowing what makes other people tick
4. **Justice** – Civic strengths that underlie healthy community life
   - *Teamwork* [citizenship, social responsibility, loyalty]: Working well as a member of a group or team; being loyal to the group; doing one's share
   - *Fairness:* Treating all people the same according to notions of fairness and justice; not letting feelings bias decisions about others; giving everyone a fair chance
   - *Leadership:* Encouraging a group of which one is a member to get things done and at the same time maintain good relations within the group; organizing group activities and seeing that they happen

5. **Temperance** – Strengths that protect against excess
   - *Forgiveness* [mercy]: Forgiving those who have done wrong; accepting others' shortcomings; giving people a second chance; not being vengeful
   - *Humility* [modesty]: Letting one's accomplishments speak for themselves; not regarding oneself as more special than one is
   - *Prudence:* Being careful about one's choices; not taking undue risks; not saying or doing things that might later be regretted
   - *Self-Regulation* [self-control]: Regulating what one feels and does; being disciplined; controlling one's appetites and emotions
6. **Transcendence** – Strengths that forge connections to the universe and provide meaning
   - *Appreciation of Beauty and Excellence* [awe, wonder, elevation]: Noticing and appreciating beauty, excellence, and/or skilled performance in various domains of life, from nature to art to mathematics to science to everyday experience
   - *Gratitude:* Being aware of and thankful for the good things that happen; taking time to express thanks
   - *Hope* [optimism, future-mindedness, future orientation]: Expecting the best in the future and working to achieve it; believing that a good future is something that can be brought about
   - *Humor* [playfulness]: Liking to laugh and tease; bringing smiles to other people; seeing the light side; making (not necessarily telling) jokes
   - *Spirituality* [religiousness, faith, purpose]: Having coherent beliefs about the higher purpose and meaning of the universe; knowing where one fits within the larger scheme; having beliefs about the meaning of life that shape conduct and provide comfort

The table represents the most updated character strengths terminology of the VIA Classification, adjusted from Peterson and Seligman (2004), courtesy of the VIA Institute.

The 24 character strengths have been viewed by many as the backbone of the study of what is "right" with people (Park, Peterson, & Seligman, 2004; Seligman, 2002; Seligman & Csikszentmihalyi, 2000), and may indeed occupy the most central role in the field of positive psychology as pleasure, flow, engagement, and other positive experiences are enabled by good character (Park & Peterson, 2009; Peterson, Ruch, Beermann, Park, & Seligman, 2007).

Character Strengths – General Concepts

Key Definitions and Concepts

Character strengths are capacities for thinking, feeling, volition, and behaving. They are the psychological ingredients for displaying virtues and human goodness.

These positive characteristics of our personality are different from other types of strength, such as talents (what we do well), interests (what we enjoy doing), skills (proficiencies we develop), and resources (external supports). While each of these areas of strength are important, character strengths are viewed as the individual's core which provide a pathway for developing the other strength areas. For example, a person may use perseverance and self-regulation to pursue a talent in music or sport, hope in developing a new skill for work, curiosity to explore areas of interest, and gratitude and kindness to tap into external resources. Talents can be squandered, skills can diminish, and resources lost, but strengths crystallize and evolve and can integrate with these other positive qualities to contribute to the greater good.

Character strengths are viewed as "who we are," in other words, they are part of our core identity. One might think of them as positive personality characteristics. In the early days of positive psychology, the character strengths were referred to as the wellsprings of a good, full life because they can be viewed as flowing out of us like a well spring in many directions.

Signature strengths are those strengths we bring forth most naturally across multiple settings and infuse us with energy. As they are core to identity, they help individuals to function at their best and maintain a sense of authenticity. In addition, these are strengths that family and friends will often nominate as particularly characteristic of the individual. Typically, these strengths appear toward the top of one's VIA Survey results. However, there is no set number of signature strengths an individual has. Conventional thinking in the early days of positive psychology suggested individuals have about five (plus or minus two) signature strengths, and researchers generally use "top 5" as a convention in studies. This is a useful heuristic as this quantity of strengths is a reasonable amount for individuals to keep in their mind; and other strengths proponents (e.g., the Gallup Organization) have taken this approach. Nevertheless, research by the VIA Institute has found that people tend to believe they have significantly more than five signature strengths, and that of those strengths that do appear in an individual's top 5, about four of these tend to be viewed by the individual as a "signature" strength.

Signature strengths research and practice are discussed throughout this chapter and book. The approach of understanding one's own signature strengths and how they are expressed in the world, as well as learning others' signature strengths and discussing/reinforcing those strengths, cannot be underscored enough. While additional research is needed, the expression of signature strengths in a strong, versatile yet balanced way may actually be connected with each of the many pathways to well-being, flourishing, and living a full life.

Practice Tip: Even Though You're "Strengths-Based," Learn the Language

These days it seems that everyone is strengths-based. When I speak to groups of psychologists, counselors, social workers, educators, teachers, or coaches, I often ask them: Who here is strengths-based? Inevitably, almost every hand goes up. This makes sense because who wants to view themselves as deficit-based? For every hand that goes up, there is a different perspective on what "strengths-based" means. For decades, professionals have been calling themselves "strength-based," yet this has almost no meaning as each professional defines this differently. For

some professionals this simply means being nice to a client; for others it means not attacking; for others it means being solution-focused, motivation-based, or goal-oriented; the explanations go on and on. The VIA Classification is a scientific-based, common language that brings these disparate approaches together.

Having a common language means communication doors open. It means practitioners have a template for thinking about and working with clients. It means clients have a new way of viewing themselves; the language serves as a guide for understanding the core of who they are. From this mutual understanding, interventions and strategies can sprout, and conversations (in which client and practitioner mutually spot strengths) emerge.

I recall in my early work as a clinical psychologist, prior to the advent of the VIA Classification, I would fumble around in describing the good qualities of my clients. I was much more versed and fluid in describing their diagnoses, assessment procedures for their problems, and plans for treating their problems. My description of their good features felt more limited and I certainly did not give the positive and negative features equal attention, as suggested as a starting point by positive psychology practitioners (Rashid, 2009). Instead, the minimal amount of positive attributes I did identify seemed to come across as awkward. For example, suggesting a depressed client who was under-appreciating the good to keep a gratitude journal felt as if there was no basis for my suggestion other than that spiritual writers suggested it was a good idea (Steindl-Rast, 1984). As a psychologist, I needed to offer interventions based in science and the research literature on gratitude had not emerged at that time.

The VIA Classification offers a "language" and a substantive approach for describing what is best in people. Try to become familiar with the contents of Table 2.1 just as you would go about learning a new language. If you were to attempt to master a new language, you would study the vocabulary, use the words in your writing and speech, observe others using the language, and study it as closely as possible. You can take the same approach in learning this "strengths language" – not only the virtues and strengths – but also the dimensions listed in brackets and the definitions. Experiment, observe, and practice.

Misconceptions

As discussed with the word "mindfulness" in Chapter 1, there are similarly a number of misconceptions that emerge when people hear the words "character" or "character strengths." The word character is often connected with "values," which is a highly subjective term that is often linked with personal, political, or religious beliefs. Moreover, the scientific study of character had been cast aside for decades after leading personality theorists proclaimed it to be too value-based to be studied empirically and should therefore be left to the study of philosophers (Allport, 1921). However, the new science of character discussed in this chapter employs both quantitative and qualitative, objective methods, and offers empirical data and applications with validated measurement tools. Researchers around the globe are now studying the character strengths of employees, college students, teachers, children, adolescents, CEOs, those with medical and psychological illnesses, and many other populations.

It was previously thought that character simply meant integrity or being authentic and honest. Taken a step further, character has been misconceived as boiling down to a finite number of traits that the individual either has or doesn't have. Approaches to character strengths are much more sophisticated now and espouse that people have many character strengths that are expressed in different degrees and combinations, depending on the context.

Another misconception is that focusing on strengths is "happiology," selfish, or Pollyannaish. This can be quickly negated because at least half of the character strengths are other-oriented (e.g., kindness, fairness, forgiveness, and teamwork), so to focus on these is to contribute to the well-being of others. Moreover, any of the character strengths can be applied to bring benefit to others. As will be discussed frequently in this book, character

strengths apply to what is best and what is worst in life. Sometimes the focus on strengths leads to positive outcomes, sometimes it does not.

Strengths Blindness

The pervasiveness of autopilot and everyday mindlessness discussed in Chapter 1 carries over to character strengths. There appears to be a pervasive strengths blindness (i.e., lack of a deep mindfulness) of one's character strengths in today's culture. What follows are four different types of strengths blindness:

1. General Unawareness of Strengths

The unawareness of character strengths might reflect a lack of self-awareness or disconnection with who one is (identity). The point is that many people find it difficult to recognize their strengths (Linley & Harrington, 2006). This includes the individuals who are stunned like deer in the headlights when asked what their strengths are at a job interview. Some of these individuals might be unreflective or lack psychological mindedness while others have simply never given the topic of their strengths much thought. I feel a wave of sadness when I asked psychotherapy clients what their strengths are and they say: "I don't know" or "I don't have any." Unfortunately, this is a fairly common response.

2. Disconnect With Meaning

Linley (2008) has reported survey research finding only 1/3 of people have a meaningful awareness of their strengths. Some individuals might be able to respond to the general question: What are your best qualities or strengths? But often the answer is not a very substantive one. Responses are often vague (e.g., "I have good qualities") or confuse character strengths with other strength domains such as interest (e.g., "I like listening to music") and talent/skill (e.g., "I'm good at baseball"). A person may say they perform better than the average person at recreational baseball; however, it is character that makes the connection with meaning and substance. In this example, it is the person's demonstration of perseverance, teamwork, and self-regulation on the baseball field that start to tell us something about this individual's strengths.

3. Seeing Strengths as Ordinary Rather Than Extraordinary

This is the taking-strengths-for-granted effect. Sometimes individuals minimize or downplay their strengths. They may take the VIA Survey and react with a response of, "Yeah, I already knew that, no big deal." It might be true that the person would have guessed some of their highest strengths, but that's far from the point. The point is that the individual has engaged in something that has potential to be a springboard for many positive outcomes and they are already moving on to another topic. They are glossing over their core traits, not actively drawing connections with strengths and their experiences, not engaging in a strengths conversation in the moment, and not actively brainstorming ways to move forward with strengths expression. The potential good and possible outcomes that can emerge from strengths use is large and quite extraordinary, thus there is a certain level of blindness that is occurring when individuals view strengths as ordinary phenomena to be passed over (Biswas-Diener, Kashdan, & Minhas, 2011). Such an approach stifles or limits oneself from digging deeper. There are always more angles that could be taken when it comes to strengths use. A given individual can be blind to the use of one of their strengths in a particular context or situation, blind to how a strength might appear in disguise, or unaware of how their strength presents in daily routines, when stressors arise, or when working toward a particular goal. In this vein, it's probably fair to say that most people could benefit from a deeper awareness of and meaning applied to their character strengths.

4. Strengths Overuse

Strengths underuse is a phenomenon that underpins each of the categories above. Strengths overuse is a fourth type of blindness. Strengths overuse occurs when an individual puts forth their strength(s) too strongly in a particular situation. A person might express so much curiosity that they become nosey or so much leadership that they appear controlling. Often, strengths overuse has an impact on relationships and the individual who is doing the overusing is unaware (i.e., blind) to this impact or at least the extent of the impact. On other occasions, the individual might be blind as to what to do about their heavy exertion of zest

at work or their overuse of teamwork that pushes their individuality to the side.

The integration of mindfulness and character strengths is one way to work with each of the types of strengths blindness.

The Strengths Paradox

There exists an interesting paradox in strengths-based work. On one hand, there are the widespread types of strengths blindness and on the other hand, when prompted, individuals are marvelous at discussing their best qualities. Often this takes individuals just a little push, such as having a discussion about a time when they were successful, strong, or at their best. When given even simply one opportunity to explore their best qualities, individuals are usually willing and able to offer something. In addition, individuals seem to have at least some natural skill in strengths-spotting – readily finding strengths in a conversation or story. I've found in workshops around the world that people well-versed in strengths and those new to strengths exhibit this skill. Participants also seem to be able to discuss the nuances of strengths easily (e.g., overuse, the role of context). This was shown in early research exploring VIA character strengths with high school students (Steen, Kachorek, & Peterson, 2003). Even very young children can readily understand each of the 24 strengths when time is taken to teach them (Fox Eades, 2008). Practitioners who encourage and reinforce strengths discussions find that clients – even those depressed or disengaged – are able to find themselves in their strengths and are able to have a strengths conversation. It is as if a new door has been opened allowing the client to see themselves and others in a new way.

I call this simultaneous existence of the unawareness of strengths along with a high potential for strengths use *the strengths paradox*.

Signature strengths can be a "game-changer" with this strengths paradox, especially when working with clients. Signature strengths can help close the gap on the strengths paradox. In every sporting event, there is often a moment when the momentum shifts to one team's favor that eventually leads them to a victory. Something happens – maybe it's a slam dunk that energizes the team, maybe it's a great touchdown pass that puts the score out of reach, or maybe it's a goal that ties the game with seconds left after being down the whole game. Similarly, signature strengths are that game changer. Even the savviest of clients can be blind to their strengths or at least forget to consider their strengths in the context of their struggles. When brought to their attention, there is often a reaction of "oh yeah, of course!"

Practice Tip: Assume the Best
Practitioners are well-equipped to focus on what is wrong about their clients and to expect the worst. We easily get caught up in the stories of negativity, suffering, and pain. However, keep the strengths paradox in mind – it is likely that with just a little push by you your client will be able to unfold powerful stories and experiences filled with character strengths.

Therefore, consider taking an approach that *assumes* there is a strengths conversation waiting, just below the surface, ready to be facilitated.

Character Strengths Principles

There are a number of core concepts relevant to the study of character. Many of these have been introduced elsewhere (Niemiec, 2013); however, additional principles have been added here as well.

Character is not singular, it is plural (Peterson, 2006). Rather than viewing character as a singular construct such as honesty or integrity, it is useful to view character strengths as being expressed in combination or as a constellation. This was expressed in a scientific dialog between the Dalai Lama and top scientists in which virtues ethicist Lee Yearly and the Dalai Lama expressed the inadequacy of compassion as the sole foundation of ethics as this would limit the human experience too severely (Goleman, 1997).

Character strengths are multi-dimensional (Peterson & Seligman, 2004). There is a complexity to character strengths in that there are notable dimensions and qualities within each. For example, kindness is more than being kind, it involves dimensions of compassion, altruism, generosity, care, nurturance, and niceness. The character strength of honesty involves dimensions of integrity and authenticity. Several of these "dimensions" are listed in brackets after many of the character strengths in Table 2.1.

Character strengths are who we are at our core. Character strengths are our true essence – the core parts of our personality that account for us being our best selves. When we think about our best qualities, it is likely we will immediately name one or more of the 24 character strengths or a construct that is closely related to them.

Character strengths can be measured. It is groundbreaking science to have a tool with good reliability and validity that measures many of the positive traits found in human beings. The VIA Survey, like any measurement tool, is imperfect, in that some scales could be improved (e.g., self-regulation), and in one instance (i.e., humility) a self-report scale may not be the best option for assessing the character strength (Davis, Worthington, & Hook, 2010). As one adage goes, *all tests are wrong, some are useful.*

Character strengths are universal (Biswas-Diener, 2006; Park, Peterson, & Seligman, 2006; Peterson & Seligman, 2004). Character strengths can be found in the most remote cultures and lands, among people whom are literate and non-literate, and in those with differing beliefs, religious affiliations, and political preferences. The creation of such a nonarbitrary classification means that, among other things, there are no culture-bound strengths, such as achievement or ambition, that are often characteristic of Western cultures (Peterson & Seligman, 2004).

Character strengths are expressed in degrees and within contexts (Fowers, 2008; Schwartz & Sharpe, 2006). How individuals express character strengths differs widely according to the person and the situation they are in. Because each person has their own unique profile of strengths, the expression will be idiosyncratic and will differ in degree. This means that two individuals might share the strength of love as their highest strength; however, that strength will likely be expressed at different frequencies, durations, and intensities at different times.

Depending on the context, one individual might call forth his or her social intelligence and curiosity when with friends; use self-regulation and prudence when eating; draw on teamwork and perseverance at work; and love and kindness with family. The degree of kindness and love the person expresses with family may differ depending on the personality of the relative: the restrained mother, jovial father, down-to-earth uncle, or un-emotional daughter. Moreover, the *situation* – a funeral home, an amusement park, or a public lecture – will also play a significant role in the strength expression. Remember that the VIA Survey tool is a *dimensional* measure; there are no all-or-none categorical distinctions in which we either have a strength or we don't.

Character strengths can be overused, under-used, or misused. Some individuals will use their strengths for malevolent purposes, as seen in the many e-mail scams in which individuals employ high creativity to make up stories to fool people into sending money or bank account information. Character strengths can also be overused and underused. It is striking that character strengths can be quickly forgotten or expressed in an unbalanced way. The overuse of curiosity can lead someone into a dangerous part of a city while the underuse of fairness may lead to problems in one's relationships. Each of the 24 strengths can be plotted along a continuum as shown with the strength of kindness in Figure 2.1. At some point in some situations, a person can express too much of a strength and it turns into an overuse in that situation and likewise at some point there is a point where the strength is being underused. Note that when a strength is overused or underused it is no longer a character strength! It is something else. In the case of kindness below, it can transform into intrusiveness or indifference.

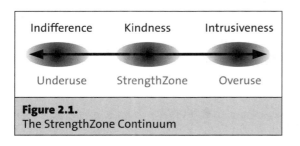

Figure 2.1.
The StrengthZone Continuum

Character deals with both "being" and "doing." Not dissimilar to the philosophical debate between "being" and "becoming," character strengths and mindfulness can be viewed in terms of being and doing. In his presentations, Jon Kabat-Zinn often makes the comment that mindfulness is about bringing the "being" back into human beings because people have arranged their lives to focus almost entirely on "human doing." Character is

both who we are (being) and the action we put out into the world (doing). When compiling a list of virtues derived by reading through each entry in a dictionary, researchers Cawley, Martin, and Johnson (2000) used linguistic criteria to determine virtues. One of their criteria was whether the virtue word fit each of these two sentences: "I ought to be ___ " and "I ought to show ___." While social evaluation terms (e.g., fame, power, beauty) do not readily fit this approach, one can ideally plug in one's signature strengths into either sentence and find a nice fit.

Good character is more than the absence of bad character. Many individuals avoid bad behavior but this alone does not mean that they are expressing character strengths to a strong degree.

Virtuous character is guided by a clear vision of what is good and admirable where the individual is able to act consistently in a way that fits the situation (Fowers, 2008). One pathway toward virtuous character, in addition to expressing character strengths according to the golden mean, is to give authentic expression to one's signature strengths.

All 24 character strengths matter. Several of the earlier principles underpin this concept that each of the 24 strengths is important and relevant for different purposes. This resembles what Fowers (2008) discusses as "unity of character."

Character strengths work is more about synthesis than analysis. Psychology has spent decades picking apart problems and the issues that life brings (i.e., analysis). Strengths work, however, is largely about connecting aspects of life together – synthesizing qualities, memories, thoughts, feelings, and strengths to elicit a whole.

Character strengths differ from other types of strengths. Human beings have many strengths, coming in different shapes and sizes. Strengths of character are different from strengths that can be called talents, skills, interests, values, or resources.

- *Talents* are strengths that are innate abilities, which typically have a strong biological loading, and may or may not be well-developed (e.g., intelligence, musical ability, athletic ability).
- *Skills* are strengths that are specific proficiencies developed through training (e.g., learning a particular trade; computing skills; researching skills).

- *Interests* are strengths that are areas or topics an individual is passionate about and driven to pursue, such as playing sports, engaging in particular hobbies, and working with arts or crafts.
- *Values* are enduring beliefs, principles, or ideals that are of prime importance to the individual. Values are the most subjective and personal of these strength categories. Values reside in cognition and affect (not behavior).
- *Resources* are the one type of strength that is external; resources are external supports, such as social and spiritual connections.

Character strengths are stable but can be developed (Borghans, Duckworth, Heckman, & ter Weel, 2008; Peterson & Seligman, 2004). A commonly held misconception is that our character – much like an engraved mark etched in stone – is immutable and unchanging. Character strengths are part of our personality, which we know is quite stable. At the same time, personality traits can shift through normative changes based on our genetics and predictable changes in our social role

(e.g., starting a family), as well as nonnormative changes. Nonnormative changes include deliberately chosen changes in our social role (e.g., joining the military), atypical life events (e.g., the experience of trauma), and deliberate interventions (Borghans et al., 2008). Normative and nonnormative changes can have an impact on our strengths.

The development of character is not a new topic, and neither is the use of intentional activity that focuses on improving character strengths. Aristotle (2000) and Saint Thomas Aquinas (1989) emphasized that virtue could be acquired through practice. One of the founding fathers of the United States, Benjamin Franklin (1962), set up a system where he placed his attention on improving one virtue per week while leaving the other virtues to "their ordinary chance." Franklin tracked his progress and journaled about his experiences. In his autobiography, he described this approach as contributing greatly to his happiness and life successes. Many others have echoed these sentiments and practices recently (see Franklin, 2009; Linley, 2008; Peterson, 2006). People can learn to be more curious,

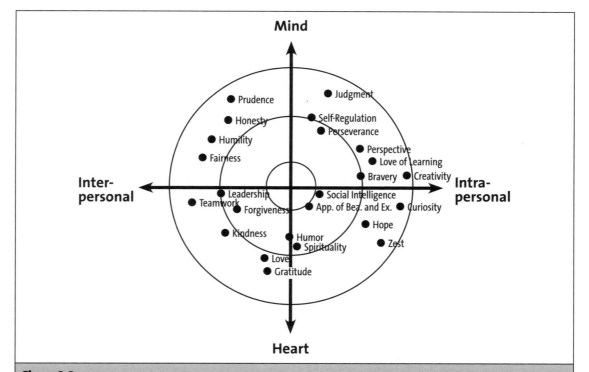

Figure 2.2
Circumplex model of the VIA Classification

Note. VIA Classification of character strengths and virtues is copyright of VIA Institute of Character. All rights reserved. Used with permission.

more grateful, fairer, or to be better critical thinkers. Overall, the key is to create new habits, which are established through practice and effort over time, allowing us to break free from routines.

Each character strength has heart, mind, interpersonal, and intrapersonal capacities. This principle is elucidated by Figure 2.2, which exhibits a circumplex model[1] offering a unique vantage point for viewing character strengths. Researcher Chris Peterson (2006) originally plotted the character strengths in this way following deployment of a scientific procedure that revealed two dimensions: a mind-heart dimension – which depicts the degree to which each strength is based in mental activities (e.g., thinking, logic, analysis) or activities of the heart (e.g., feelings, emotions, intuitions) – and an intrapersonal-interpersonal dimension which depicts the degree the strength focuses attention on oneself or others in order to express it. While some strengths are clearly more mind-based (e.g., judgment/critical thinking) and some more heart-oriented (e.g., love), each character strength is so multifaceted that it can be conceptualized from each quadrant of the circumplex model. For example, consider gratitude, which is depicted as the strongest "heart strength" in this model, an individual may feel genuine and deep appreciation for someone's kindness (heart), have grateful thoughts (mind), express thanks to someone (interpersonal), and feel grateful for one's good health (intrapersonal).

Virtues are corrective and expressive (Goleman, 1997; Yearley, 1990). Virtues and certain character strengths can serve to correct a temptation or a vice (e.g., self-regulation can counterbalance impulsivity; zest can correct sloth; humility can counterbalance hubris). At the same time, virtues and character strengths are often an expression of what is best in the individual.

---

[1] The character strengths are plotted according to the findings of one type of factor analysis. The circles are there for aesthetic purposes and to help orient the viewer visually; they do not have meaning beyond that. Strengths that are closer together on the graph are more likely to easily co-occur (e.g., consider the ease of expressing creativity and curiosity together), while strengths that are further apart are more likely to be traded off, in that it's less likely although not impossible that the individual would regularly express both at the same time (e.g., consider bravery alongside the caution of prudence).

Strengths-Spotting

Strengths-spotting is one of the best initial activities to help clients engage their strengths. Strengths-spotting can be done with any of the 24 strengths; however, taking notice of an individual's signature strengths is likely to be more obvious than spotting other strengths in action. This is because observers can look for energy, enthusiasm, and excitement as a sign that a strength might be present. Such energy will not always be present when an individual is expressing a lesser strength. Use the VIA Classification "language" in Table 2.1 to facilitate discussion.

There are two levels of strengths-spotting: (1) Spotting strengths in the actions of others and (2) spotting strengths in the actions of oneself. These levels can occur in any order; however, people commonly report that it's easier to spot strengths in others than in oneself. Therefore, one's relationships are a good place to start.

Spotting one's own strengths is also referred to as the self-nomination of strengths. While some research has found benefit to the self-nomination of strengths by using a list of the 24 strengths with definitions (e.g., Peterson & Seligman, 2004; Proctor, Maltby, & Linley, 2009), it is not a validated measure of character strengths. Thus, the VIA Survey and VIA Youth Survey remain the most thorough, validated options and should be considered the first-line approaches for identifying character strengths. In 2013, both the VIA Survey and the VIA Youth Survey were substantially reduced in terms of the number of questions yet have maintained good psychometric properties.

Practice Tip: Spot Strengths in Others

At your next work meeting or family gathering, enter the environment wearing "strengths goggles." This means walk in with a mindset to look for strengths as they occur. Spot your co-worker asking lots of questions (curiosity) or collaborating on a project (teamwork). Notice when your mother puts her arm around you when she speaks (love) or when your brother keeps the family entertained with a funny story (humor).

After you spot the strength(s), if the timing is right, tell the person how you value their strength use. Express your appreciation.

Name the strength that you saw them use and share the rationale for your observation. Examples of strengths-spotting in others:

- "John, I was impressed by how well you kept your cool during that heated debate at our meeting yesterday. That took a lot of self-control on your part!"
- "Mom, you seem to always offer me warmth and kind words at just the right time. This is exactly what helps me feel cared for and supported. I want you to know how much I value your love."

Practice Tip: Spot Strengths in Yourself

There are many activities you can do to identify your character strengths. In addition to taking the VIA Survey, consider the following:

- *You at your best* (Seligman, Steen, Park, & Peterson, 2005). Think of a time when you were at your best. It might be a time when you were particularly successful or happy. Write out or share the experience with someone – tell it like a story with a beginning, middle, and end. What character strengths did you use? What character strengths are most evident in the story as you tell it?
  - Whether we choose to play the "humility card" or not, we all have times in our life when we have done something really well. In other words, we have all performed "better than ordinary" at one time or many times in our life.
  - When you write down the story, consider the role you played in bringing about a positive outcome? What did you do that was particularly successful or useful to someone? After you write out this experience, go back and read through the story; as you read it through, circle the words or phrases that relate to the use of one of the 24 character strengths.
  - Listen to Track 3 of the attached CD for an example of this you at your best exercise, which includes spotting strengths in yourself.
- *Someone who "gets" you.* Think about a time when someone noticed something good about you in which that sharing took

you completely off-guard. This person really seemed to "get you" in a way that made you feel totally understood. What did this person see in you? What did they "get" about you? What character strengths were they seeing in you? How did it feel and what impact did it have on you?

  - When I lived in St. Louis, I went to breakfast once a month with a 70-year-old nun named Sr. Marilyn. We had wonderful conversations about spirituality, living life fully, and expressing meaning and purpose in life. In each conversation, Sr. Marilyn found a way to comment on a positive quality I was expressing or that she had witnessed in me in the previous months. These comments addressed my signature strengths and what mattered most to me. I was often quite surprised when she made comments about my character, even though I was quite familiar with my signature strengths. To hear someone directly express such observations offers a different angle or perspective, as well as carries weight in terms of validation of the behavioral aspects of one's character.
- *Monitor yourself for a day.* Choose an ordinary day in your life. Go about your day as you typically do but with one change: Set an alarm or smart-phone alert to signal you every 30 minutes. When you hear the alarm, pause, and ask yourself: "What character strengths was I just using?" Keep a log for one day or a half-day in which you write down the strengths and how you were using them, along with the time of day. What stands out to you as you review your log? What patterns emerge?

Character Strengths Research

The benefits of virtue and strength have been written about for centuries by philosophers and theologians, as well as by contemporary figures such as Roger Walsh (1999), Blaine Fowers (2008),

Lee Yearley (1990), and of course, the Dalai Lama (Dalai Lama & Cutler, 1998), to name a few. Science, however, has been slow to put these adages to the test. Positive psychology offers a direct pathway for researchers to become involved in the study of character strengths and virtues.

Scientists have found that there are indeed many benefits to using strengths, just as the great thinkers that preceded them had predicted. Strengths have been found to predict well-being over and above self-esteem and self-efficacy, and have been linked to increased happiness, well-being, work satisfaction, work engagement, meaning, self-efficacy, self-esteem, goal achievement, positive affect, vitality, and lower perceived stress (Govindji & Linley, 2007; Linley, Nielsen, Gillett, & Biswas-Diener, 2010; Littman-Ovadia & Davidovitch, 2010; Littman-Ovadia & Steger, 2010; Park et al., 2004; Proctor, Maltby, & Linley, 2009; Wood, Linley, Maltby, Kashdan, & Hurling, 2011).

Researchers have begun to study the underlying mechanisms that explain "why" character strengths use is connected with well-being. Linley and colleagues (2010) found that signature strengths use helps individuals make progress on their goals and meet their basic psychological needs for autonomy, relationship, and competence. Forest and colleagues (2012) concluded that signature strengths use allows individuals to experience harmonious passion which develops when an activity becomes part of a person's core identity and they can express it without any constraints.

Despite the stability of strengths over time, it is becoming clear that character strengths can be systematically and deliberately developed (Biswas-Diener et al., 2011; Louis, 2011). Several studies have evaluated the practice of expanding and developing character strengths through the intervention of using one's highest character strengths – often called signature strengths – in new ways each day. In contrast to comparison groups, this intervention has resulted in a variety of benefits from increased work satisfaction and

Table 2.2.
Character strengths associations noted in Peterson and Seligman (2004)

Character Strength	Positive Correlates
Creativity	Openness to new experiences; cognitive flexibility
Curiosity	Positive affect; willingness to challenge stereotypes; creativity; desire for challenge in work and play; goal perseverance; adept at making complex decisions; excitement/enjoyment/attentiveness; engagement and achievement in academic settings; sense of subjective well-being
Judgment	Adept at problem solving; increased cognitive ability; more resistant to suggestion and manipulation; more effective in dealing with stress
Love of Learning	More adept at navigating obstacles/challenges; autonomy; resourcefulness; increased sense of possibility; self-efficacy; healthy, productive aging; more likely to seek/accept challenges; decreased levels of stress
Perspective	Successful aging; life satisfaction; maturity; open-mindedness; even-temperedness; sociability; social intelligence
Bravery	Prosocial orientation; internal locus of control; self-efficacy; ability to delay gratification; tolerance for ambiguity/uncertainty; capacity to assess risk; capacity for reflection; involvement in socially worthy aims; capacity to create and sustain high quality connections with others
Perseverance	Achievement/goal completion; resourcefulness; self-efficacy
Honesty	Positive mood; life satisfaction; openness to new experience; empathy; conscientiousness; capacity for self-actualization; agreeableness; emotional stability; effort/goal attainment

Character Strength	Positive Correlates
Zest	Autonomy; connection with others; goal attainment
Love	Positive relationships with others; healthy balance between dependency and autonomy; positive social functioning; higher self-esteem; less susceptibility to depression; capacity to cope with stress
Kindness	Overall mental and physical health; longevity
Social Intelligence	Smooth social functioning; life judgment; lower levels of aggression; lower incidence of substance abuse
Teamwork (framed as citizenship)	Social trust; positive view of human nature
Fairness	Perspective; self-reflection; cooperation; leadership; altruism; prosocial behavior
Leadership	Cognitive skills/intelligence; flexibility/adaptability; emotional stability; internal locus of control; integrity; interpersonal skills; creativity/resourcefulness
Forgiveness	Prosocial behaviors; agreeableness; emotional stability; lower levels of anger, anxiety, depression, and hostility
Humility	Perspective; forgiveness; self-regulation; capacity to attain self-improvement goals
Prudence	Cooperativeness; interpersonal warmth; sociability; assertiveness; positive emotion; imaginativeness; curiosity; insightfulness; physical health; longevity; optimism, internal locus of control; high achievement/performance; lower levels of anger expression
Self-Regulation	High levels of academic achievement; self-esteem; self-acceptance; capacity to control anger; secure interpersonal attachments; high levels of satisfaction with social relationships; lower levels of anxiety and depression; perceived by others as more likable/trustworthy
Appreciation of Beauty & Excellence	Openness to experience; altruism; devotion to others/larger community; capacity for change/self-improvement
Gratitude	Positive emotion; life satisfaction; optimism; prosocial behavior; increased cardiovascular and immune functioning; longevity; lower levels of anxiety and depression; openness to experience; agreeableness; conscientiousness; less neuroticism
Hope	Achievement; positive social relationships; physical well-being; active problem-solving; lower levels of anxiety and depression; conscientiousness; diligence; ability to delay gratification
Humor	Positive mood; capacity to manage stress; creativity; intelligence; less neuroticism
Spirituality	Self-regulation; lower levels of substance abuse; positive social relationships; marital stability; forgiveness; kindness; compassion; altruism; volunteerism, philanthropy; happiness; sense of purpose; life satisfaction; capacity to cope with illness and stress

sense of meaning to increased happiness and decreased depression, with effects lasting as long as six months in some studies (Gander et al., 2012a; Linley et al., 2010; Mitchell, Stanimirovic, Klein, Vella-Brodrick, 2009; Mongrain & Anselmo-Matthews, 2012; Peterson & Peterson, 2008; Rust, Diessner, & Reade, 2009; Seligman et al., 2005). The use of character strengths have been applied in many different ways, ranging from work with youth (Madden, Green, & Grant, 2011), to use of movies in which the strengths of cinematic characters can serve as an emotional inspiration as well as a role model for strengths in action that can be emulated by viewers (Niemiec & Wedding, 2014).

Each of the 24 character strengths has an array of research describing it and examining it. A comprehensive review of the correlates, consequences, development, and enablers of each character strength can be found in *Character Strengths and Virtues* by Peterson and Seligman (2004). This is the original work outlining the VIA Classification. Table 2.2 outlines many of the main correlations associated with each character strength found in the literature up to 2004. Some strengths have had far more scholarly inquiry than others – for example, creativity has been studied for decades and is the focal point of at least two scholarly journals, while humility has only had a handful of studies, although this has grown significantly in the last few years.

Character Strengths Practice

How to Practice With Strengths

Following the advent of the VIA Classification in 2004, I became intrigued by how practitioners could make practical use of the 24 strengths. Like an explorer, I set out to discover the approaches that were being used. I tracked the work of leaders in the strengths world, read the predominant books at the time, and most importantly, observed practitioners who took a strengths-based approach. While not overtly stated, the general process practitioners took followed three phases, simply worded as aware-explore-apply (Niemiec, 2013). First, practitioners help clients become aware of their existing strengths; next, time is spent discussing, reflecting, and better understanding one's strengths

use; finally, action is taken and the client applies their new knowledge to a problem, the task-at-hand, or the formulation of a new goal.

This process model will be discussed next in more practical detail, and is used in the Mindfulness-Based Strengths Practice (MBSP) program, which is reviewed in Section III.

Phase 1: Aware

All change begins with awareness. Many people are not aware of their best qualities, and those that are aware may readily take their strengths for granted. Simply asking the question "What are my highest character strengths?" offers a shift in the right direction. Placing one's attention on strengths to cultivate greater self-awareness clearly involves mindfulness.

A component of this phase is to take the VIA Survey in order to attain a valid measure of one's top character strengths. As another awareness building exercise, individuals confirm their signature strengths through questioning each of their top strengths (e.g., top 10). These questions involve the core features of signature strengths:

- Does the strength come naturally without any effort?
- Do family and friends readily observe this strength in me?
- Is it core to who I am? In other words, does it feel like the real me when I express it?
- Is the strength highly energizing to use?
- Do I express this strength across settings and adapt it easily in many situations?

Example: Mary Jane is the parent of two young children. She is struggling in her marriage, trying hard to keep her full-time job, and is constantly feeling the stress of life weigh her down. When Mary Jane was asked "What are your best qualities?" she gave a blank stare. She was blind to her signature strengths. She took the VIA Survey and discovered her signature strengths were fairness, curiosity, kindness, and judgment/critical thinking. In many ways this was a re-discovery for Mary Jane. She had once known she had these wonderful qualities but over time life simply "got in the way" and her character strengths eroded – she forgot about them and hence forgot to use them in her life. By the time her children came along, her personal strengths were far from her mind. The good news, which Mary Jane quickly realized, was that she could tap back into these strengths right away. Her strengths began to soar and her confidence as a parent re-emerged.

Phase 2: Explore

This phase involves digging in and investigating how and when a client expresses their strengths. It involves considering when the strength was used in the past, what strengths the client tends to use in various situations of their present lifestyle, and how they might use their strengths more in the future.

- How have I used this strength when I was at my best?
- What does it look like for me to express this strength?
- When and where do I use this strength in my daily life?
- How have I used this strength at times of stress and upset?
- What happens if I express too little of this strength? When does that usually occur?
- What happens if I express too much of this strength? When does that usually occur?
- What benefits does this strength bring me and others?

Phase 3: Apply

This is the action phase. After proper exploration, discussion, and reflection on the client's strengths, the third phase of the strengths process involves impacting behavior and embedding strengths into the life routine. The approach here is to help the client set goals with their character strengths; specific interventions are discussed throughout the rest of this chapter.

One of the most popular positive psychology interventions is identifying top strengths and then using one signature strength in a new way each day. Research has found that individuals who use one of their signature strengths in a new way each day experience a number of benefits, such as an increase in happiness and a decrease in depression for a sustained period of time (e.g., Seligman et al., 2005; Gander et al., 2012a).

Encourage your client to take action with one of their signature strengths. The practice involves expanding the use of strengths and deploying the strength in a novel way each day. For example, if the individual chooses curiosity, they could take a different route home and explore a new area or neighborhood. If they choose perseverance, they could complete a small project that they have been putting off. The idea is to stick with the practice for a couple weeks. Table 2.3 lists two practical examples for each of the 24 character strengths as a starting point and reference guide.

The aware-explore-apply model can be used in any profession or population; however, it is not the only model proposed to work with strengths. Strengths-based models, philosophies, and practices can be seen across professions, including counseling (Smith, 2006), social work (Saleebey, 1996), school counseling (Galassi & Akos, 2007), psychotherapy (Wong, 2006), coaching (Biswas-Diener, 2010; Linley & Harrington, 2006; Whitmore, 2002), and business (Buckingham & Clifton, 2001).

In summary, the main concept in working with character strengths is to practice using them, thinking about them, discussing them, and spotting them in others. The more a client can make the practice a routine, the more strengths will be in their consciousness ready for deployment and use. The next two sections review interventions: general practices that can be applied to any of the 24 character strengths followed by specific interventions tailored to each strength.

General Strength Interventions

When exploring character strengths or working with clients on strengths use, it is useful to have some guide posts. In other words, everyone needs a "road map" at one point or another. ROAD MAP serves as an acronym for the several ways one can dig deeper into character strengths – Reflect, Observe, Appreciate, Discuss, Monitor, Ask, and Plan.

Each of these action verbs can be applied to any of the 24 character strengths in the VIA Classification. A general approach can be taken, such as reflecting on past strengths use and appreciating the strengths of others. Or, a specific approach can be taken and one or more strengths can be targeted, such as discussing the strength of curiosity with a friend or planning ways one might use more fairness in life.

This template is intentionally general in order to provide broad application to any strength. What follows is a ROAD MAP for character strengths use:

Table 2.3
Using Signature Strengths in New Ways

Creativity	Think of one of your problems and two possible solutions. Present the solutions nonverbally as an act or mime to someone.
	Turn an inanimate object (e.g., like paperclips, toothpicks) into something meaningful.
Curiosity	Try a new food for the first time, preferably from a culture different than your own.
	Take a different route home and explore a new area or neighborhood.
Judgment (critical thinking):	Watch a political program from the opposite point of view of your own, and keep an open mind.
	Ask one or two clarifying questions of someone who has a different approach to life or different beliefs than you (e.g., a vegetarian).
Love of learning	Read some of the original works of Gandhi online.
	Consider your favorite subject matter. Do an Internet search and surprise yourself by deepening your knowledge about the topic.
Perspective	For one of your interactions today: First, listen closely. Second, share your ideas and thoughts.
	Consider the wisest quotation you have come across. Think of one way you can live more true to that quote.
Bravery	Take on a new adventure or hobby that fits with one of your areas of interest.
	Consider one of your personal fears. Take one small, healthy action toward facing it right now.
Perseverance	Complete a small project that you have been putting off.
	Set a new goal today, then list two potential obstacles that may come up and ways that you will overcome them.
Honesty	Write a poem that expresses an inner truth.
	Contact a family member or friend whom you have told a "partial" truth and give them the complete details.
Zest	Exert your energy in a unique way – jump on a bed, run in place, practice yoga or body stretching, or chase around a child or pet.
	Express your energy through an outfit, pair of shoes, and/or accessories that are striking and befitting of your personality.
Love	Surprise somebody with a small gift that shows you care (e.g., flowers; a specialty coffee).
	Tell someone about a strength you saw them use and how much you value it. Words of affirmation are a powerful, verbal force for the expression of love.
Kindness	Put coins in someone's parking meter that has run out of money.
	Stop by a hospital or nursing home and offer to visit with someone who is lonely.
Social intelligence	Start up a conversation with someone whom you normally would not say much to other than typical pleasantries. This person might be the person at the checkout counter, a telemarketer, or a new employee.
	Express a feeling of frustration, disappointment, or nervousness in a healthy, direct way that someone can easily understand.

Teamwork	Spot and express appreciation for the strengths expressed by one of your team members.
	Savor a positive team interaction from the past by replaying it in your mind; share it at a team meeting.
Fairness	Look for beings (e.g., people, animals) that are cast aside or typically held in disgust and go out of your way to treat them right.
	Include someone in a conversation who is typically excluded from groups or is a newcomer.
Leadership	Discuss with someone who reports to you about how they can align their top character strengths more in their work.
	Gather and lead a group to help support a cause you believe in.
Forgiveness	Consciously let go of a minor irritant or a grudge.
	Give yourself permission to make a small mistake.
Humility	Consider an interaction that typically involves you doing more talking/sharing and flip it to where the other person talks/shares more.
	Ask someone you trust to give you feedback on your struggles and growth areas.
Prudence	Before you make a decision that is typically very easy, take one full minute to think about it before you take action.
	Write down your plans for each hour of the remainder of the day, no matter how trivial.
Self-regulation	The next time you feel irritated or nervous today, pause and breathe with the experience for a count of 10 breathes.
	Monitor all the food and drinks you put in your body. Write it down on a tracking sheet.
Appreciation of Beauty & Excellence	Go outside and stand still in a beautiful environment for 20 minutes.
	Listen to a song or piece of music that is viewed as extraordinary; allow yourself to marvel at the talent that went into producing it.
Gratitude	Tell someone "thanks" who deserves it and is typically not recognized.
	Share your appreciation on a post-it note that you put on someone's desk as a surprise or send it in a spontaneous e-mail.
Hope	Consider a problem or struggle you are having. Write down two optimistic, realistic thoughts that bring comfort.
	Watch a movie that promotes a message of hope and think about how the message applies to your life.
Humor	Do something spontaneous and playful when you are with at least one other person (e.g., saying something silly or telling a funny story or joke).
	Watch a classic comedy show you haven't seen before and laugh as much as possible.
Spirituality	Read about a religion/spirituality different from your own and look for ways in which the core messages parallel one another.
	Contemplate the "sacredness" of this present moment. Allow yourself to find meaning in the moment.

- **R**eflect: Take time out to think about ways you have used strengths in your past successes and your struggles. When you were at your best, what strengths did you use? At times of high stress, what strengths did you call forth to help you push forward? Consider how you have recently used your bravery or your curiosity. What strengths have you deployed today?
- **O**bserve: Just be, sit and observe your surroundings. Use mindfulness to gently hold your attention on what you take in with your five senses. Rather than trying to spot any strength in particular, simply observe your environment and the people around you with curiosity and interest. What strengths pop up?
- **A**ppreciate: Tell others about how you value their strengths. Name the strength that you see them express and share the specific rationale for how you saw them display the strength in action.
- **D**iscuss: Communicate with others about your strengths. Allow "strengths of character" to be your topic of conversation. When with your family, talk about what the family's core strengths have been over the years; when you are with friends, tell them about your burgeoning curiosity or the ways you've expressed your creativity at work in the last week.
- **M**onitor: Self-monitoring is one of the best researched techniques in all of psychology. It involves closely tracking internal experiences and behaviors across some unit of time (e.g., each hour, each morning, each day). It is commonly applied to dietary intake, exercise, and emotions. Track your strengths use in a log or journal by monitoring and writing down your use of signature strengths, lower strengths, or particular strengths you want to enhance.
- **A**sk: Get feedback from your family, friends, co-workers, and neighbors on the strengths you use. What strengths do others see that you don't see? Maybe others see a lot of creativity and forgiveness in you that you were not aware of. What strengths do you see in yourself that others also report you show? Knowing this will help you see how well your perception of yourself lines up with your actual behavior.
- **P**lan: Want to boost one of your strengths? Set a goal around the strength you'd like to display more often. The general idea is to turn your use

of strengths into a routine. It might be helpful to set up reminders and environmental cues (e.g., post-it notes) to prompt yourself.

This road map will help clients get started and make substantial progress on their strengths journey. Of course, no map can contain every pathway and landmark, so be sure to encourage clients to veer from this map, take some side-roads, and create their own path as they explore and express the best parts of themselves.

Specific Strength Interventions

Research has also revealed strategies for boosting each of the 24 character strengths. Some character strengths have a robust number of findings that can be used to improve the strength (e.g., perspective), and for others, the research is still developing; however, expert opinion is available (e.g., humility).

Creativity. Practicing divergent thinking is one of the most important research-based interventions to boost creativity. When facing a problem, brainstorm multiple alternatives rather than one solution to the problem (Scott, Leritz, & Mumford, 2004).

Curiosity. Curiosity can be built by consciously paying attention to and tracking things in one's daily environment that have not been noticed before or things about familiar people that have gone unnoticed. The key is to encourage being "actively curious," asking lots of questions, and making new, mini discoveries (Kashdan, 2009). In a more formal way, an individual may take an approach of naming three novel features of any activity that they are doing.

Judgment. Seeking and considering other viewpoints is the cornerstone of judgment/critical thinking. When one is having a discussion with a person with an opposing viewpoint, take an approach of asking at least one clarifying question. The approach should be one that involves "collecting information" rather than "evaluating information." This approach is contrary to what people typically do, as individuals are nearly two times as likely to seek information that supports their attitudes, beliefs, and behaviors than to seek information that is contradictory to their views (Hart, Albarracin, Eagly, Brechan, Lindberg, & Merrill, 2009).

Love of Learning. To build love of learning, it's important to identify where the highest interests in learning are and then work to discover the preferred ways of learning about that subject, whether it is self-initiated, through reading, Internet searches, courses, hands-on experiences, peer learning groups, or viewing video clips or documentaries. The learning interest should be pursued by systematically digging deeply into the material (Covington, 1999).

Perspective. An intervention that has been shown to boost wisdom-related knowledge is to imagine having a conversation with a wise person about a problem. Imagine the full dialog in terms of questions asked, responses given, the nuances of the discussion, and any advice that would be offered (Glueck & Baltes, 2006).

Bravery. Research is finding that one of the most common ways people can increase their bravery is to focus on the outcome of the courageous act. In other words, focusing on the beneficial outcome of a brave act rather than focusing on fears can increase the likelihood of acting bravely (Pury, 2008).

Perseverance. Reframing setbacks or failures as learning opportunities and ideas for growth can boost the strength of perseverance. Setbacks can be viewed as providing useful information so that the individual can overcome obstacles, be less inclined to "give up," and persist toward their goal (Dweck, 2006).

Honesty. Honesty can be increased by limiting the degree to which one moves around or avoids the truth, such as making excuses, rationalizing, minimizing behavior, not taking responsibility, and condemning authority (Staats, Hupp, & Hagley, 2008).

Zest. Sharing the positive events that occur in one's life and relaying positive experiences with those one cares for is a general way to boost enthusiasm, energy, and vitality (Lambert, Gwinn, Fincham, & Stillman, 2011).

Love. Loving-kindness meditation is an effective way to experience and boost the strength of love (Fredrickson, Cohn, Coffey, Pek, & Finkel, 2008). This form of meditation provides a way to consciously tap into one's inner resources of love through imagery and affirmative statements of one's capacity for love and to acknowledge the power and beneficial effects of love in the world (listen to Track 6 of the attached CD for an example of this type of meditation).

Kindness. Some research has found there are benefits of practicing several random acts of kindness in one day (Lyubomirsky, 2008). Encourage clients to look for opportunities to conduct random acts of kindness and consider how they might infuse variety into the kind acts committed each week.

Social Intelligence. Studies have linked emotional intelligence, a dimension of social intelligence, with mindfulness (Bauer, McAdams, & Pals, 2008; Schutte & Malouff, 2011). It is possible that social intelligence might improve through the practice of mindfulness, in which one tunes in closely to the feelings of oneself and others, facial expressions, one's environment, and the social context.

Teamwork. In order to become a better team member, it is important to notice and express positive emotions (e.g., gratitude, joy, hope) to other team members. In addition, it's important to take an open-minded and curious stance in understanding others' points of view as opposed to only advocating for one's own opinions (Losada & Heaphy, 2004).

Fairness. Imagining and appreciating the differences of others can boost the strength of fairness. Perspective-taking, cultural awareness and sensitivity training, and role-playing are ways to develop a more "other-focused" perspective, particularly when facing complex moral dilemmas (Peterson & Seligman, 2004).

Leadership. In addition to competently using one's strengths, leadership requires highly developed organizational skills. This takes planning and goal-setting. Consider ideas and opportunities in which one can practice taking a leadership role in activities, groups, or organizations, even if the task seems minor or trivial (Peterson & Seligman, 2004).

Forgiveness. There are many ways to boost forgiveness. One method is to write about the benefits one has experienced following an experience in which one was interpersonally hurt (McCullough, Root, & Cohen, 2006).

Humility. One intervention suggested by experts is to look for humility exemplars among family, friends, philosophical lore, movies, or spiritual readings. One can then create a "Hall of Humility," that is a listing of all those individuals most respected for their humble nature, and then reflect and discuss how these learnings might be applied into daily life (Worthington, 2007).

Prudence. Practice conducting cost-benefit analyses of problems. Write out the costs and benefits of taking a particular action and the costs and benefits of not doing that action, resulting in four quadrants. Review the results to consider the most practical decision (Miller & Rollnick, 1991).

Self-Regulation. Research has found that the best way to build this character strength is to exercise some area of discipline on a regular basis. Self-monitoring is one pathway. Consider a behavior one wishes to change (e.g., eating more healthy, exercising more, managing finances better) and begin to track it with honest detail (e.g., keeping a food diary or an exercise log). Continue to closely monitor the behavior while slowly making changes (Baumeister, Matthew, DeWall, & Oaten, 2006).

Appreciation of Beauty & Excellence. Research has shown that keeping a beauty log can enhance an individual's engagement with beauty around them. The key is raising one's consciousness of beauty. When something beautiful is seen or felt, whether it is from nature, is human-made (e.g., artwork), or is the virtuous behavior of others (i.e., moral beauty), write down the accompanying thoughts and feeling in a log or journal. This can increase this character strength as well as the strength of hope (Diessner, Rust, Solom, Frost, & Parsons., 2006).

Gratitude. Counting one's blessings is one of the most widely researched interventions to boost gratitude. It involves reflecting on one's day and tracking the good things that happened throughout the day. The formal approach typically involves writing down three of these good things that occurred, why one is grateful for them, and what role one played in the experience (Emmons & McCullough, 2003; Gander et al., 2012a; Seligman et al., 2005)

Hope. One research-based strategy that has been shown to boost hope is the "best possible self" exercise. This involves imaging a future in which one is bringing one's best self forward (King, 2001; Meevissen, Peters, & Alberts, 2011; Peters, Flink, Boersma, & Linton, 2010; Sheldon & Lyubomirsky, 2006). This is visualized in a

way that is pleasing and realistic. In addition, one considers the character strengths needed in order to make that image a reality.

Humor. Some research has found that keeping track of the humorous and funny things that happen each day is a way to boost this strength. Writing down three funny things that occurred throughout the course of the day can build awareness and increase the use of humor (Gander et al., 2012a).

Spirituality. Consider someone that can be viewed as a wise, spiritual role model. Researchers describe this as taking an approach of "observational spiritual learning" (Oman, Shapiro, Thoresen, Flinders, Driskill, & Plante, 2007; Plante, 2008). The model could be someone from a book or movie, someone in the public eye, or a person in one's life. Reflect on how this person has conducted their life in a way that is spiritually driven and meaning filled.

Practice Tip: Takeaway Tip-Sheet

- Many times the strengths transformation for people seems to happen when they realize character strengths can be viewed as mechanisms or processes that can be employed in daily life. Like mindfulness, they can be tapped into at any moment. While appreciating the positive outcomes of strengths is important, seeing strengths as the actual mechanisms in life offers a different angle.
- Lead with your signature strengths.
- All 24 character strengths matter! Learn the VIA strengths language fully. Take a look at the Figure 2.3 graphic of this language. You might copy and post this image somewhere in your environment where you can be reminded of the importance of all 24.
- Working with strengths is an ongoing process toward mindful competence.
- Never stop practicing strengths-spotting.
- Never get "locked-in": This research is young so stay psychologically flexible to new ideas and interventions.
- Learning often occurs gradually, then suddenly
- As you learn, keep going deeper (explore your strengths and then explore them some more)

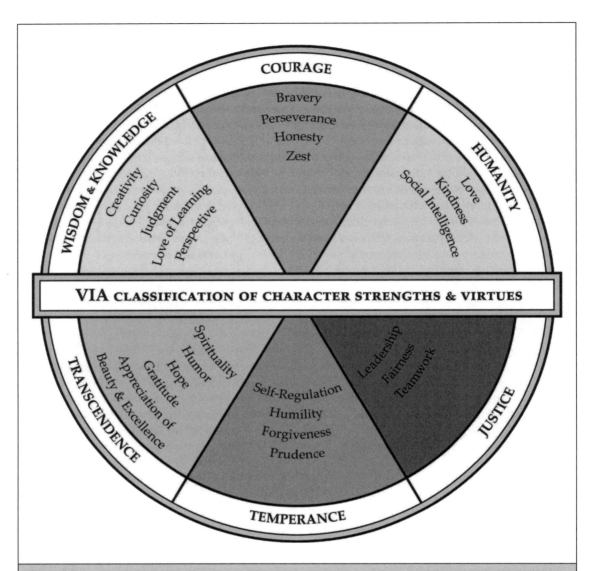

Figure 2.3

VIA Classification graphic

The VIA Classification is copyrighted material of VIA Institute on Character, 2004. Used with permission. www.viacharacter.org. Duplication of this image requires permission from the VIA Institute and a reference to Niemiec (2012).

Section II: Integration

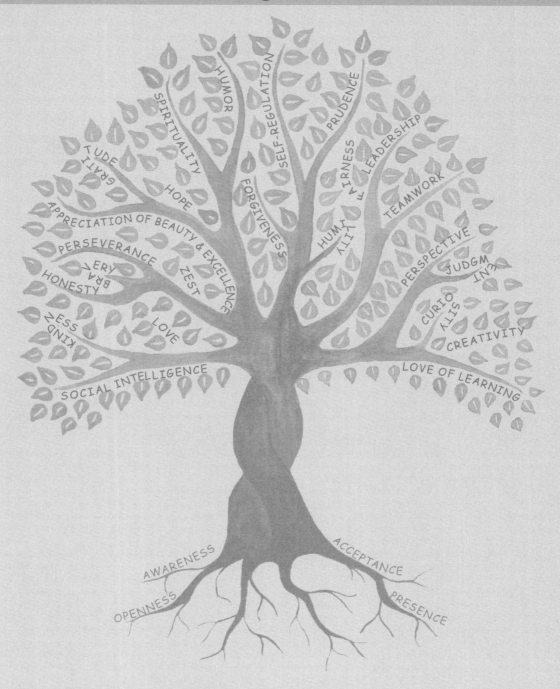

Chapter 3

The Integration of Mindfulness and Character Strengths

We can't understand what is happening to 'something' if we aren't looking. But nothing is going to happen to that 'something' if we don't look deeply. That's why so many things with incredible potential go unnoticed because nobody bothers to look.

Filmmaker Alejandro Gonzalez Iñárritu
commenting on his film *Biutiful* (2010).

Chapter Snapshot

This chapter offers rationale for the integration of mindfulness and character strengths. It highlights programs and areas that have previously integrated these two areas and discusses recent mindfulness-based interventions and the relevance of character strengths therein. The empirical links between mindfulness and each of the 24 character strengths is reviewed. Directions for future research are offered.

Opening Story[1]

Two virtuous, solitary monks walk together in silence, making their way from their monastery to the closest nearby store, several miles away down a windy dirt path. After walking a few miles, the monks come upon a babbling brook. On the other side is a woman carrying a large bag and appearing hesitant and fearful at the brook's edge. The younger monk, recalling his vow of silence and commitment to have minimal contact with the outside world, swiftly crosses the brook and passes by the woman keeping his eyes on the path in front of him. The older monk follows the young monk across the brook. Upon reaching the other side, he gives pause, turns to the woman and asks if he can assist her. He lifts the woman and carries her across the brook. He and the young monk then continued their journey. About a mile down the road, the young monk stops and turns to the older monk, angrily exclaiming, "How could you pick up that woman? I can't believe you disregarded our vows." "Brother," said the elder monk, "I let that woman go back at the creek and you are still carrying her with you."

This story represents a blend of mindfulness and heartfulness, of wisdom and character strength. As we face increasingly complex, conflicted, or challenging circumstances, the use of mindful awareness, along with our strengths of character, becomes pivotal. We come to understand it's not enough

---

[1] This classic story has been shared in many forums and has seen various minor adaptations. One version of this story can also be found in Kornfield and Feldman (1996).

to just be mindful, we must point that mindfulness at something; it's not sufficient to simply know our character strengths, we must use them in a balanced way, with mindful care. The integration of mindfulness and character strengths is an art-form that can be learned and has the potential to have a profound impact on our lives.

Why Integrate? Rationale

The image on the cover of this book offers a representation of the integration of mindfulness and character strengths, expressing themes of distinctiveness, similarity, mutual benefit, interdependence, interconnection, and synergy.

When leading Mindfulness-Based Strengths Practice (MBSP) groups, I offer a description of this image as a metaphor for the work ahead:

> Picture this: Two, tall trees growing side by side as they branch out toward the limitless sky. With solid trunks that twist around each other, each tree has an extensive root system spreading several yards long and wide. Some of their roots intertwine and begin to depend on one another as they nourish one another, becoming one in the same; other roots go their separate ways, extending deeper and deeper. The trees are of similar height and are so close to one another that their branches interconnect. As time goes on, the branches from each tree weave in and around one another. This occurs so seamlessly that when the passerby gazes up at the trees, their tops have become one.

> Mindfulness and character strengths are like these two great trees, separate but connected, independent yet interconnected, synergistic and mutually supportive. Their expression in the world is often viewed as though they are unique entities, yet there is a potential in each person to bring them together in a harmonious way that benefits oneself *and* others. Each has a deep root system; some roots are shared and others distinct. Those who practice mindfulness and character strengths taste a unique fruit that positively impacts their health and well-being, and brings great benefit to those around them.

The process of this integration occurs both automatically as well as within our conscious control. In cognitive behavioral therapy the emphasis is on changing the content of thoughts and in interpersonal therapy the emphasis is on understanding and finding new ways to relate to others; however, in mindfulness practices the focus is on changing the relationship one has to one's thoughts, body, and feelings. This is understood

through the underlying mechanisms of mindfulness which involve cognitive defusion (a term used in Acceptance and Commitment Therapy, ACT) or decentering (a term used in Mindfulness-Based Cognitive Therapy, MBCT), which refer to seeing thoughts as mental events passing through the mind rather than paying attention to the content of the thoughts. In addition, mindfulness involves taking a compassionate, gentle, and accepting approach toward one's mind and body. This offers a new way of relating to oneself.

The integration of mindfulness with strengths practice allows for the individual to become more aware of not only negative/troubling thoughts and feelings but also to become more aware of positive thoughts, emotions, and behaviors. MBSP offers a wide, biopsychosocial, whole-person focus in which all mental events and experiences are important rather than solely aspects of the self which are troubled. The mindful focus on one's strengths, or active recall of one's strengths, along with sustained attention in one's moment-to-moment experiences, activates cognitive processes (e.g., reappraisals and metacognition) that help individuals accept negative experiences more adaptively. In this way, MBSP potentially aligns with *all* aspects of ourselves (positive and negative) coherently and meaningfully in our life narratives.

Put simply, mindfulness opens a door of awareness to who we are and character strengths are what is behind the door since character strengths are who we are at our core. Mindfulness opens the door to potential self-improvement and growth while character strengths use is often the growth itself.

As discussed in earlier chapters, mindfulness and character strengths share similar features, including the following three ways of viewing each:

- *States:* Individuals might have moments of passing awareness (e.g., being struck by the blue of the sky), just as one might experience a strength in a brief, transient way (e.g., gratitude at Thanksgiving or when someone offers a gift). Both mindfulness and character strengths are states that can be initialized and developed through particular practices, such as deliberate intervention. This relates to the view of building mindfulness or a particular character strength as one might develop a skill through practice.

- *Traits:* Character strengths are also referred to as character traits, or aspects of our personality that are relatively stable across situations over time. In addition, researchers have found that some people are more naturally strong in mindfulness, just as the extravert easily expresses talkativeness in a social interaction. Such mindfulness occurs across situations for some individuals more than others and is referred to as being high or low in trait mindfulness.

- *Higher-order processes:* Conceptually, each can be viewed as a meta-process that can be layered onto one's current orientation in working with people (e.g., applying a strengths focus in psychotherapy or mindfulness in how one approaches and conducts health coaching). Individuals can be mindful of their own mindfulness and can deliberately apply this awareness to other processes (e.g., consciously applying mindfulness to one's creativity). Character strengths, too, can act as a meta-process for operating or opening up other strengths, e.g., using one's prudence strength in order to carefully deploy gratitude or hope. In this vein, researchers have discussed a number of strengths that might serve as a master (or meta) character strength although there is no consensus on this topic. Two examples are perspective/wisdom (Schwartz & Sharpe, 2006) and self-regulation (Baumeister & Tierney, 2011; Baumeister & Vohs, 2004).

Despite the universality and natural interconnection of mindfulness and character strengths, not much has been written on their integration. Ruth Baer and Emily Lykins (2011) explored the connections between mindfulness and various domains of positive psychology, including character strengths, virtues, well-being, and optimal functioning. My colleagues, Tayyab Rashid and Marcello Spinella, and I discussed one-half of the conceptual foundation of this integration as we examined how character strengths can be used

to bolster the practice of mindfulness (Niemiec, Rashid, & Spinella, 2012). Finally, I've discussed character strengths interventions to serve as pathways for mindful living and for practicing the five mindfulness trainings taught by Thich Nhat Hanh (Nhat Hanh, 1993; Nhat Hanh & Cheung, 2010), which is also discussed later in Chapter 4 (Niemiec, 2012).

Previous Integration of Mindfulness and Character Strengths

For centuries Tibetan Buddhism has widely taught and practiced meditation with two main virtues at its core – wisdom and compassion. These are the focus of many Tibetan Buddhist teachings and direct practices, and it is believe these can be developed through meditation. Moreover, the majority of philosophers and spiritual leaders in Buddhism and Buddhist psychology emphasize these virtues and related constructs (e.g., loving-kindness). Pema Chodron (1997), the Dalai Lama (Dalai Lama & Cutler, 1998) and Thich Nhat Hanh (2009) all emphasize mindfulness and compassion/kindness. Also relevant to this discussion are the paramitas discussed in different schools of Buddhism (Tibetan, Theravada, Mahayana). Paramitas refers to the culmination of certain virtues; in Buddhism, virtues such as honesty, serenity, energy, and patience can be cultivated along one's life as pathways toward purification, with the goal of enlightenment.

In his ongoing dialogs with Western scientists, the Dalai Lama explained the connection between happiness and strengths and suffering and vices:

> Both the happiness that I strive for, and the suffering that I wish to be free of, are results. Recognizing that, one seeks out the causes that lead to these results: to well-being, or to grief and suffering. One pursues the causes that lead to happiness, and one avoids the causes that lead to suffering and mental afflictions. The vices fall into the latter category, while the virtues fall into the former (Goleman, 1997, p. 170).

The integration of values and mindfulness is also of relevance to this work. One program that has explicitly linked values, mindfulness, and approaches designed to boost acceptance is ACT. This is an empirically-supported approach for a number of problems and it emphasizes values clarification and value-directed action/behavior, among other elements (Hayes et al., 1999; Wilson et al., 2010). The concept of values overlaps with character strengths, although important contrasts can be made. Values encompass thoughts and feelings but do not inherently address the behavior a person expresses. A person might have a value for family and a value for creativity, but this does not speak to whether they (behaviorally) spend a significant amount of time with family, prioritize family over work, or whether they use their creativity regularly in their daily life. Character (or character strengths) fills in the void where values end; in addition to encompassing cognition and emotion, character encompasses volition and behavior as well. Thus, character strengths can map onto both values and value-directed action. One study trained school teachers on human values education and mindfulness skills and compared this group with a control group (Delgado, Guerra, Perakakis, Viedma, Robles, & Vila, 2010). The mindfulness and values group, in comparison with controls, improved significantly on attention quality, anxiety, depression, worry, negative affect, stress, emotional comprehension, and reactivity per physiologic measures.

While philosophers, religious leaders, researchers, and practitioners have noted some slices of the connection between mindfulness and character strengths over the decades, no systematic program has emerged. At the same time, mindfulness programs have not omitted positive traits from their programs. Quite the contrary, some programs explicitly include meditations that focus on one particular strength (e.g., kindness/compassion), as well as helping participants engage in practices that would naturally increase a particular strength (e.g., perspective/wisdom).

In Mindfulness-Based Stress Reduction (MBSR), Kabat-Zinn (1990) offers seven core attitudes cultivated by mindfulness practice (the first seven are noted below), while Shapiro et al. (2002) add five additional mindfulness attitudes to the original list. These researchers explain that these are important qualities of both the intention and commitment of mindfulness practice because they are brought to the practice itself and, in turn, are cultivated through the practice of

mindfulness. Note that many of these attitudes are character strengths or dimensions of character strengths:

- Nonjudging
- Nonstriving
- Acceptance
- Patience
- Trust
- Openness/beginner's mind
- Letting go
- Gentleness
- Generosity
- Empathy
- Gratitude
- Loving-kindness

In Mindfulness-Based Cognitive Therapy (MBCT), a number of the program benefits listed below (Segal et al., 2002) appear to be closely related to strengths of character (noted in brackets):

- Observe negative thoughts with curiosity and kindness (curiosity, kindness, judgment/critical thinking, self-regulation).
- To accept themselves and stop wishing things were different (forgiveness, perspective).
- To let go of old habits and choose a different way of being (forgiveness, bravery, perseverance).
- To be present in the moment and notice small beauties and pleasures in the world (curiosity, appreciation of beauty & excellence).

It appears that mindfulness and character strengths positively impact one another. Increased amount of time spent using strengths has been found to correlate significantly with mindfulness (Jarden, Jose, Kashdan, Simpson, McLachlan, & Mackenzie, 2012). There are a number of theoretical and empirical links connecting mindfulness and specific character strengths in the VIA Classification. Some character strengths are inherent in mindfulness itself, e.g., curiosity and self-regulation (Bishop et al., 2004), some character strengths correlate with mindfulness, e.g., creativity, judgment (Sugiura, 2004), while others have been found to be outcomes of mindfulness practice, e.g., hope/optimism (Carson et al., 2004). The VIA Classification structure of six virtue categories – wisdom, courage, humanity, justice, temperance, and transcendence – provides a good framework for discussing these connections. While major meta-analyses of mindfulness and character strengths are currently in progress, what follows is a review of the empirical connections between mindfulness and each of the 24 strengths. Please note that for the purposes of this exploration and review, a couple examples of studies involving different types of meditation/mindfulness are included, such as transcendental meditation and mindfulness conceptualized by Ellen Langer, who emphasizes the cognitive aspects of mindfulness.

Wisdom Strengths

The cognitive-oriented strengths are called wisdom/knowledge strengths in the VIA Classification (Peterson & Seligman, 2004) and include *creativity*, *curiosity*, *judgment*/critical thinking, *love of learning*, and *perspective*/wisdom. For decades Ellen Langer (1989; 2006; 2009) has drawn connections between mindfulness and most of these cognitive strengths, particularly creativity, curiosity, and learning, as her approach to mindful learning involves taking a stance of creative problem-solving and openness towards novelty. In this vein, mindfulness entails open, assimilative "wakefulness" to cognitive tasks such as the creation of new categories – something underscored in the character strength of creativity. Mindfulness has been found to reduce worry by increasing the perceived quality of problem-solving, which is important for effective critical thinking (Sugiura, 2004). This is particularly relevant to the strengths of judgment and creativity, the latter of which is strongly characterized by divergent thinking – finding multiple ways to solve problems (Scott et al., 2004). Researchers have found that certain types of meditation practice can lead to particular aspects of creativity. For example, an approach to meditation involving the open monitoring of the present moment has been found to promote divergent thinking, thus facilitating a variety of new ideas (Colzato, Ozturk, & Hommel, 2012). In randomized controlled trials of transcendental meditation, creativity increased significantly at 6-month follow-up among Chinese high school students in a meditation group and was replicated in Chinese junior high school students (So & Orme-Johnson, 2001). Among un-dergraduate students in a Zen meditation training group, significant gains in creativity were found relative to a group taught relaxation techniques (Cowger & Torrance, 1982).

Curiosity is one of the two factors measured by the popular Toronto Mindfulness Scale (Lau et al., 2006) and has been noted as a central aspect of the operational definition of mindfulness since it is viewed as an important attitude one might take toward sensations, cognitions, and emotions (Bishop et al., 2004). This mindfulness-curiosity link is discussed at length in Kashdan (2009), and is robustly demonstrated in a couples intervention in which mindfulness was used to teach couples to be open and curious, to build self-kindness, manage negative feelings, and align with core values; and the couples participated in novel and interesting things together and appreciated what one another had previously overlooked (Carson et al., 2004; Carson et al., 2007). The combination of curiosity and mindfulness has been linked with an approach of less defensiveness (Kashdan, Afram, Brown, Birnbeck, & Drvoshanov, 2011). Research has connected mindfulness to receptivity to a wide range of ideas, values, and activities (Brown & Ryan, 2003; Costa & McCrae, 1992), which parallels open-mindedness, a dimension of judgment, as well as openness to experience, a dimension of curiosity. Furthermore, mindfulness teaches one to avoid evaluations, thereby facilitating the character strength of open-mindedness/judgment (Hayes & Feldman, 2004). There are a number of cognitive biases that impact the character strength of judgment/critical thinking. One study found that those who practiced a brief mindfulness mediation demonstrated less of a negativity bias (Kiken & Shook, 2011), which parallels good critical thinking.

Flow is a psychological state that accompanies activities where attention is sharply focused and the sense of time fades (Csikszentmihalyi, 1997). Because flow also involves a decrease in self-consciousness, mindfulness cannot be related throughout the entire flow experience. When in flow, individuals are engaged in an activity and when engaged it is likely strengths are being used (Seligman, 2002). The love of learning strength is particularly relevant here as such engaged learning is likely to be expressed through the state of flow. When people learn with mindfulness, they are more likely to enjoy the learning experience and their performance increases (Langer, 2009). One of the positive effects of brief mindful awareness practices found with college students is that the majority of students report mindfulness had a positive effect on their learning (Yamada & Victor, 2012).

Many mindfulness practices have a wisdom component built into the meditation practice. Perspective (wisdom) is offered as an explicit or implicit approach in most mindfulness programs. In DBT, this is called promoting "wise mind" (Linehan, 1993), while in Mindfulness-Based Eating Awareness Training a formal "wisdom meditation" is employed, and wisdom is suggested as an outcome of the approach (Kristeller, 2003; Kristeller & Hallett, 1999). Another example is the "expanded awareness" component of the 3-minute breathing space used in MBCT (Segal et al., 2002); as well as the wider perspective approach Kabat-Zinn (1990) promotes in the body scan exercise of MBSR. Since these wisdom strengths are cognitively oriented, it is also relevant to note that mindfulness improves cognitive abilities, such as working memory and executive functioning, and can improve the distribution of limited brain resources (Slagter et al., 2007). However, it is possible that these cognitive benefits may only present for some individuals. A link between mindfulness and perspective taking has also been made (Block-Lerner, Adair, Plumb, Rhatigan, & Orsillo, 2007).

Courage Strengths

The courage-oriented strengths of *bravery, perseverance, honesty*, and *zest* involve the exercise of will to accomplish goals and overcome opposition (Peterson & Seligman, 2004).

While not the subject of rigorous research, it would be virtually impossible to exclude bravery when discussing the application of mindfulness with chronic pain or deep emotional turmoil. Indeed, to use mindfulness to directly face deep suffering takes a high degree of bravery. Sustained focus over time can also facilitate inhibition of emotional expression. It can be argued that this inhibition allows the individual to reappraise the painful experience or memory (Bridges, Denham,

& Ganiban, 2004), which involves enacting the character strength of bravery.

Mindfulness, specifically the nonreacting and nonjudging aspects, has been found to predict increases in persistence (perseverance), as evidenced in a difficult laboratory test (Evans, Baer, & Segerstrom, 2009). Most of the studies done on mindfulness showing clinical effectiveness have been done over several weeks requiring participants to engage in a daily practice of meditation (e.g., Hoffmann, Sawyer, Witt, & Oh, 2010). While not directly measuring this strength, such practice clearly requires perseverance. In addition, sustained focus, volitional control, and elaborate processing during mindfulness (Lutz, Brefczynski, Johnstone, & Davidson, 2008) underscore perseverance.

The strength of honesty is characterized by dimensions of authenticity and integrity. Authenticity has been found to correlate positively with mindfulness (Lakey, Kernis, Heppner, & Lance, 2008; Levesque & Brown, 2007). The former set of researchers also found that higher scores on mindfulness and authenticity related to lower levels of verbal defensiveness. Furthermore, mindfulness is connected with knowing one's true or real self (Carlson, 2013) as one is encouraged to accept all emotional experiences, regardless of their valence, intensity, and perceived utility (Whelton, 2004). Those higher in mindfulness were more likely to behave consistently with their feelings and actions (Chatzisarantis & Hagger, 2007); said another way, a strong expression of mindfulness might be related to integrity.

Thich Nhat Hanh has defined mindfulness as keeping our attention alive in the present moment, in other words, mobilizing enthusiasm and energy for the here and now. Vitality, i.e., zest, has been found to benefit physical and psychological health in a number of studies, one in particular was undertaken by Reibel et al. (2001), in which subjects completed an eight-week MBSR program and were required to practice 20 minutes of meditation per day. Mindfulness has been associated with a decrease in fatigue in a number of studies (e.g., Kaplan, Goldenberg, & Galvan-Nadeau, 1993; Surawy, Roberts, & Silver, 2005), and while this should not be viewed as a certain increase in zest/vitality, it represents the concept that participants had to use mindfulness to shift toward a direction of greater energy.

Humanity Strengths

The strengths of *love*, *kindness*, and *social intelligence* are viewed as the humanity strengths in the VIA Classification, those interpersonal strengths that help individuals tend and befriend others, most typically in one-on-one relationships (Peterson & Seligman, 2004). Higher levels of trait mindfulness have been associated with higher levels of relationship satisfaction and management of relationship stress in two studies (Barnes, Brown, Krusemark, Campbell, & Rogge, 2007). The strength of love is manifested strongly in close relationships in which individuals can show both the capacity to love and to be loved. Mindfulness-Based Relationship Enhancement (MBRE) is a structured eight-week couples program that favorably impacts couples' closeness, as well as levels of relationship satisfaction, autonomy, relatedness, acceptance of one another, and relationship distress (Carson et al., 2004). A qualitative study of MBRE found that mindfulness not only contributed to relationship health but also to the durability and resilience of relationships (Bohy, 2010).

There is a developing literature over the last decade on a type of mindfulness practice called loving-kindness meditation and the closely related practice of self-compassion. Research has found that the practice of loving-kindness meditation can lead to long-term benefits (15-month follow-up after intervention concluded) for boosting personal resources such as resilience and social support (Cohn & Fredrickson, 2010). Standard loving-kindness meditations involve the individual bringing a mindful awareness to their strength capacity of love through the cultivation of positive emotion and imagery (Salzberg, 1995). It is also relevant to note Daniel Siegel's (2007) work on the neurobiology of mindfulness and mirror neurons, which are implicated in the process of interpersonal attunement when individuals in relationship "feel felt" by one another.

Dan Goleman reports some of the earlier studies of loving-kindness conducted by David McClelland in which subjects watched a film about Mother Teresa caring for those in need while others watched a film depicting Nazis in Germany. There was a brief rise in T-cells in the immune systems of those watching the film about Mother Teresa, and this increase lasted longer if the individuals spent time practicing loving-kindness meditation after the film (Goleman, 1997). Several scientists have examined the neural responses of individuals practicing loving-kindness meditation (Brewer, Worhunsky, Gray, Tang, Weber, & Kober, 2011; Hofmann et al., 2011; Lee et al., 2012; Lutz et al., 2008). Kristeller and Johnson (2005) proposed a two-stage model: The first stage involves disengagement from typical patterns of self-defeating or self-indulgent reactions, while the second stage involves focused attention on the capacity for love, altruism, and compassion. Research shows a number of benefits that result, such as increased hope and decreased anxiety (Sears & Kraus, 2009), increased social connectedness (Hutcherson, Seppala, & Gross, 2008), and increased positive emotions, improved mood, greater curiosity, self-compassion, and the building of personal resources such as resilience and social support (Cohn & Fredrickson, 2010; Fredrickson et al., 2008). A pilot study of loving-kindness meditation documented success in increasing positive emotions and decreasing the symptoms of schizophrenia (Johnson et al., 2011).

Kindness, when directed outward toward others, is fundamental to the practice of mindfulness as it involves the heartfelt experience of empathizing with another person (Goldstein, 2003; Salzberg, 1995). By increasing one's emotional awareness and acceptance, mindfulness might be expected to increase one's kindness. Social interactions involve many somatic and autonomic reactions to socially-relevant stimuli, such as subtle changes in facial expression and prosody (e.g., Dimberg, Andréasson, & Thunberg, 2011). Increased awareness of interoceptive cues could increase one's perception of these subtle emotions and build further motivation for compassion. Mindfulness has been shown to boost empathy. A study of premedical and medical students showed that 8 weeks of mindfulness training increased empathy (Shapiro, Schwartz, & Bonner, 1998). Another study of psychotherapy trainees showed that mindfulness meditation not only increased empathy, but this, in turn, led to greater improvement in their clients (Grepmair, Mitterlehner, Loew, Bachler, Rother, & Nickel, 2007).

Kindness can also be directed inward in the form of self-compassion. Kristin Neff (2003a; 2003b) developed the Self-Compassion Scale, which includes subscales of mindfulness, common humanity, and self-kindness, and reverse-scored subscales for self-judgment, isolation, and over-identification. Her research has found that self-kindness has most of the benefits of self-esteem with fewer drawbacks, and the practice of self-compassion has been correlated with many psychological benefits including increased optimism, curiosity, social connectedness, emotional intelligence, wisdom, and mastery of goals, to name a few (Neely, Schallert, Mohammed, Roberts, & Chen, 2009; Neff, Rude, & Kirkpatrick, 2007; Neff & Vonk, 2009). Self-compassion also served as a buffer against negative comparisons, and resulted in less self-criticism and perfectionism. Higher levels of self-compassion have been an outcome of mindfulness practice in a number of populations (Proulx, 2008; Shapiro, Astin, Bishop, & Cordova, 2005). Germer (2009) and Gilbert (2009; 2010) have also written extensively on the topic, created structured programs to develop compassion and self-compassion, and report numerous benefits of these practices.

Self-compassion has consistently been found to relate to higher well-being (Barnard & Curry, 2011). Other research has identified important gender differences in how self-compassion can help or hurt relationships. Baker and McNulty (2011) found that for men high in conscientiousness, self-compassion was connected with a greater motivation to offer constructive problem-solving and greater marital happiness, while the opposite was the case for men low in conscientiousness; for women, self-compassion never seemed to harm the relationship.

The character strength of social intelligence has some interesting connections with mindfulness. Mindfulness encompasses both awareness of attention as well as awareness of the background radar of situations; in other words, mindfulness helps in the monitoring of both inner and outer environments (Averrill, 1992; Mayer, Chabot, & Carlsmith, 1997). This is consistent with aspects of emotional intelligence, a core dimension of the social intelligence strength. Higher mindfulness has been associated with greater emotional intelligence (Bauer, McAdams, & Pals, 2008; Schutte

& Malouff, 2011), and, in turn, emotional intelligence explains the connection mindfulness has with higher positive emotion, lower negative emotion, and greater life satisfaction (Schutte & Malouff, 2011). In a mindfulness treatment program for irritable bowel syndrome, emotional intelligence was formally taught as a core part of the course, where emphasis was placed on individuals learning skills for differentiating body sensations from emotions (Ljótsson et al., 2011). Indeed, the skill of using mindfulness to observe, allow, and accept emotions and distinguish them from body sensations is a common component of mindfulness training (Segal et al., 2002). Mindfulness allows for genuine expression of emotion in which one is neither under-engaged or over-engaged with feeling (Hayes, Wilson, Gifford, Follette, & Strosahl 1996; Hoeksma, Oosterlaan, & Schipper, 2004).

Adding to this area of improved emotional management, mindfulness facilitates a way for individuals to cultivate a deep respect for, rather than avoidance of, emotions, enabling the appreciation and honor of emotions (Khong, 2011); and associations between mindfulness and a decrease in both rumination and the behavioral, emotional, and cognitive components of aggression have been found (Borders, Earleywine & Jajodia, 2010). Mindfulness may also lead to improvements in affective forecasting (being able to accurately predict emotions in the future), as was found in one experiment of young adults who forecasted their feelings for the weeks after a presidential election (Emanuel, Updegraff, Kalmbach, & Ciesla, 2010). As another benefit to the strength of social intelligence, various aspects of mindfulness (acting with awareness, acceptance without judgment, observing, and describing) have been positively associated with expressing oneself in various social situations (Dekeyser, Raes, Leijssen, Leysen, & Dewulf, 2008). Trait mindfulness helps people to avoid making negative social comparisons and gain more accurate information about themselves. Mindful social comparisons could, in the end, also help people gain more accurate information about themselves, helping them to truly learn and create. Trait mindfulness exerts a positive influence on individuals' perceptions of performance (Djikic & Langer, 2007; Langer, Delizonna, & Pirson, 2010). Improved social perception was found in a mindfulness group over a mindless group when viewing positive, negative, normal, and deviant people on video; the mindfulness group more accurately perceived gestures and physical characteristics (Langer & Imber, 1980).

Justice Strengths

The character strengths of the virtue of justice include *teamwork*, *fairness*, and *leadership* and are considered to be civic strengths that help individuals connect in groups (Peterson & Seligman, 2004). Although little research has been done connecting these strengths with mindfulness, the conception is that these strengths would be linked to specific training areas of mindfulness, namely the areas of mindful speech/listening and the domain of bringing greater mindfulness toward issues of social injustice and oppression (Peterson & Seligman, 2004).

One dimension of teamwork is citizenship, which is a concept frequently studied in work settings as organizational citizenship behavior. Mindfulness was found to interact with qualities such as hope and resilience to foster positive emotions which then led to greater citizenship and organizational change (Avey, Wernsing, & Luthans, 2008). In an unpublished research study, Silberman (2007) studied 102 students who were administered the VIA Survey and a mindfulness instrument. The strength of teamwork/citizenship was among the significant correlations with mindfulness, in addition to perspective, social intelligence, bravery, honesty, and self-regulation.

The use of mindfulness in the arena of social justice, fairness, and peace to create greater societal well-being is not a new concept, however, empirical studies are lacking. DeValve and Quinn (2010) discussed an application relating to mindfulness and justice as they related specific practices of the Zen monk and peace activist Thich Nhat Hanh pertaining to police officers working in the criminal justice system and the community. For decades, Nhat Hanh has spoken of the use of mindfulness to promote peace and nonviolence, the latter of which fairness might be considered a dimension of. An older study on the effects of transcendental meditation found that duration of meditation practice correlated with higher scores on scales of moral development (Nidich, Ryncarz, Abrams, Orme-Johnson, & Wallace, 1983), a concept closely linked with the strength of fairness (Peterson & Seligman, 2004). More recently, researchers found similar findings that MBSR led to improvements in moral reasoning and ethical decision making at two-month follow-up (Shapiro, Jazaieri, & Goldin, 2012).

Boyatzis and McKee (2005) draw a strong theoretical connection between the use of mindfulness and the resonant leader. The synergy here is the use of mindfulness to build resilience by becoming more self-aware as a leader, taking stock in one's values at work, and fostering self-renewal and life balance (McKee, Boyatzis, & Johnston, 2008). In a study that explored trait mindfulness in supervisors (i.e., leaders), researchers found mindfulness was connected with employee well-being and performance (Reb, Narayanan, & Chaturvedi, 2012).

Temperance Strengths

The VIA Classification defines the temperance virtue in terms of *forgiveness*, *humility*, *prudence*, and *self-regulation*, each of which are strengths that help protect individuals from excess and vices (Peterson & Seligman, 2004). One study found a connection between mindfulness and different types of forgiveness such as self-forgiveness, other-forgiveness, and situational-forgiveness (Webb, Phillips, Bumgarner, & Conway-Williams, 2012); these researchers suggest that the expression of forgiveness may open up resources to allow for additional energy to be invested in mindfulness. Unforgiveness is associated with greater anger and rumination (e.g., Barber, Maltby, and Macaskill, 2005), while mindfulness, on the other hand, emphasizes a quality of "letting go" and reduces rumination and provides an adaptive means for dealing effectively with an emotion like anger, apart from acting on it impulsively or suppressing it. Furthermore, in a study of college students, mindfulness meditation increased forgiveness (Oman, Shapiro, Thoresen, Plante, & Flinders, 2008). Research has also found the combination of forgiveness with gratitude to positively correlate with acceptance (Breen, Kashdan, Lenser, & Fincham, 2010).

Heppner & Kernis (2007) explain mindfulness as a process of quieting the ego or detaching feelings of self-worth from everyday affairs. Quiet ego is a multi-dimensional construct that involves objective self-awareness, interdependence with others, compassion, and growth/wisdom (Wayment & Bauer, 2008; Wayment, Wiist, Sullivan, & Warren, 2011). In addition to the strengths of perspective and kindness, being able to let go, e.g., quiet, one's ego as well as taking a realistic approach, objective self-awareness is an important quality of a true humility. Indeed, mindfulness allows individuals to perceive performance in an authentic yet humble way (Langer et al., 2010; Djikic & Langer, 2007).

It is evidenced from a meta-analysis of 29 studies by Giluk (2009) that there is a strong association between mindfulness and conscientiousness, the latter of which has parallels with the character strength of prudence.

The self-regulation of attention is part of the core definition of mindfulness (Bishop et al., 2004). Mindfulness, even brief meditations, seems to serve as quick and efficient methods for boosting self-control among those who are low in this strength (Friese, Messner, & Schaffner, 2012; Papies, 2012), but mindfulness can also be beneficial for those who are high in this strength as marked by high self-discipline (Bowlin & Baer, 2012). Shapiro and Schwartz (2000) discuss how self-regulation is based on feedback loops that can be enhanced through attention, and how therefore all self-regulation strategies involve the cultivation of attention. Not surprisingly, those high in mindfulness compared with those low in mindfulness have been found to exhibit greater attentional control and concentration (Kee & Wang, 2008). Masicampo and Baumeister (2007) discuss how mindfulness therapies can be viewed as a form of self-regulation exercise. The authors note that mindfulness interventions are similar to self-regulation interventions in that both require the individual to alter and control the response of the self. Mechanisms of mindfulness that may be distinguished from self-regulation, however, include nonattachment, exposure, and metacognition. Masicampo and Baumeister report how some scholars note mindfulness facilitates self-regulation and well-being while others claim the reverse is the case.

Taking the connection further, mindfulness could be described as an overarching human strength that is strongly linked with human well-being (Masicampo & Baumeister, 2007; Wallace & Shapiro, 2006) and the ability to adaptively regulate one's feelings and actions (Baliki, Geha, Apkarian, & Chialvo, 2008; Eisenberg & Spinrad, 2004). Rather than perceiving psychological phenomena as fixed, a mindful disposition encourages us to treat them as transitory and impermanent (Kabat-Zinn, 1990; Segal et al., 2002). Such a disposition, however, is not developed overnight. It requires repeated effort – usually through regular meditation practice (self-regulation practice) – which allows individuals to move towards a healthier regulation of feelings and actions (Kabat-Zinn, 1990). Baumeister and colleagues have found that self-regulation can operate like a muscle in that it is a limited resource and strength that can be depleted or built up and developed with practice (Baumeister et al., 2006; Muraven & Baumeister, 2000). In flexing the self-regulation muscles, a mindful disposition offers new insights by enhancing cognitive flexibility, which decreases the individual's need to control or alter one's environment and experiences; the individual then moves towards more acceptance and genuine appreciation (Chambers, Gullone, & Allen, 2009).

Transcendence Strengths

The transcendence strengths are viewed as *appreciation of beauty and excellence*, *gratitude*, *hope*/optimism, *humor*, and *spirituality*/religiousness, which help the individual forge connections outside of themselves and with the larger universe (Peterson & Seligman, 2004).

Individuals might connect with beauty in nature, in art, or through moral beauty (observing virtuous acts). Cattron (2008) found that engagement with beauty correlates with mindfulness; engagement with artistic beauty correlated higher with mindfulness than natural beauty or moral beauty. Increased awareness of sensory perceptions may also lead one to have an increased appreciation of beauty. Sharpening of sensory awareness can enhance experiences of sights, sounds, and touch. Another study found an association between connection with nature and both well-being and mindfulness (Howell, Dopko, Passmore, & Buro, 2011).

Gratitude is a strength that relates to mindfulness through the development of greater awareness. Gratitude involves the ability to notice, appreciate, and savor the elements of one's life (Emmons & McCullough, 2003). Intentionally applying attention to savor and increase enjoyment of experiences has been noted to relate to many aspects of well-being, including increased happiness, optimism, and decreased hopelessness, depression, guilt, and anhedonia (Bryant & Veroff, 2007). By increasing awareness of experiences and one's subjective reaction to experiences, mindfulness makes one more prepared to respond to positive events with gratitude. Significant increases in optimism were also found among inmates who practiced intensive mindfulness meditation while incarcerated (Bowen et al., 2006). Other studies have found a connection between mindfulness training and optimism (Carson, Carson, Gil, & Baucom, 2004) and hope (Sears & Kraus, 2009).

Direct empirical links between mindfulness and humor are rare. However, one is not hard-pressed to find connections made by venerable meditation luminaries. For example, meditation teacher and Buddhist monk Henepola Gunaratana (2002) advises to take a light-hearted approach to mindfulness meditation and not turn it into a "grim endurance contest." Such an approach involves not taking oneself too seriously so as to not get quickly lost in habitual patterns of mind.

Given the relevance of mindfulness meditation to humility, gratitude, forgiveness, and perspective, one might predict that mindfulness relates to spirituality. These strengths have been connected to many spiritual and religious traditions across culture and time. The sense of a larger perspective and meaning that is inherent in these and other strengths would lend itself to some form of spiritual or existential development. Indeed, studies have showed that mindfulness training leads to an increase in spirituality (Birnie, Speca, & Carlson, 2010), particularly in having a sense of meaning (Carmody et al., 2008). Increases in both state and trait mindfulness were associated with increases in spiritual-

ity, and both of these, in turn, were associated with fewer psychological and physical symptoms. Goldstein (2007) employed an intervention studying sacred, spiritual moments in which experimental group participants practiced mindfulness daily and turned their attention to the sacredness in an object they considered holy or precious with resulting benefits to well-being. MBRE was found to benefit couples' spirituality and optimism/hope strengths (Carson et al., 2004). In addition to reduced psychological symptoms, MBSR has been found to lead to an increase in spiritual experiences (Astin, 1997; Geary & Rosenthal, 2011; Shapiro et al., 1998). In a study of maturity, mindfulness and spirituality were related to maturity and their combination was stronger than either one alone. In the workplace domain, regular meditation practice related to higher workplace spirituality (Petchsawang & Duchon, 2012).

Benefits of Integrating Mindfulness and Character Strengths

Building off this inherent connection initiated elsewhere (Niemiec et al., 2012) and considering the research just reviewed, the merging of mindfulness and character strengths offers a number of distinct and promising benefits. Here is an overview of why the integration of mindfulness warrants further investigation:

- Offers individuals who practice mindfulness a way to deal with obstacles and barriers that naturally emerge during mindfulness practices.
- Gives mindfulness practitioners concrete tools to widen perspective and deepen practice.
- Provides mindfulness practitioners a language to capture positive states and traits, many of which are organic outcomes of mindfulness.
- Elicits a greater awareness of the positive potential within us, and, taken a step further, offers a pathway to explore and develop character strengths. As Cloninger (2007) explains, character develops through growth in self-awareness as individuals gain life perspective through meaning and satisfaction. He notes that extensive empirical work has shown that

movement through stages of development can be described in terms of steps in character development.

- Creates a positive synergy of mutual benefit that can foster a *virtuous circle* of positive impact. Mindful awareness boosts strengths use which, in turn, enlivens mindfulness. A similar concept is what is known as upward positive spirals (Fredrickson, 2001). This synergy might be what underlies successful positive interventions. After finding success in boosting well-being with nine positive psychology interventions that involve character strengths, Gander et al. (2012a) hypothesize that this success might be attributed to mindfulness and the broaden-and-build theory (Fredrickson, 2001).

- Fosters individuals' ability to respond appropriately and successfully in different contexts; that is, the integration may promote psychological flexibility (Kashdan & Rottenberg, 2010), help individuals find balance and practical wisdom in situations (Schwartz & Sharpe, 2006), and engender a growth mindset (Dweck, 2006; Louis, 2011).

- Facilitates increased self-awareness and potential for change activation by bringing one's character strengths more clearly into view. As Carlson (2013) describes, mindfulness serves as a path to see oneself as one really is.

- Offers an anchor to the practice of character strengths as individuals often are uncertain what direction to take and how to work with strengths.

- Motivates individuals to use their signature strengths more, which is particularly relevant since some research has found that only 1/3 of individuals have a meaningful awareness of their strengths (reported in Linley, 2008); and for those that are aware, there may be the issue of strengths blindness (Biswas-Diener et al., 2011); that is, taking one's strengths for granted and downplaying them as ordinary. Mindfulness may be the ideal approach for remedying the "taking-strengths-for-granted" effect.

- Provides a pathway for balanced character strength expression and a way to practice bringing them to fruition. Mindfulness can serve as a way for individuals to attend to the golden mean of character strengths (Chapter 2)

and therefore manage strengths overuse and underuse.

- Helps individuals get off the "hedonic treadmill," which states that humans quickly adapt to the good or bad that is experienced in life. This theory states that individuals eventually return to baseline levels (i.e., a particular set point) of happiness (for example, lottery winners become happier in the moment but return to the level of happiness they had prior to winning; Brickman & Campbell, 1971). However, studies have shown that other happiness theories (e.g., authentic happiness theory) better explain well-being than this set-point theory (Headey, Schupp, Tucci, & Wagner, 2010). In addition, Ed Diener and colleagues (2006) have offered several revisions to the hedonic treadmill theory, showing that humans have multiple happiness set points and that these set points can change under some conditions. In addition, Lyubomirsky (2008) has added the impact of intentional activities in having a lasting effect on happiness and shares several empirically validated activities that involve strengths, such as practicing gratitude and kindness. Mindfulness and character strengths align with these suggestions that boost happiness and potentially help to counter the habitual nature of adaptation (i.e., hedonic treadmill).

- Gives a direct and indirect boost to many strengths at once. The character strengths "inter-are," meaning that, in reality, one strength cannot be expressed without using other strengths. For example, how can a person practice cultivating gratitude without employing the strengths of perspective (e.g., reflecting back on their day with a wider lens when counting one's blessings) or bravery (e.g., using courage to deliver a gratitude letter to someone)? Each strength has elements of the others within it, and moreover, each strength requires the use of other strengths to deploy it. Thus, mindfulness focused on boosting one strength is automatically assisting other strengths to some degree.

- Offers a counterbalance to the human tendency to focus on and become impacted by what's wrong or bad (i.e., "bad is stronger than good"; see Baumeister, Bratslavsky, Finkenaeuer, & Vohs, 2001).

Many of these and related concepts are explored further in later chapters that discuss in detail the practice of integrating mindfulness and character strengths.

This integration naturally elicits a variety of questions with practice implications. A couple of general practice questions are important to consider before moving forward to the next two chapters that focus on practice:

- Can individuals practice mindfulness without character strengths?
  - It depends. It is possible to practice mindfulness without *signature* strengths use (depending on which strengths are highest for a given individual). However, it seems impossible to be mindful and have no strengths use. In part this is because certain strengths are inherently part of the mindfulness process itself (i.e., curiosity, self-regulation).
- Can an individual use their character strengths without mindfulness?
  - Absolutely, but not without some loss of competent use. The first step in working on the development of character strengths is awareness, therefore, to be more skilled and savvy with strengths use, mindfulness is important.

Future Directions

Despite the large number of studies cited in this chapter, there are more empirical questions to be grappled with than there are answers. For example, is it possible that any of the 24 character strengths can be developed with mindfulness? If so, to what degree can they be developed over time? Does the focus on particular strengths lead to improved mindfulness-group engagement (e.g., MBSR, MBCT, MBSP) and, in turn, better outcomes? Is the integration of these two areas a key for improving the maintenance of long-term mindfulness practice? How much does mindfulness help individuals spot strengths in others, enhance individual strengths, and express value in the strengths of others? Ultimately, these are empirical questions that warrant attention in this arena of integration. My hypothesis is that the integration of these areas is a recipe for flourishing – for greater engagement in work, higher sense of meaning and purpose, higher physical and psychological well-being, and improved relationships. Early pilot data (see Chapter 6) supports this hypothesis.

Chapter 4

Practice I: Strong Mindfulness (Bringing Strengths to Mindfulness)

The one who sits in solitude and quiet has escaped from three wars: hearing, speaking, and seeing; yet against one thing shall he continually battle: that is, his own heart.

Anthony of Egypt, 3rd century monk

 Chapter Snapshot

The focus of this chapter is on using character strengths to create a solid mindfulness practice. This is referred to as "strong mindfulness," which applies to any instance in which character strengths are being used to support or enhance mindfulness practices. Just as mindfulness practices extend far beyond the cushion, strengths can be applied during and outside of formal meditation periods. There are a number of ways this unfolds. Three overarching manifestations will be covered:

- The use of character strengths to "supercharge" or reinvigorate meditation practices, such as activities of daily life (e.g., mindful walking, mindful driving).
- The use of character strengths to manage or overcome common barriers and obstacles in practicing mindfulness (e.g., mind wandering).
- The use of character strengths interventions to support principles of mindful living (e.g., reverence for life). These health-based principles were formulated by the Zen monk, Thich Nhat Hanh, and are widely referred to as the Five Mindfulness Trainings.

 Opening Story[1]

There was a king who believed if he could figure out the best answers to three questions, he would become a better, fairer ruler. The questions were:

- Who are the most important people?
- When is the best time to do things?
- What is the most important pursuit?

The king searched far and wide, speaking with countless people, but could not find any satisfactory answers. He decided to travel to the mountains and find the old wise hermit who lived there and

---

[1] This story has been shared in different works with minor adaptations. Two previous versions of this story can be found in Martin and Morimoto (1995) and Young-Eisendrath (1996).

might have some ideas. After days of searching, he found the hermit outside his hut, working in his garden. The old man was quiet, barely saying a word to the king. The king studied the hermit for awhile, watching his effort and hard work. Noticing the hermit's energy dwindling, the king offered to help and took a shovel and began to dig. He asked the hermit the three questions. The old man seemed unmoved by the questions and continued to work.

The king continued to work, helping the frail hermit who could not keep up his stamina. Toward the end of an afternoon of working in the garden, they heard a strange noise followed by a cry coming from the woods. The men hurried over toward the commotion. They found a soldier lying on the ground, wounded and in pain. The king picked him up and took him to the hermit's hut and tended to his wounds. The soldier was hungry and thirsty; the hermit and king fed the man and brought some fresh water from a nearby stream. They arranged a warm bed for the soldier to rest.

The king awakened the next morning to the soldier sitting next to him.

"What's wrong?" asked the king.

"I'm ashamed and so sorry, your majesty," exclaimed the soldier.

"I don't understand."

"Your majesty, when I learned that you would be traveling to an isolated region, I plotted to take my revenge on you. You see, many years ago you banished my family from its farmlands, and we no longer could make enough money to survive. We have suffered greatly for many years, and one of my sons died from a lack of food. I then vowed revenge. While I waited in the woods for your return, one of your men found me and stabbed me. I fled but would surely have died without your help yesterday."

The king apologized to the soldier for his careless actions years ago, restored his lands, and the soldier returned home. The king turned to the hermit:

"Well, it seems that you cannot answer my questions, so I will turn my search elsewhere."

"Take notice," laughed the hermit. "You already have your answers."

"What?"

"Look at the actions of your day. Working in the garden with me ended up saving your life. The most important pursuit in that moment was helping me dig. When you were tending to the soldier's wounds and getting him water, he was the most important person to you in that moment and the most important pursuit was caring for him."

"The present moment is the only time you have," continued the hermit. "The most important person is always the person you are with, and the most important pursuit is contributing to the happiness of that person."

Common Mindfulness Practices

This section discusses examples of mindfulness practices typically found in mindfulness programs. Each serves as an opportunity to deepen one's connection with the present moment and cultivate stronger mindfulness in daily life.

In order to engage in the practice, many character strengths are employed, such as self-regulation, perseverance, self-kindness, curiosity, and perspective, to name a few.

Raisin Exercise

A common exercise done in the first session of many mindfulness programs is what is typically referred to as "the raisin exercise," created by Kabat-Zinn (1990). It has become such a standard in mindfulness programs that it could be viewed as the quintessential mindfulness exercise. This practice involves taking several minutes to eat one (or more) raisins while fully engaging all of one's senses. The practice is explicitly designed to tap into participants' "beginner's mind," which means to see things as if for the first time; participants approach each raisin as if they are noticing it and eating it for the first time. This exercise also tends to promote the process of savoring (Bryant & Veroff, 2007), although savoring involves deliberately attempting to prolong a positive experience whereas mindfulness involves observing whatever is going on in the experience and not attempting to prolong or eliminate it. Participants use their curiosity to explore the raisin and begin to use self-regulation as they are instructed to bring their attention back to the raisin when their mind wanders.

One study randomly assigned subjects to a group that practiced mindful eating with a raisin, a group that ate a raisin without mindfulness instructions, and a no-task group (Hong, Lishner, & Han, 2012). Individuals were then offered anchovies, wasabi peas, and prunes to sample. Those subjects in the raisin group who sampled food expressed a higher enjoyment level of the food they sampled than those in either of the other two groups. Researchers did not find an impact of mindfulness on the likelihood of individuals trying different foods.

Body Scan and Mindful Yoga

Mindfulness of the body is another core practice taught early on in mindfulness programs because not only is the body something very concrete to attend to, it is something that is quickly taken for granted and even viewed as foreign by many individuals. Often individuals are not very tuned into their body until something is wrong with it – being sick with the flu, stubbing one's toe, or suffering from a physical illness. Such physical afflictions bring people's attention immediately to the body, and, moreover, they elicit a desire to want to change the experience. Careful, mindful attention to the body, just like taking 10 minutes to eat one raisin, delivers a certain level of surprise and appreciation to participants. Individuals quickly understand that mindfulness is something much more than simply sitting still with good posture.

Being curious and interested in the body is explicitly part of the body scan practice, as is using self-regulation with breathing, and concluding

with taking a wider perspective – generating a sense of oneness with the body. Kabat-Zinn (1990) has referred to the latter as connecting with the body as-a-whole or whole-body-breathing. Shapiro et al. (2002) report that oneness motivation (a positive sense that one is part of a larger whole) and trust increased during a course of mindfulness in a controlled trial. Listen to Track 2 of the attached CD for the Body Mindfulness exercise.

Mindful yoga is another practice frequently used in mindfulness programs, especially MBSR but also MBCT and MBRE. Mindful yoga invites participants to be accepting of their body as it moves, stretches, and holds postures. Participants build a more acute perception and inner ear, so to speak, for their body's needs and limitations but also its wonders and beauties. Mindful yoga and the body scan also place a strong emphasis on the character strength of kindness turned inward. Taking an understanding, gentle, and compassionate approach with one's body is a core part of meditation practice (Brahm, 2006).

In a study comparing the effects of the body scan, mindful yoga, and sitting meditation, researchers divided participants into one of the three groups and offered guided meditation and discussion for three, 1-hour sessions (Sauer-Zavala, Walsh, Eisenlohr-Moul, & Lykins, 2012). While all three practices elicited improvements in self-compassion, psychological well-being, and rumination, differences between groups were also noted. They found that mindful yoga was associated with greater psychological well-being, that sitting meditation and mindful yoga were both related to decreases in emotional regulation problems, and that sitting meditation was connected with taking a nonevaluative stance more than the body scan. In another study, participants who practiced the body scan meditation, compared to those in a control group, improved in their accuracy of body perceptions (Mirams, Poliakoff, Brown, & Lloyd, 2012).

Breathing Space Exercise

The 3-minute breathing space was initiated in MBCT (Segal et al., 2002) and is essentially a shortened version of sitting meditation or mindful breathing practice. This meditation is used repeatedly in MBCT and involves three steps: awareness of the present moment, concentration on the breath, and expanded awareness on the breath and the whole body/mind. In MBCT groups, I've found this to not only be an effective exercise but also participants tend to report this as one of their favorite experiential exercises because it can easily be threaded into busy daily lifestyles.

The 3-minute breathing space has been adapted in MBSP by maintaining the three phases, each lasting for approximately one minute each; however, greater emphasis is placed on the core character strength that is naturally involved at each phase: curiosity in the awareness phase, self-regulation in the concentration phase, and perspective in the expanded awareness phase. Each of these strengths is natural to the meditation component at each phase and the emphasis on each serves as a way of boosting each of these three strengths. Therefore, this is called the character strengths breathing space in MBSP programs. Listen to Track 4 of the attached CD to hear the character strengths breathing space.

In a study comparing mindful breathing, loving-kindness, and progressive muscle relaxation, mindful breathing practice was related to more decentering than the other two groups (Feldman, Greeson, & Senville, 2010). The researchers add that mindful breathing may help to reduce individuals' reactivity to repetitive thoughts. This points to the importance of maintaining the simplicity of mindfulness – the act of focusing attention on one's breathing. It might be that this helps the individual keep a more watchful stance on their thinking to better enable decentering as opposed to other practices where mental energy is exerted to focus on something in particular, such as a loving image or specific meditation phrases (as in loving-kindness meditation) or on tensing and relaxing specific muscle groups (as in progressive muscle relaxation).

Practice Tip: 3 Strengths in 3 Minutes

It is common for individuals to struggle with regular meditation practice or to not want to put in extra time. The character strengths breathing space exercise is a brief mindfulness meditation adapted from the 3-minute breathing space used in MBCT. For individuals struggling with meditation, this exercise can be presented as a reframe in that the individual is simply practicing working on three character strengths. This becomes a useful heuristic in that all that the individual needs to remember is curiosity, self-regulation, and perspective. Individuals begin to see this as the practice of curiosity for the present moment, followed by the practice of self-regulation of one's attention on the breath, and conclude with the practice of taking a wider perspective.

Mindful Speech and Mindful Listening

Listening and speaking to others with mindfulness is one of the most challenging mindfulness practices, fraught with obstacles and interpersonal barriers. That said, it is also one of the most rewarding. The majority of mindfulness practices, despite their frequent occurrence in group settings, are solitary activities (there are exceptions such as mindful yoga with one's partner in MBRE).

A healthy, mindful communication is one in which both parties are attempting to relate and connect with one another. *Mindful speech* involves speaking with one's honesty strength and generally can be described as concise, specific, direct, and from the heart; it means to let go of speaking that includes tangents, disclaimers, rationalizations, hurtful comments, and extra repetitions. *Mindful listening* means to give one's full attention to the listener with genuine kindness/compassion; this involves setting aside the impulse to react or to think of ways one might respond while the other is talking (i.e., self-regulation).

Mindful communication is in stark contrast with an "I–It" relationship in which individuals treat each other like objects, attempting to one-up the other or win the conversation. Rather, as philosopher Martin Buber explained, the communication should pursue an "I–Thou" relationship in which individuals accept the other person as they are, not as they want them to be (Buber, 1958). This kind of conversation in which individuals show interest in learning about the other has two goals – to improve the relationship and to increase the understanding of the topic at hand (Kahn, 1995). Imagine taking that approach with those whom you disagree, those whom you make difficult joint decisions with, and those whom you love the most. Taking just the first goal, what if the driving force of every interaction you had with people in your life was that each conversation – each present moment – would serve to improve your relationship with them? When we are mindfully present in our conversation, we are heading in that direction – we are staying present to who the person is and giving them the space to express their best self (character strengths). No doubt this involves the mindful use of a number of heart-oriented character strengths.

Because our autopilot tendencies around other people are so well-worn, the practice of mindful listening/speaking can benefit from setting up a framework for mutual practice. Many years ago I was working with a young woman in psychotherapy for depression and relationship distress. One of the practices I encouraged her to employ each day is described in Box 4.1. She returned the following week energized and excited. She explained how it opened new doors for her and her boyfriend; they began to ask one another about their needs during the day, more frequently offered undivided attention to one another (rather than listening while watching television), spent more time together, and felt better about their relationship. Her boyfriend was so intrigued that he requested to attend a future therapy session to learn more.

Increased mindfulness during interpersonal communication allows for greater attention to others' verbal and nonverbal cues as well as one's own reactions to these cues, an increased ability to nonjudgmentally listen, and an opportunity to tune into one's personal patterns during conflict. Longitudinal studies have found that trait mindfulness predicts higher relationship satisfaction and more constructive responding to relationship stress (Barnes, Brown, Krusemark, Campbell, & Rogge, 2007); trait mindfulness also predicts lower emotional stress responses during conflict discussion and post-conflict, while state mindfulness relates to better communication quality during the discussion. The impact of mindful listening and speech is also evident in MBRE, which has led to a number of relationship improvements

---

Box 4.1. An Intervention for Mindful Speech and Mindful Listening

Ideally, each member of the couple will first express some motivation to improve the communication in their relationship. The couple should then schedule a time each day to practice this exercise for one week. A good amount of time to start with is 15 minutes per day. It is useful for the couple to agree to some basic rules, such as setting aside all electronic devices, sitting together in a quiet space where you can be alone, refraining from talking when the other person is talking, and following a structure such as the following:

- Flip a coin to determine who speaks first. A timer is useful so that you don't have to monitor your watch. Mindful breathing should be implemented by both individuals during each role. This is encouraged during periods of silence, transition, while listening, and in between sentences.
- (5 minutes) Person A speaks while Person B listens. Person A practices the principles of mindful speech and shares something from his or her day that happened or some positive, negative, or neutral event. Person B practices the principles of mindful listening.
- (5 minutes) Switch roles. Person B is now the mindful speaker and Person A is now the mindful listener.
- (5 minutes) Open-ended practice of mindful communication back-and-forth. During this time, each person practices what they've been learning in a way that more closely simulates typical, real-world interactions. Thus, they are immediately practicing the underlying principles of a "new way" of communicating.
- Conclude for the day or repeat.

and insights, including greater relationship satisfaction, closeness, autonomy, acceptance of one other, and less relationship distress; benefits were maintained at a 3-month follow-up (Carson et al., 2004; 2006; 2007). This indicates that greater mindfulness practice on a given day was associated with better relationship quality and stress coping for several consecutive days. Other research involving qualitative reports from physicians undergoing mindfulness training indicate improvements in mindful listening and greater self-awareness (Beckman et al., 2012). Higher levels of mindful observation/listening have also been associated with greater engagement and empathy (Dekeyser et al., 2008).

Mindful Walking

Mindful walking is a great joy for those who practice mindfulness regularly, and it can serve as an easy transition for those new to mindfulness or those intimidated by the seemingly daunting task of sitting still on a cushion or chair for extended periods of time. Another immediate benefit of mindful walking is that it is "meditation in motion," therefore those who might be more anxious or tense have the opportunity to gently "walk off" their tension with their movement. At the same time, mindful walking is equally vulnerable to our autopilot mind and our tendency to become lost in thought. In fact, if an individual is practicing mindful walking outdoors, those newer to mindfulness are likely to be drawn into the visuals of the natural environment, which may become distractions leading the individual to lose focus on attending to both the internal (posture, gait, balance, thoughts, feelings, sensations) and the external.

The practice of mindful walking is a core practice in many mindfulness programs, including MBSR (Kabat-Zinn, 1990) and MBCT (Segal et al., 2002). One mindful movement program for older breast cancer survivors led to improved quality of life through reduced fear and increased mindfulness (Crane-Okada et al., 2012). While there is little research focusing only on the practice of mindful walking, movement-based therapies such as tai chi have been found to have a positive impact on mindfulness (Caldwell, Harri-

son, Adams, Quin, & Greeson, 2010; Nedeljkovic, Wirtz, & Ausfeld-Hafter, 2012). Reviews of studies of tai chi programs have revealed additional benefits; however, most of these studies need more rigorous investigation and control groups (Logghe et al., 2010; Zhang, Layne, Lowder, & Liu, 2012).

Behavioral activation, such as increasing one's movement or walking, has been linked with increased energy and well-being (Mazzucchelli, Kane, & Rees, 2010; Ryan & Frederick, 1997). Consequently, this connects with the character strength of zest, which has dimensions of enthusiasm, energy, and vitality and is expressed as individuals become more active and consciously aware of their movement. As individuals increase their activity level, their energy and mood typically improves, which becomes a reinforcing virtuous circle leading to more zest and energy to engage in further activity.

In MBSP groups, when individuals practice mindful walking with slow, deliberate steps, this more acute observation leads them to "stop and smell the roses," or in other words, take notice of and appreciate beauty they had previously overlooked. Table 4.1 relays examples of how each of the 24 character strengths might become a natural part of mindful walking, at one time or another. My formal walking meditation practice has transferred into some aspects of my daily life. One of the most personal areas has been the sacred act of walking my son to sleep each night. I've done this almost every night since his birth, and he is now two years of age. In Table 4.1, I describe some of the phenomena related during these walking meditation experiences with my son. Each of these did not occur in every instance of mindful walking, however, they almost always occurred in combination with one another. In most cases, the character strength enhanced the quality of the mindfulness. Each strength, in turn, can boost the joy and vibrancy of the walking. For example, taking notice of beauty can be uplifting and enlivening and therefore motivate the individual to return to mindful walking the next day. At the same time, each character strength has the potential to become distracting, pulling the individual away from pure mindfulness. For example, being too focused on beauty can draw the person away from the present moment of noticing one's sense of balance while walking.

Table 4.1
Mindful Walking with the 24 Strengths and a Newborn

Creativity	Particularly relevant in the early months, I merged every creative pathway of soothing I could think together into a conglomeration of gentle walking, including swaying, change of walking speed, rhythmic singing, variations of "shhh'ing," and patting in downward motion.
Curiosity	Focusing on the novelty and newness of the new person I was holding but also the newness of the experience of walking with him.
Judgment	While walking, being open to taking a completely new approach to movement based on the infant's needs in the moment.
Love of Learning	Applying new learnings from books, websites, and other parents as to the best ways to help walk a newborn to sleep.
Perspective	Viewing the big picture of how my life, previously without a child, had culminated to that specific moment-in-time of walking.
Bravery	Facing distress (e.g., a crying baby), uncertainty, and confusion head on, and not avoiding these challenges as they become more intense.
Perseverance	Rising beyond obstacles of my own fatigue, stress from the day, or struggles my son may have been having, and continuing forward with gentle, peaceful walking.
Honesty	The honesty dimension of authenticity is expressed as I expressed love and care, staying true to myself and my priority role as a father.
Zest	To walk with mindfulness and love holding my son naturally infused me with energy and enthusiasm. Stressors faded, fatigue diminished, vitality surged.
Love	Warm love was expressed in the gentle, secure holding of my son closely, with tenderness.
Kindness	Tapping the compassion dimension of kindness, I often recited a particular "chant of compassion" (not in English) while walking.
Social Intelligence	While walking, part of the moment-to-moment observing involved taking notice of my own and my son's emotions and responding appropriately.
Teamwork	My son and I are one on these walks. Anything I do has an effect on him; anything he does has an effect on me. We are a team that works together toward a common intention (e.g., sleep, calmness, presence).
Fairness	I practice fairness by given my son undivided, nondistracted attention. It would be unfair to him if I were to pull out my I-Phone and start playing chess, responding to a text message, or checking my e-mail while walking.
Leadership	As the adult, there is leadership responsibility in that the walking leads to the comfort and, in most cases, the slumber of my son. I thus take action accordingly and make decisions during the walking to reach particular outcomes.
Forgiveness	There is a constant letting go – a letting go of stress, of body tension, of expectations, of thoughts, and of other plans when engaging fully in the moment of each step during the walking.

Humility	The mindful walking experience is an honor to do and to be part of. I feel humbled to have the privilege and responsibility of this act of caretaking for another human being. There is a felt sense of this humility during the experience.
Prudence	Each step is taken with carefulness and caution, especially since most walking is done in the dark and there are often toys scattered on the floor. I focused on the mindful placement of each foot and the weight of my body shifting from foot to foot.
Self-Regulation	When the mind wandered, bringing the attention back to the breath, back to my body's movement, back to the weight of my son in my arms, back to his precious face, etc. (back to what is happening in the present moment).
Appreciation of Beauty/Excellence	Taking notice of his beauty while walking as well as the excellence and precision of each careful step.
Gratitude	Very profound and emotionally felt during each walk, particularly related to the perspective strength noted above. Often gratitude was expressed verbally.
Hope	Taking notice that each step of holding my son and walking mindfully is a wonderful, positive moment, there is hope for the next step to equally hold such joy … and then the next hour, next day, and future years with him.
Humor	Playfully pretending to trip while walking which, in the later months of his first two years, could turn cries into bursts of laughter (perhaps this can be called "mindful tripping"?)
Spirituality	Each step mattered; each step was sacred. It was the ultimate engagement with the preciousness of life (see the section First Mindfulness Training later in this chapter).

Mindful Driving

Mindful driving involves bringing a curious and open approach to one's internal and external experiences while operating a vehicle (Niemiec et al., 2012). This is one of the areas of daily life that has received the least attention in the mindfulness literature, indicating there is rich potential for the exploration and practice of mindful driving, though there are some meaningful exceptions where it has been referred to (Honore, 2005; Nhat Hanh, 1992). Due to the pragmatic challenges of live practice, it is typically not addressed in formal mindfulness programs aside from being part of discussion exercises. In addition, many mindfulness programs encourage participants to choose one routine activity they do every day and consciously bring mindfulness to this activity. Driving is a common activity for participants to choose for this homework exercise. When it is chosen, participants often return dismayed as to how mindless they have been with their driving and the ease at which they slip into autopilot.

Mindless driving is indeed commonplace. About a half-century ago, Eric Berne (1964), author of *Games People Play* and father of transactional analysis, described mindful awareness as eidetic perception, which involves being unusually aware and vivid as one lives in the here and now. He posed the question: "Where is the mind when the body is here?" (p. 179), and reflected on this in the case of driving. He noted several categorical observations:

- *The jerk:* Berne described this individual's main preoccupation as being on time and how it would appear to the boss if they were late. This person only takes notice of their surroundings in that they are obstacles to reaching one's destination. He describes this individual as the most mindless of drivers.

- *The sulk:* This individual focuses on collecting excuses when running late. Thus, any attention to the present moment is focused on looking out for injustices and rationalizations they can contrive to help with their excuses.
- *The natural driver:* This is the individual who treats driving like a science or an art and weaves in and out of traffic. This individual feels connected with the vehicle but is unaware of their surroundings except when they add scope to the craft of their driving.
- *Aware:* This is the mindful driver who is living in the present moment, present to the motion of the vehicle and to the surroundings. Berne offers the story of two men traveling to work by subway and one man suggests they take the express train and save 20 minutes. The friend agrees and when they arrive at their stop 20 minutes early, the friend steps out of the train and sits down on a bench. When asked what he is doing, the friend observes, "Since we saved twenty minutes, we can afford to sit here that long and enjoy our surroundings" (p. 180).

To become the "aware" driver is a particular challenge due to a myriad of internal and external stimuli available when a vehicle is in motion. Internally, individuals might notice muscle tightness, mind wanderings to thoughts of the day at work, emotional irritations, leftover feelings of disappointment from the day, and fear or excitement in driving; externally, individuals might notice the sizes, shapes, colors, depth, and movement of other cars, objects alongside the road and in one's environment such as trees, buildings, other roads, and the sky, and nearby objects such as the dashboard and speedometer; vehicle noises, smells, and the tactile sensation of the steering wheel and the body in the seat might also be noticed. Ultimately, the individual may cultivate a sense of perspective and appreciation for the enormous "machine" that the driver is in charge of.

Researchers are at the very beginning of the study of the impact and relationship between mindfulness and driving. One study using a driving simulator in the lab found that mindfulness and concentration levels were significantly related to situational awareness while driving (Kass,

VanWormer, Mikulas, Legan, & Bumgarner, 2011). The researchers speculate that mindfulness training might impact actual driving performance by improving mindful awareness of one's environment. Another study found that individuals lower in mindfulness reported more texting while driving (Feldman, Greeson, Renna, & Robbins-Monteith, 2011).

In mindfulness programs, individuals can be encouraged to consider the character strengths that accompany a practice of mindful driving. Two strengths in particular that can be focused on are prudence and social intelligence (Niemiec et al., 2012). Prudence refers to having wise caution, attending to the short-term effects of one's actions, and making sound, practical decisions. This can counterbalance the anonymity and tendency of some individuals to be cavalier behind the wheel, leading to an overuse of bravery and an underuse of prudence and kindness/empathy for others. To the latter strength, mindfulness participants frequently note the importance of being aware of the potential role of emotions and the social realities of others (e.g., some drivers' behavior might be a reaction to an upsetting stressor or emergency in their life). This involves the use of the social intelligence strength. Deploying the strengths of kindness, e.g., letting others into one's lane, and forgiveness, e.g., giving other drivers the benefit of the doubt when they cut you off and therefore letting go of ensuing tension, can help individuals feel good in the moment and therefore open up internal resources for improved mindful attending. The alternative is to narrow one's attention to another driver's behavior, and for some individuals this may lead to a cascade of distressing thoughts and intense emotions. In such instances, individuals may benefit from deploying the strength of self-regulation to manage emotions and impulses.

I recall a therapy client of mine who had made enormous progress in one-on-one mindfulness-based strengths work. His relationships had improved, his depression had lifted, and his anxiety had lessened. However, the trappings of autopilot can be particularly strong. One day, following a stressful day in his chemistry lab, he was driving home from work and upon getting cut off by another driver, he snapped. He became so upset that he lost hold of any memories of his mindfulness practice and chased the perpetrator several miles to his house, culminating into a yelling match that eventually was softened by a group of neighbors walking by. While no one was hurt in the incident, my client had placed himself, the other individual, and other drivers at risk. What is particularly ironic about the story is that my client's highest character strength was self-regulation, the least common character strength around the world (Park et al., 2006). In many areas of his life, he had successfully used his signature strength of self-regulation to connect with others, accomplish very difficult tasks, and become happier in life. However, this did not mean he was always mindful and balanced in his expression of the signature strength. After this incident, he added mindful driving to his routine. He practiced mindful breathing, used his perspective and appreciation of beauty/excellence strengths to tune into his external surroundings, and recited the following mindfulness meditation by Thich Nhat Hanh (1991) each time he got into the front seat of his car:

> Before starting the car;
> I know where I am going;
> The car and I are one
> If the car goes fast, I go fast.

Mindful Consuming

Mindful consuming refers to being aware of everything that we take into our bodies, in addition to the obvious of eating and drinking, but also the consumption of media, books, video games, magazines, movies, television programs, and websites (Nhat Hanh, 1993; Nhat Hanh & Cheung, 2010). Mindful consuming involves a combination of multiple strengths, such as gratitude, appreciation of beauty, kindness, self-regulation, and perspective, to name a few (Niemiec et al., 2012). Consumption is a normal part of living in society, and, as such, is subject to patterns of mindlessness and autopilot. Without much thought, we can forgo self-regulation and prudence and gorge ourselves at a dinner buffet or curiosity can take over as we flip television channels watching various programs when we should be working or completing a household chore. The excesses of materialism and consumerism relate inversely to

many areas of our well-being (Sirgy, 1998), while mindfulness seems to relate to less materialism and to a greater emphasis on our personal values. Adolescents and adults with higher well-being report more ecologically responsible behavior (Brown & Kasser, 2005), which together relate to higher trait mindfulness and an orientation toward values. Mindful consumption parallels approaches in simple living (e.g., one approach is called voluntary simplicity; Elgin, 1993), involving a way of life that emphasizes downshifting from heavy consumerism and materialism toward a lifestyle that is self-sufficient, balanced, and ecologically friendly.

Research has consistently found that improvements in the self-regulation of one area (e.g., exercise, eating, financial management, posture control) improves the general capacity to self-regulate thus impacting the other areas of self-regulatory functioning (Baumeister et al., 2006). This means that potentially improving one area, such as mindful eating, can automatically lead to improvements in other self-regulation activities, such as becoming stronger in having an exercise routine, more mindful financial management, more mindful shopping behaviors, and so forth. Further research is needed to flesh out the complex role of various mindful activities in relation to this important character strength capacity. It is interesting to explore how mindfulness can assist in monitoring and managing consumer behaviors. The mindful consumption of movies, i.e., the selection and viewing of positive psychology movies that might be used to inspire character strengths, positivity, and meaning in viewers has been discussed at length (Niemiec & Wedding, 2014).The use of specific character strength exercises to promote healthy, mindful consuming is a subject explored later in this chapter.

Managing Obstacles

One of the biggest challenges of mindfulness practices, such as formal meditation, is the management of obstacles that emerge during and around the practice. Countless individuals who embark on meditation retreats, attend classes, or begin meditation on their own give up fairly quickly because of frustrations, difficulty managing their mind, physical discomfort, apathy, and a number of other hurdles their body-mind presents them. This can be compounded in that mindfulness programs are not always explicit about teaching behavioral changes unless such changes are needed in order to maintain a mindfulness practice (Baer & Lykins, 2011).

This topic of dealing with obstacles is so important that it is the focus of Session 2 of MBCT (Segal et al., 2002) and of Session 3 of MBSP, discussed in Chapter 9. There are a number of character strengths that can be deployed to address barriers and consequently build and maintain a strong practice (Niemiec et al., 2012).

The most common obstacles to mindfulness practice noted by participants in MBSP are mind wandering, forgetting to practice, and being too busy to practice. Additional common barriers noted in mindfulness programs include boredom, physical discomfort, and distraction with sounds. In many cases, one or more of these obstacles can lead to the individual feeling discouraged or disinterested and consequently giving up the practice. I will review several of these obstacles and discuss the potential for character strengths use with each.

When individuals face barriers and problems during meditation, mindfulness teachers typically normalize the experience and encourage the individual to stick with it and to try to see things clearly. This is good advice and can help individuals transcend obstacles; however, for many this is not enough, too vague, or too difficult. Individuals pursue meditation often with false hopes and unrealistic expectations for a quick fix, immediate enlightenment, or a swift pathway to inner peace. While there is no shortcut, the integration of character strengths into mindfulness practice can help individuals transcend obstacles more quickly. This can amount to a "mini success" that then becomes empowering. Character strengths offer more clarity to what the individual is trying to reach; they are a label of insight that can be just the clarity a meditator needs to move forward or transcend an obstacle. Consider the person who realizes they are underusing their strength of perseverance with their persistently wandering mind, or the person who realizes they are overusing curiosity and love of learning by getting lost in every new thought or idea their mind comes up with. Such labels can serve as the catalyst for shifting to a more balanced mindfulness practice.

In this way, character strengths may act as a "supercharger," sometimes helping individuals leap over stubborn obstacles that have long been troubling. They expedite one's focus on the present moment. Such exact language brings the meditator to the point at hand, offering more substance than a phrase such as "keep going," "just try," "just do it," or "let's manage this better." While these phrases are positive, they may lead individuals to eventual helplessness if progress is not made. Instead, these phrases can be shifted to strength-based language which, when focused on, may become a positive, unplanned outcome (e.g., focusing on kindness happened to lead to an outcome of greater altruism). In addition, character strengths are qualities that naturally reside in the meditator so it is often a matter of simply turning one's attention to them. MBSP participants remind themselves to "use a signature strength," "find bravery at this painful moment," and "use perseverance despite feeling fatigued." Practitioners offering advice along these lines emphasize "your" since these are capacities the client already has, e.g., "use your creativity to consider a new way to handle that obstacle."

What follows are common obstacles to mindfulness practices and recommendations about ways to use character strengths to overcome or better manage them. Note that individuals always need to reconcile whether it's best to deploy one's signature strength(s) or to use a specifically recommended strength (e.g., perseverance) to respond to a given obstacle. The argument for signature strengths, regardless of which of the 24 the individual is highest in, is that these are the most energizing and easy for the individual to deploy; the argument for tapping a specific character strength in which the individual might be low in (e.g., bravery to deal with a difficult emotion) is that consciously targeting a strength offers an efficient, direct pathway. Many of these obstacles are linked with one another and have some conceptual overlap, but they are nevertheless pulled apart to offer a wider array of examples pertaining to strong mindfulness.

Mind Wandering

No doubt the most common obstacle individuals encounter is mind wandering. Mind wandering can be particularly frustrating because it is very frequent and pervasive during mindfulness practice, among both new and established meditators. In addition, research has found that people are less happy when their mind wanders (Killingsworth & Gilbert, 2010). The advantage more experienced meditators have is the insight, acquired over time and with repeated practice, that mind wandering truly is normal, natural, and not a sign of failed mindfulness. Experienced meditators draw on this wisdom to persevere with self-kindness despite wandering attention. This is an important obstacle to address directly because some individuals may begin to associate mindfulness with mind wandering which sets up a negative reinforcement cycle and discourages people from practicing (Niemiec et al., 2012).

When I've presented on the integration of mindfulness and character strengths in Asian countries where meditation is more commonplace, there is a similar reaction to mind wandering. The individuals explain that they experienced a disarray of thoughts and that some of the time they hadn't been aware that the mind was away from the present moment. Then, over time, individuals settle in and at least catch their mind wandering a bit more efficiently, allowing them to focus on the task at hand, which in this case, was to zero in on one of their character strengths. The same dynamic occurs in the West. Mind wandering is not an Eastern or Western phenomenon, it is a human phenomenon. One of the key reminders, especially for those newer to mindfulness, is to normalize the experiences of the wandering mind.

Meditators typically spend more time focusing on what's wrong (e.g., "My mind keeps wandering off") rather than focusing on what's right (e.g., "I continue to bring my mind back to the

Table 4.2
Character Strengths and Mind Wandering

Perspective	Each time one becomes aware that the mind has trailed off, this can be described as a success because it's another instance of mindful awareness.
Curiosity	Becoming fascinated about the nature of the mind and how automatic and mysterious the process of mind wandering is.
Love of learning	Making note and registering the content of where the mind is going off to. Certain themes or ideas that are repeated might be fodder for deeper learning and investigation following a meditation period.
Perseverance	Seeing mind wandering as an "opportunity" for growth. Pushing oneself onward in mindfulness practice, repeatedly moving beyond the obstacles that emerge.
Hope	Keeping a positive outlook no matter how intense the mind wandering becomes during a particular session. One might remind oneself that mind wandering is not a "permanent" state.
Kindness	Approaching oneself with gentleness and care, allowing frustration to soften with self-compassion.
Humility	Noting that mind wandering will occur and that there's no such thing as total mind control. Thus, one might view one's mind from a stance of humbleness and awe.
Self-regulation	Reminding oneself that each time one uses self-control to bring attention to the breath that one is strengthening the "muscle" of self-regulation.

present moment"). This emphasis on errors dampens motivation. Eventually, many meditators give up out of frustration. It is more productive to build on the successes and what is going right.

Because mind wandering is so pervasive, it can take multiple character strengths to manage it. See Table 4.2 for examples of several character strengths and the role they may play in handling the obstacle of mind wandering, either alone or, more likely, in combination with one another.

Forgetting to Practice

Forgetting to practice mindfulness can sometimes be a symptom of another obstacle (e.g., the real issue is a lack of motivation or perhaps a lack of understanding why one would want to practice). When forgetfulness is the real issue, then the use of prudence – being planful, setting short-term goals, being conscientious to follow through with plans – is likely to be helpful. Making a list of answers to the question, "Why practice mindfulness?" and posting it in a prominent place is another prudent strategy.

Not Enough Time/Too Busy

> You should sit in meditation for 20 minutes a day, unless you're too busy; then you should sit for an hour.
>
> Old Zen saying

The busy-ness of life is a reality every person must face. It is important to remember, however, that not only are our bodies busy doing many activities, our minds are experiencing the busy-ness as well. This elevates the stress that we take on and can lead us to feel unfocused and unsettled. Thus, our minds and bodies need time to be present, to focus on breathing, to focus on "just one thing."

Brief mindfulness meditations offer a starting point that many busy individuals find reasonable. Brief meditations are receiving increasing attention in research studies. One brief mindfulness exercise discussed in several places in this book is the 3-minute breathing space practiced in MBCT (Segal et al., 2002), referred to as the character strengths breathing space in MBSP. The brevity of this exercise is appealing to those newer to mind-

fulness and those who frequently report the "not enough time" obstacle. The practice of this exercise with regularity can develop into a good practice habit that is later expanded upon and adjusted.

While prudence is a crucial strength that is employed when planning and structuring one's days or weeks, prudence can also come in the form of simply being realistic about what is possible with what one has going on in one's life. Practitioners, too, must work with where the client is at. When I lived in New York in 2000, I recall many mornings in which I simply did three minutes of meditation before going to work. I sat down in a sacred space in my apartment and practiced mindful breathing and letting go. Even though many of these meditation periods were only one to three-minutes long, it "felt" to me as if this had a big impact on my day. I judged this by examining Mondays when I had to attend a difficult, all-day meeting filled with individuals who were quick to criticize and berate those who expressed a difference of opinion. These were difficult days; however, over the months I noticed a difference in finding greater joy and peace with those who were more critical and I felt a deeper acceptance of my limitations on those days in which I kept my commitment to mindfulness practice (regardless of the time length) as compared to those days when I omitted mindfulness altogether.

A similar story occurred in my work with a middle-aged man who was suffering immensely with unique physical symptoms (spontaneous vomiting) and body pain. He had medical and psychological evaluations from the most prominent institutions in the United States (e.g., Mayo Clinic; Cleveland Clinic). No cause or successful medical treatment was determined. The one approach that he found successful, however, was any form of self-regulation practice. In our therapy sessions, I taught him medical hypnosis, mindfulness, and relaxation, all geared to assisting in his symptoms and to helping him make the most of his very full life. He found significant success working in my office but for several weeks he refused to practice any self-regulation strategy at home. Rather than continue to push him to listen to the 20-minute recordings we made or the 30-minute CDs he had purchased, I shifted to work with him where he was at: "Is there any amount of time you'd be willing to agree to practice this week?" He thought for a moment and said: "Yes, I'd be willing to meditate in my basement apart from my family for two minutes. But not two minutes per day, just two minutes this week." Knowing the tiny fraction of time 2 minutes is out of a possible 10,080 minutes in a week, I nevertheless was pleased that he had shifted from "not enough time" to "I am willing to make time." "Great, go for it," I said. He returned one month later and had indeed done two, and only two minutes. He felt good about his commitment. Each month he slowly upped the quantity, eventually getting it to a comfortable daily practice. In order to combat this obstacle of resistance and client time constraints I had to use self-regulation to balance any expectations or impulses I had of wanting my client to do more quantity of practice. He, too, had to enlist a number of character strengths such as bravery, perseverance, self-honesty (about the importance of the practice), self-regulation, and prudence in order to overcome the obstacle.

Troubling Thoughts

In addition to a general running commentary of autopilot thinking, another barrier of thinking nests within or alongside this commentary – that of negative self-talk. Having a harsh inner critic is exceedingly common. In addition, individuals may have morbid thoughts, distressing thoughts, condemning thoughts, and various thoughts that attack oneself and others. The thoughts can also be directed to one's meditation practice, e.g., "I knew I was a nonmeditator," "Mindfulness is not for me," "I can't do this, I'm no good at it," and "I don't know what I'm doing when I'm sitting here." A vast majority of these thoughts are those that individuals do not want to "own" or identify with. The important aspect of mindfulness, namely the decentering aspect, is the teaching that one does not own one's thoughts, that thoughts are not facts, and that thoughts are best viewed as mental events that can be observed as passing through the mind rather than as descriptors of one's character (Segal et al., 2002; Teasdale, 1999).

Such teaching helps generate the character strength of perspective, which involves having self-knowledge, understanding larger patterns of meaning, and taking the wider view of situations. This approach of dis-identifying with the thinking can elicit other character strengths such as humility, humor, and love, in which one does not have to take oneself so seriously. Turning a typical other-oriented strength such as forgiveness, love, or fairness toward oneself is another way to take a wider, meta-view with one's thinking. This might involve being fair with oneself by challenging unfair, harsh, or unwarranted thoughts that attempt to recycle; using self-forgiveness to let go of pressures involving high expectations; and offering loving-kindness to oneself even when one's thoughts say that one does not deserve love. Take another look at the circumplex diagram in Figure 2.2 in Chapter 2, which outlines strengths of the heart, mind, interpersonal, and intrapersonal and allow this to give you additional ideas in applying strengths in different ways.

Discomfort

Discomfort comes in many forms but the two most commonly discussed types are physical and emotional. Who wants to face discomfort and pain? It's a natural human tendency to pursue what gives us pleasure and to avoid what causes pain. Thus, mindfulness is often the exact opposite of not only what individuals commonly do but also is distinct from many traditional Western approaches that treat suffering by attempting to numb it. This is because core to the practice of mindfulness is nonavoidance – facing discomfort, ailments, and suffering directly. This rallying call to our inner strength of bravery is one of the most challenging aspects of mindfulness. Clients who work with and work through discomfort are demonstrating psychological courage (Putman, 1997), and it is frequently beneficial to label such strength in the client. One of my chronic pain clients framed his use of mindfulness and bravery as "finding the peace within my body's sensations." Kabat-Zinn (1990) often refers to mindfulness for pain management as learning to work with the sensations and to work around the edges of the pain.

An approach of acceptance – also referred to as allowing and letting be – stands in stark contrast to the natural human inclination to want to fight off or control pain and other displeasures. Christopher Germer (2009, p. 28), a prominent self-compassion teacher, explains that acceptance is a process that involves several, not-necessarily-linear, stages:

1. Aversion – resistance, avoidance, rumination
2. Curiosity – turning toward discomfort with interest
3. Tolerance – safely enduring
4. Allowing – letting feelings come and go
5. Friendship – embracing, seeing hidden value

Survivors of trauma who practice meditation are likely to face a number of challenging obstacles relating to emotional discomfort and troubling thoughts, especially when memories of the trauma emerge during practice. A large constellation of character strengths (the individual's signature strengths and other strengths) will be necessary to help the individual "ground" themselves in the present moment, bravely face their challenges, gain perspective to see the bigger picture, and offer self-kindness. With one client who had experienced several horrifying traumas, we began the mindfulness practices with the "mountain meditation" described by Kabat-Zinn (1994). This practice involved helping her ground herself in the present moment by embodying the sturdy and solid qualities of a mountain that was unfettered by the natural elements. Thus, she was taking on a posture, belief, and image of "strength" from the onset while using her self-regulation to anchor her attention to her breathing and to her mountain image.

Fatigue and lowered energy is another form of discomfort and certainly can become a significant obstacle to mindfulness practice. The calling forth of one's zest and enthusiasm becomes crucial, even if the amount brought forth is small. Zest corresponds closely to the Buddhist concept of *viriya*, which can be translated as energy or enthusiasm (Kuan, 2008). Mindfulness involves striking a balance with one's energy effort – to avoid overdoing and underdoing – each of which can be an Achilles' heel to pain, fatigue, and various medical conditions. When the individual becomes aware that tiredness or lethargy are emerging, greater enthusiasm is needed in one's practice; similarly, in contemplative traditions, zest is applied to avoid the state of lethargy and apathy called *acedia* (Norris, 2008).

Lack of Motivation

Individuals can quickly learn how to meditate, but it's the internal factor of motivation – the "wanting" to practice – that makes the difference in terms of sustaining a practice. Even though an individual might highly value meditation, sometimes practicing it is the last thing they want to do.

In his lectures, meditation teacher Ajahn Brahm (e.g., Brahm, 2006) offers a poignant example of how fear can serve as a powerful motivator, especially motivation toward shifting into deeper states of meditation. He recalls walking barefoot in the jungles of Thailand at night and trying hard not to step on a snake. With every step, his mindfulness was razor sharp, driven by a fear of not getting bitten. In another story he describes waking up from sleep to discover a very poisonous, large centipede on his chest (i.e., a species that causes excruciating pain for several hours to those who are unfortunate enough to be bitten by one). Brahm explains that these fear examples led him to very deep meditation later that evening or day because the mind was hyper-aware and very focused. The emotion of fear becomes a powerful driving force that can push through internal obstacles of mindlessness and help the meditator become focused after they are already on the cushion. Other somewhat dramatic examples can jolt us into awareness and motivate us into deeper meditation. Chapter 1 reviews several of these moments of mindfulness, such as mystical experiences, weddings, funerals, and rites of passage.

These events and fear-based experiences are not always at our beck-and-call to help motivate us to get to the cushion or to go deeper when we are already practicing. However, motivation to reach one of our signature strengths – to allow our mind to be with what is best in us – can serve as a motivator at any time of need. Our character strengths can be that major source of motivation. Individuals avoiding the practice who are aware of the benefits of meditation might be drawn to practice as a means to improve one of their strengths. Thus, they can view mindfulness as an opportunity to engage one of their signature strengths. For example, a person high in creativity may be drawn to sit in the quiet and watch the various new ideas that pop up in their mind, while the individual high in spirituality may be drawn to the creation of a sacred space where they can "just be." Like fear, the potent energy of signature strengths can be a motivating factor in one's practice.

Sounds as Distractions

Sometimes, when practicing mindfulness, the mind focuses in on a sound, and it is difficult to let it go. Managing sounds can present as a particularly vexing issue for individuals. General recommendations are to use the sound as a "bell" of mindfulness that helps one tune in closely to the present moment; similarly, mindfulness teachers often advise individuals to allow the sound(s) to become part of one's present moment experience – to take notice of sounds but to give equal weight to noticing other stimuli in one's environment. The latter concept relates to the use of the strength of fairness in that the meditator should not give extra attention to any one stimulus, but instead to take notice of what is emerging in the environment, let it go, and attend to what else is emerging.

In my mindfulness community, an issue emerged when some members were repeatedly arriving late to the weekly meditation gathering. This began to cause a problem for certain members who were already sitting quietly and peacefully and felt the sound reverberations from the newcomers settling in were a significant disruption to the community energy. A discussion and exchange of ideas emerged for handling the situation:

- One person exercised the strength of prudence offering an idea to set up chairs in a different area of the building so that latecomers could sit and meditate and when there was a transition, could then join in the group.
- Another person used kindness and creativity by encouraging all members to be more perseverant with their timeliness and offered to play a recording of a meditation chant to start off the event, allowing individuals to deepen their meditation and the latecomers to settle in and not disturb the others.
- A third person used the strengths of judgment (looking at the situation from different angles) and perspective (seeing the bigger picture).

They offered the following points of wisdom to individuals already meditating to help them personally manage the obstacle of sounds:

- When we hear a noise, we can notice the sound without attempting to label it. We can let the sound pass through us and not stop at the interpretation level of our minds. Might we look deeply? We can be aware of our reaction to the sound we have labeled as a person enters the meditation space. What is our direct experience? Is there judgment? Annoyance? Criticism? Anxiety? Is there aversion and/or a sense that "this should not be happening"? Or is there excitement and curiosity about who might be joining the group, or relief that it wasn't you arriving after the bell? We can note "liking" and "disliking" and the desire to "peek."
- Does my reaction to having my peace disturbed create more peace?
- We can note our body's reaction at the level of sensations. Are we tight in the chest, clenching our jaws, butterflies in our stomach? We can note what stories we are making up about why the community member is arriving late. Might we link our desire and craving to have our meditation time a certain way as a cause of our suffering? Might we see how our monkey mind has taken us away from the present moment?

All three responses are equally valid and show the breadth of ways that character strengths might be catalyzed in such situations of distraction and irritation.

The Conditions Aren't Right

Like the challenge to accept sounds that occur during meditation, there can be other "conditions" of the present moment that one does not want to accept (e.g., the environment is too hot or cold). When one of my mindful eating groups was preparing to eat lunch by first practicing mindful breathing and attending to hunger cues, one client, James, became frustrated. He claimed that he was unable to eat or enjoy his food if it was not piping hot. James' mind was so focused on having to eat his food in a certain way (one specific condition) that he lost complete touch with his body, his hunger cues, and why he was in the group in the first place!

Accepting the realities of the present moment means there must be a good deal of letting go (i.e., forgiveness) of what does not appear right or correct. After all, meditation is about letting go, not trying to get more or keep things the same. Individuals can exert prudence and plan for a particular situation as much as possible but ultimately must also be humble to what other people and the situation might present.

Final Comment

When I reflect on handling obstacles with strength, I naturally reflect on those people who gracefully handle perhaps the greatest of all life obstacles – death and dying.

I think of my supervisor, friend, and mentor from many years ago, the late Dr. Bob Wilke, who was dying of a brain tumor and asked me to work with him on mindfulness through his dying process. It was one of the things I was most privileged to do in my life, especially considering he knew at least 10-times more about meditation and related fields than I did. Each time we got together, I, the student, had become the teacher, and I reviewed mindful breathing, loving-kindness meditation, and other mindfulness and strengths practices. He attempted to be aware of and let go of distressing thoughts about dying or the doctors who couldn't do enough amidst numerous other thoughts and feelings relating to gratitude, love, wisdom, and care. He named some of these from moment to moment as he slowly began to lose touch with the present moment and his memory became more and more affected as the days went on. Yet, in this extreme situation of a tumor tearing through his brain, he continued to deploy a sense of fairness, kindness, humility, and most of all, love, to himself, to me, to his family, and to others.

For reflection: Who in your life faced the reality of their death with grace and mindfulness? What character strengths were part of the process?

Setting the Stage for Mindful Living[2]

My actions are my only true belongings.
Thich Nhat Hanh

A strong mindfulness is not only one that uses strengths to overcome obstacles in mindfulness practice and one that adds support to activities of daily living (e.g., mindful driving), but also one that uses strengths to directly enhance mindful living. The best way to envision the well-worn phrase, mindful living, is through the lens of principles or trainings in mindful living. This can be found in the Five Mindfulness Trainings of the humble and influential monk Thich Nhat Hanh (referred to by his students as "Thay," which is Vietnamese for "teacher"). With over 100 books and a Nobel Peace Prize nomination to his credit, Thay's work has been instrumental in the fields of mindful living, meditation, spirituality, health, violence management, and peace, to Buddhists and nonBuddhists alike. The wisdom and applicability of his teachings may lead practitioners and researchers in positive psychology to think of Thay as a close colleague. It is only a matter of time before each of his teachings will have scientific support, in addition to their wide applicability. Here are a few examples of some of the core themes of Thay's teachings that align closely with positive psychology and character strengths. These themes lay the groundwork for the discussion of the Five Mindfulness Trainings and strengths interventions which follows.

Internal Conditions for Happiness

Individual well-being relies more upon internal conditions such as compassion, joy, and the pursuit of community, positive relationships, and

---

[2] Portions of this section come from Niemiec (2012), published in the *International Journal of Well-Being*, which appears in the references, and is the original source. I am grateful to the journal's editor, Aaron Jarden, who not only championed the publication of the article but who graciously allows authors to retain copyright.

personal growth than external conditions such as money, status, and image. As Thich Nhat Hanh (2009) has often noted, we already have more than enough conditions to be happy. He is referring to those internal conditions that we can turn to within ourselves in any present moment. This is consistent with cognitive-behavior therapy research, mindfulness-based interventions, and happiness research findings that there are better outcomes for intrinsic goals (e.g., I want to have a closer relationship with my spouse) over extrinsic goals (e.g., I want to make more money) (Kasser, 2006). Character strengths can be viewed as many of those important "internal conditions" that are already present in everyone and that are pivotal for setting intrinsic-oriented goals.

The Middle Way

Echoing the Buddha, who spoke of practicing "the Way," Thich Nhat Hanh (1998) emphasizes the application of diligence among extremes such as those of austerity and sensual pleasure, and emphasizes finding balance in one's practice of the Five Mindfulness Trainings rather than forcing oneself to be "perfect" or rigid in the application. Similarly, Aristotle (2000) articulated this as the "golden mean," the balance between excess and deficiency in one's life activities in working, learning, playing, loving, and serving; this balance then leads to the ultimate goal of personal happiness. In strengths psychology, this can be referred to as finding a balance between overuse and underuse of character strengths (Biswas-Diener et al., 2011; Grant & Schwartz, 2011; Linley, 2008), e.g., for bravery, the middle way is the balance between recklessness and cowardice, while for curiosity, it is the balance between nosiness and lack of interest.

Watering the Seeds

All 24 character strengths matter. This important principle emphasizes how each strength is a capacity in individuals that can be developed with practice. Thich Nhat Hanh (1998) describes the practice of "watering the seeds" of virtue and those wholesome, interior elements rather than

unwholesome seeds of suffering and violence (e.g., watering kindness rather than anger). This is likened to the nourishing of any of the 24 character strengths' "seeds" through deliberate intervention and mindful care. While all strengths matter, it might be that "watering" one's highest strengths elicits the greatest benefit. Research on signature strengths – those most authentic, natural, and energizing to the person – has revealed a strong connection with happiness (e.g., Gander et al., 2012a; Madden et al., 2011; Mitchell et al., 2009; Mongrain & Anselmo-Matthews, 2012; Peterson & Peterson, 2008; Rust et al., 2009; Seligman et al., 2005).

Interbeing

Thich Nhat Hanh (1998) offers the word "interbeing" to refer to the mutual relationship and interconnection of things. Also described as "interdependent co-arising," this teaching describes how causes and effects co-arise and

> [...] everything is a result of multiple causes and conditions. The egg is in the chicken, and the chicken is in the egg. Chicken and egg arise in mutual dependence. Neither is independent. (Nhat Hanh, 1998, p. 221)

Thay also offers the example of how we can gaze at a tree and see how a cloud, the rain, and the soil are part of the tree, because without the cloud, rain, and soil, there wouldn't be a tree to grow. Thus, there is interbeing among these elements. This teaching can be applied to the 24 character strengths in that all of the character strengths are linked with one another; the strengths do not function in isolation nor are the strengths independent of one another – the expression of one of these virtuous qualities likely affects the others to some degree. For example, when a person is offering deep forgiveness to another, they are also expressing perspective, bravery, kindness, spirituality, humility, and so forth. Scientists have performed intercorrelation matrices on the VIA character strengths and naturally each strength positively correlates to some degree with the others (there are no negative correlations among the 24). When focusing on a character strength in order to practice a mindfulness training, it is likely other character strengths are deployed and impacted.

Mindful Living With the Five Mindfulness Trainings

One of Thay's most popular teachings is the Five Mindfulness Trainings, which are a modern-day re-formulation of some of the Buddha's core messages. The Five Mindfulness Trainings are Reverence for Life, True Happiness, True Love, Loving Speech and Deep Listening, and Nourishment and Healing (Nhat Hanh, 1993; Nhat Hanh & Cheung, 2010). These provide pathways to a life of greater joy, engagement, better relationships, and meaning. Indeed, these are not only a recipe for mindful living but present a striking vision for a global ethic. The potential impact of the trainings on individuals, relationships, and society is significant. Consider a world in which more people, groups, and organizations bring careful intentionality to what they are doing, listen to one another with more compassion, and reflect more deeply on the impact of healthy and unhealthy choices on oneself and on others. For a full commentary on an earlier version of the trainings, see Nhat Hanh (1993), or for the most recent revision of the trainings discussed in this section, see Nhat Hanh & Cheung (2010) or go to www.plumvillage.org/mindfulness-trainings/3-the-five-mindfulness-trainings.html.

In the original work describing the VIA Classification, Peterson and Seligman (2004) describe an immediate connection between character strengths and the Five Mindfulness Trainings. They suggest that the first (Reverence for Life), second (True Happiness), and fourth (Loving Speech and Deep Listening) mindfulness trainings connect closely with the humanity and justice strengths, and that the third (True Love) and fifth (Nourishment and Healing) mindfulness trainings connect closely with the temperance and courage strengths. What follows is an attempt to take this connection a couple levels deeper.

Thich Nhat Hanh makes it clear that each of the Five Mindfulness Trainings are ideas to work toward (i.e., trainings) rather than final ideals to achieve or commandments one must or should follow. He offers an apt metaphor of the North Star, which can help to guide or direct individuals in a particular direction though one can never make it to the destination. The individual variance for how a person might go about the journey of practicing each training is significant. Some individuals take a formal, systematic approach, delving into the trainings one-by-one in their personal study or through study with their mindfulness community, while others approach the trainings more informally, focusing on where their particular needs and interests are at present.

But, what are the mechanisms that make the journey with the mindfulness trainings possible? What ingredients in ourselves can we turn to in order to manifest mindfulness and the Five Mindfulness Trainings more strongly? One answer lies in our strengths of character. I will draw some important connections between character strengths and the mindfulness trainings and offer practical suggestions that will help deepen the understanding and practice of mindfulness.

After a person becomes more aware of their character strengths, how might they use them to deepen their experience of the Five Mindfulness Trainings? Here are some practical ways that character strengths might impact, inform, and enhance one's use of each mindfulness training. An attempt is made to offer science-based suggestions, but each should be viewed as a preliminary idea that warrants further scientific inquiry, especially in terms of its potential impact on the mindfulness training; each intervention is offered to help encourage and support the mindfulness practice of individuals and communities.

Mindfulness Training #1: Reverence for Life

The first mindfulness training, *Reverence for Life*, begins:

> Aware of the suffering caused by the destruction of life, I am committed to cultivating the insight of interbeing and compassion and to learning ways to protect the lives of people, animals, plants and minerals (Nhat Hanh & Cheung, 2010, p. 210).

This training also encourages the cultivation of openness, nondiscrimination, and nonattachment to views. It directly invites individuals to increase their kindness/compassion strength to a level that moves the focus on oneself to a focus on others, namely all living beings. The strength of fairness appears to be an underlying principle for this training. Those high in this character strength navigate their lives through principles of equity and justice for all. Such an approach is the basis for a healthy, global community, which this mindfulness training emphasizes.

> **Practice Tip: Use Strengths to Support the First Mindfulness Training**
> - When one finds oneself gravitating toward dualistic or exclusiveness in thinking, call upon the judgment/critical thinking strength to consider multiple viewpoints (Tetlock, 1986). Combining this with the fairness strength can help one see all sides of an issue, and to find a sense of balance and a common middle ground.
> - Use the bravery strength to speak against acts of killing in the world, even those that appear benign, such as deliberately stepping on a spider on the sidewalk. To mindlessly "squash" any form of life is to subtly rehearse a cognitive and behavior routine of apathy and disregard for living beings.
> - Build the appreciation of beauty strength by training oneself to see beauty wherever one looks; keep a "beauty log" in which one regularly writes about the wonders of the life and beauty of plants, animals, and even the moral acts of beauty witnessed in others (Diessner et al., 2006).

Mindfulness Training #2: True Happiness

The second mindfulness training, *True Happiness*, begins:

> Aware of the suffering caused by exploitation, social injustice, stealing, and oppression, I am committed to practicing generosity in my thinking, speaking, and acting (Nhat Hanh & Cheung, 2010, p. 210).

This training also encourages the individual to see a connection between one's own happiness and suffering, and the happiness and suffering of others. It emphasizes a focus on generosity and understanding, with less of a focus on external conditions that are superficial in nature, such as fame, wealth, and material possessions. While the thrust of this training speaks against obvious,

anti-societal behaviors such as stealing, oppression or exploitation of the less fortunate, there are subtle examples of this training to examine. For example, people can *steal* someone's idea by not giving due credit, upstage someone at a business meeting ("stealing someone's thunder"), or steal someone's time by monopolizing a conversation. The impact of inaction – not helping those in real need and those being oppressed in society – deserves deep contemplation in the context of this training.

> **Practice Tip: Use Strengths to Support the Second Mindfulness Training**
> - The simplest answer is: Give. Giving, being generous, and volunteering are core components of the kindness character strength, and when expressed, have a positive impact on both the giver and the receiver (Luks, 1991; Post, 2005).
> - Be grateful. The research surrounding the benefits of expressing the strength of gratitude is mounting. Research shows that people who are grateful are often more communal, altruistic, happy, and less materialistic. Gratitude also engenders a deep sense of appreciation for what one already has in life (Emmons & McCullough, 2003; Seligman et al., 2005).
> - Teamwork and leadership: There are important benefits to taking a "we" approach as to an "I" approach (Son, Jackson, Grove, & Feltz, 2011), and indeed these two justice-oriented, civic strengths focus on what is best for the larger group. One can consider how these play a role on a small scale with a small project in one's life, and then shift the focus to a wider audience.

Mindfulness Training #3: True Love

The third mindfulness training, *True Love*, begins:

> Aware of the suffering caused by sexual misconduct, I am committed to cultivating responsibility and learning ways to protect the safety and integrity of individuals, couples, families, and society – cultivating loving kindness, compassion, joy and inclusiveness – which are the four basic elements of true love (Nhat Hanh & Cheung, 2010, p. 211).

This training calls for a mindful sexuality and a strong degree of commitment in our relationships. Another aspect of this training involves protecting children from sexual abuse and whenever possible keeping the institution of "family" together. Here, it is the perspective/wisdom strength that needs to be called forth to allow for the wider view of life and what is truly important. This involves calling forth both strengths of the heart and strengths of the mind in order to overcome desire, cravings, and drives that can lead to rash choices, superficial outcomes, and destruction of relationships.

Practice Tip: Use Strengths to Support the Third Mindfulness Training

- Build the strength of prudence. Prudence, sometimes called "cautious wisdom," is an important strength to use when it comes to sexual desire. If one is uncertain about a relationship, one should use prudence to conduct a cost-benefit analysis. What are the costs and benefits of the action that is about to be taken? What are the costs and benefits of not taking the action? (Rollnick & Miller, 1995). In addition, one might use one's heart-oriented strengths (e.g., curiosity) by asking for others' feedback about one's relationship partner and listening closely without judgment to the feedback.
- When in doubt, a general guideline is to be honest and authentic in all relationships. Integrity involves allowing who one is at the core to be aligned with what one expresses to others at work, home, and socially. This strength of honesty/integrity usually requires the strength of bravery (being brave enough to share who one is) to face any sexual improprieties in one's life (past or current), and/or to speak against any sexual misbehaviors witnessed against children, adolescents, or adults.
- Combat mindlessness with perspective and social intelligence. It's easy to fall into autopilot in our relationships (Segal et al., 2002) with close others; therefore, it is important to periodically check in on ourselves with questions such as: How

might I commit more to my relationships? Is there anything I've been avoiding with anyone? Applying these ideas requires attending to the "golden mean" of strengths and virtues – using strengths at the right time, to the right degree, in the right situation. This requires a bigger picture perspective and the social intelligence strength – being aware of one's own feelings, others' feelings, and the social nuances of the context one is in (Schwartz & Sharpe, 2006).
- Embed a loving-kindness meditation into one's meditation or mindful living. Involving imaging, loving statements, and positive reminiscing, loving-kindness practice expands love and improves health on an individual level (Cohn & Fredrickson, 2010; Salzberg, 1995), but it is likely there are further benefits extending to the fostering of healthy relationships.

Mindfulness Training #4: Loving Speech and Deep Listening

The fourth mindfulness training, *Loving Speech and Deep Listening*, begins:

Aware of the suffering caused by unmindful speech and the inability to listen to others, I am committed to cultivating loving speech and compassionate listening in order to relieve suffering and to promote reconciliation and peace (Nhat Hanh & Cheung, 2010, p. 211).

This training invites a focus upon the practice of mindful speech and deep listening. No doubt compassion/kindness is a core strength used in these practices. Curiosity is also important as research has found that being curious in social relationships can lead to stronger, more intimate relationships than those who do not take an open, curious approach (Kashdan, McKnight, Fincham, & Rose, 2011).

Practice Tip: Use Strengths to Support the Fourth Mindfulness Training

- Learn to offer active-constructive responses when someone shares good news. This involves a mix of the strengths of love (providing warmth and genuineness in the response), social intelligence (detecting the person is sharing something that's important to them), and humility and self-regulation (to not have to share your good news too but to help the person who is sharing to savor the moment). Research has shown this type of responding is important for successful relationships and it is likely to improve mindful speech and deep listening (Gable, Reis, Impett, & Asher, 2004; Reis et al., 2010).

- Learn to empathize when someone shares bad news or appears to be suffering (Batson, Chang, Orr, & Rowland, 2002). Listen with eyes and ears of compassion: What might they be feeling? As one takes notice of what the other person is feeling, can their emotions be felt as well? If so, one can share this. Compassion is to suffer with and to be with the person; it is a type of kindness strength that can be offered to loved ones. While listening, one might ask oneself, "Where is the person coming from? What are they saying or trying to say? What is the essence or core message that they are expressing?" For example, a woman yelling at her husband for being late for a dinner date might be feeling – at her core – disrespected and unloved.

- Practice forgiveness when someone close causes one harm. This does not mean forgetting their actions, nor condoning what they have done, but letting go of one's own suffering. Research reveals that writing about the personal benefits that have resulted from someone's harmful actions leads to greater forgiveness than writing about the trauma of the harmful act (McCullough et al., 2006). The strength of forgiveness is closely linked and impacted by the use of other-focussed compassion in which one listens deeply to the suffering of others and considers the humanity of the offender (Witvliet, DeYoung, Hofelich, & DeYoung, 2011; Witvliet, Knoll, Hinman, & DeYoung, 2010).

Mindfulness Training #5: Nourishment and Healing

The fifth mindfulness training, *Nourishment and Healing*, begins:

> Aware of the suffering caused by unmindful consumption, I am committed to cultivating good health, both physical and mental, for myself, my family, and my society by practicing mindful eating, drinking, and consuming (Nhat Hanh & Cheung, 2010, p. 212).

Consuming goes beyond food and drink to the consumption of websites, movies, television programs, video games, books, magazines, and conversations. This training is about taking care of one's whole self and being a mindful consumer. Core to this training are the strengths of self-regulation and prudence. Embedded in this mindfulness practice is the strength of perseverance, as the practice of not consuming alcohol or violent media images/messages is not just something to be done once or twice but is an ongoing practice requiring perseverance. This strength involves overcoming obstacles that emerge and reframing them as growth opportunities (Dweck, 2006).

Practice Tip: Use Strengths to Support the Fifth Mindfulness Training

- Self-monitor daily healthy and unhealthy eating and drinking habits. Create a detailed food and drink log. This self-regulation strategy is a key health habit. Interestingly, research has found that the regular practice and improvement of one behavior involving self-regulation improves other behaviors involving this strength. For example, improving one's self-regulation with food improves one's self-regulation in other areas, such as exercise, mindfulness, or even managing finances (see Baumeister et al., 2006).

- Track the nonedible products that one's consciousness consumes. Set a watch alarm to beep one time per hour; when it beeps, take notice of what one's consciousness is taking in – a television commercial, a radio program, a website, a video game, a personal conversation, a book, etc. Ask oneself: Is this product or experience right now having a positive or negative effect on my consciousness? What feelings and thoughts am I experiencing in the present moment in light of this current stimulus? This type of mindful consuming approach involves the use of many character strengths and can be applied to any form of media or art (e.g., Niemiec & Wedding, 2014).

• Set a health goal that is of personal value (Sheldon & Kasser, 1998). Make the goal something reasonable that one can commit to 100%, even when the going gets tough. The character strengths that appear to be most associated with goal-setting are hope, perseverance, and prudence. Be prudent to select a goal that is reasonable, be perseverant when the going gets tough, and generate hopeful thoughts about your ability to achieve the goal and to develop alternate pathways to get there.

Strategies for Building a Strong Mindfulness Practice

As a review, what follows are some practical suggestions for using character strengths to enhance mindfulness practices.

Allow Signature Strengths to Point the Way

With virtually any mindfulness practice, one can likely support one's practice or give it a boost by turning to one's highest signature strengths (Niemiec et al., 2012). If an individual has a signature strength of curiosity, they might take an approach of deliberately seeking novelty as they practice mindful sitting, driving, or eating. This will allow curiosity to peak. If kindness or love

is the person's signature strength, they can direct love or kindness inward as they practice the body scan or mindful yoga.

Use Character Strengths to Combat Obstacles

Those interested in maintaining any kind of mindfulness practice will encounter a myriad of obstacles that can distract or deter the practice. At one point or another, individuals will likely need to call upon perseverance to foster an energy of pushing through barriers, as well as the strength of bravery (whether it's a signature strength or not) to face discomfort and body tension directly. In some instances, the obstacle may be daunting and seemingly impossible (if not inappropriate) to face directly with mindfulness alone. However, when the individual faces the suffering with their own inner resources, the obstacle often appears more manageable.

Those interested in being systematic can take each of their top 5–7 character strengths and address them one at a time with a particular mindfulness barrier. You might flesh out these ideas in a journal or experiment with the practice in your mindfulness practice. See Table 4.2 earlier in this chapter for examples of how various strengths can be applied to managing mind wandering.

Use the Full Capacity of Character Strengths

When considering how character strengths can be used to combat obstacles of mindfulness practices, it is instructive to recall the definition of character strengths – capacities for thinking, feeling, and behaving in ways that benefit and support both self and others. Therefore, consider how any strength can be expressed in one's thinking, feeling, *and* behaving in relation to mindfulness. For example, behaving in a way that is zestful yet prudent might assist mindful walking; during sitting meditation, thinking of certain words such as perseverance and hope and considering perseverant and hopeful thoughts may serve as timely reminders for completing a meditation exercise; and tapping into the emotions of bravery and honesty to face challenges head on can often be what is needed to grow through difficult periods of meditation practice.

Identify and Label Character Strengths That Rise Up

When one is practicing mindfulness, the individual focuses on whatever is arising in the present moment in one's thinking, feelings, and actions. This material may often be character strengths-related. Individuals can therefore notice and label certain thoughts as kind or humble, or an emotion of hope or gratitude, or an idea for "prudent behavior" and file it away in their mind as an insight for potential future action. This act of labeling strengths in one's thinking and feeling may open up additional energy resources for mindfulness work. For example, it has been hypothesized that the act of forgiveness frees up additional resources, which could serve as extra energy that could be invested in mindfulness (Webb et al., 2012). There is a potential two-fold benefit in that one is letting go of the taxing nature of a grudge or revengeful feeling and on the other hand there is the naturally energizing experience of the character strength of forgiveness.

Consider the Causes of Good Meditation

What are the causes of your meditation when it goes well? We are quick to wonder about the causes of problems. When we receive a diagnosis, we want to know what caused it. When we have an argument with someone new, we reflect on what caused it. We seem to spend less time thinking about the causes of the good things that

happen to us. What might be the cause of that person's smile at you or their compliment of you? What was the cause of that successful meeting?

Likewise, what causes a good meditation experience? What causes you to practice mindfulness? What causes you to care about mindful living? There are likely many conditions that underlie your meditation/mindfulness practices. Inevitably, many character strengths are part of the causal benefits. Identifying these strengths might open up a variety of opportunities in the future, such as combating obstacles, building perspective on what is most important, and enhancing motivation toward greater mindfulness.

Take Stock With Mindfulness

When we give ourselves space to separate from routine, remarkable awareness can take place. For example, when I take a trip by myself to give a workshop I feel the longing that comes from separation from family. Then, perhaps on the plane or walking in the airport, in the space of the novel present moment, I begin to take stock on my life. Whether the day is positive, negative, or neutral I am often filled with gratitude. I see the wider perspective and appreciate the goodness in my life. I am encouraged to go deeper, to continue to return to the present moment, over and over. Thus, it is mindfulness that opens me up to character strengths, which then reinforce and strengthen my mindfulness practice. Thus, "taking stock" can facilitate a virtuous circle.

Other Practices

MBSP has a number of practices that support the building of a strong mindfulness practice. Review the group exercises and suggested homework exercises offered in Chapters 6–14.

Chapter 5

Practice II: Mindful Strengths Use (Bringing Mindfulness to Strengths)

Without great watchfulness a person does not advance in even a single virtue.

Father Agathon (one of the early desert fathers)

 Chapter Snapshot

Mindful strengths use refers to the use of mindfulness to enhance or bring balance to the practice of character strengths. Mindfulness can serve as a process that directs and supports our strengths use. It helps our ability to "see" our character strengths and those of others in a way that is clearer and less biased. It offers an opportunity to water our character strengths seeds and enhance our ability to express strengths in a balanced way that benefits ourselves and others. It is a mechanism of exploration and serves as a meta-process for character strengths, opening up new avenues of growth. The practice of character strengths presents many nuances to which greater mindfulness can help improve navigation; these include strengths overuse and underuse, signature strengths, the golden mean, strengths combinations and collisions, hot button issues, strengths-spotting, and strengths re-appraisals.

 Opening Story

As the expression goes, avoid talking about politics and religion at gatherings involving family or friends. In such situations, we are vulnerable to reactivity and a vicious circle of negative comments and hurt feelings. I've been on the side of unskillful reactivity too many times ... enough to want to take action to make a change. What follows is such an approach of conscious responding rather than habitual reactivity.

A couple years ago, I had an encounter with a friend who baited me with some negative comments about my political affiliation. The standard fare for us involved me falling for the trap: I would attack his political party in retaliation. And back and forth we would go with the same 'ol story – you attack my political ideals then I'll attack yours and we'll continue until someone gets hurt (at least emotionally). In the end, nothing would have changed about our beliefs. Nobody would miraculously have swayed the other side. Yet, perhaps there would be a new wedge placed in our relationship.

This game is a visceral experience. When our ideals are attacked, it can feel as though some ferocious beast is suddenly waiting to be unleashed from inside us. But, I decided to take a different approach with my friend. This time, when my friend attacked my political ideals, I stopped in mid-

> sentence, catching my strong desire to react. I considered my character strengths. I also felt a craving for mindful communication. What strengths were needed in this moment?, I asked myself. How might I play any of my character strengths to respond in a balanced way?
>
> I took a moment to breathe mindfully. I told my friend that our conversation seemed to be heading in the direction of previous conversations of attack and regret, thus a change of conversation would probably be best. My response was simple yet was coming from a position of strength. Mindfulness had centered me in the present, allowed me time to deliberately consider and call forth strengths, and helped me gather myself so I could speak with care and genuineness.

Below the surface, one can find a panoply of character strengths in this story. As situations become more complex, the number of character strengths that need to be accessed increases. Here's a peek at the character strengths that were involved in the situation and are typically useful in other situations that are hot button topics:

- *Love* and *perspective*: These two strengths are often needed in combination together. I needed to step back and see the bigger picture, reminding myself of my love and care for this friend and the fact that our relationship is about much more than a different political viewpoint. The perspective strength served to remind me that one cannot jump into another's mind and change their view so acting from that agenda is pointless.

- *Curiosity* and *judgment* (critical thinking): If one is going to have a political conversation, these two strengths should be at the forefront. Curiosity means one will ask questions in which there is a genuine attempt to understand the other's views rather than gain more information for an attack (Kashdan, 2009). Judgment refers to allowing oneself to see multiple angles of the same issue while staying open to new possibilities.

- *Love of learning:* Taking a growth mindset, which is a view that any obstacle or difference can be seen as an opportunity for learning and growth, underpins this strength. This type of mindset is linked with success and positive relationships (Dweck, 2006).

- *Kindness*, *fairness*, and *forgiveness*: It's useful to remember that these are core "other-oriented" strengths in all of us. They involve our letting others have their views. If everyone was on the same side, life would be a bore. Viewing someone who has offended oneself in a compassionate way has been found in research studies to be linked with forgiveness and positive emotions, so it ultimately serves oneself and others well (Witvliet et al., 2011). This also involves social intelligence and empathy to be aware of the impact of one's words on the feelings of others.

- *Bravery:* Courage can be used, but in a different way than one typically expects. Most people in these situations consider an attack to be the brave approach because they are not stepping down and are speaking their mind. Indeed, that is one of many ways to exert bravery. But, isn't the "higher road" a path made manifest by courage? Isn't it brave to allow discomfort within oneself while walking away to preserve a relationship?

This example indicates a quick "one-two approach" in which mindful awareness is the first step and character strengths use is the next step. In this way, one might imagine mindfulness as opening a door that suddenly gives view to a long corridor of doors. Mindful awareness is that first door that must be opened. Then, the individual has many options for the next door they might choose. For example, if a person is angry and they become mindful in the moment that they are angry and of the cause of their anger, then they have opened the first door – an opportunity to change or dig deeper has been opened. What will the individual do next? Which door will they choose among the corridor of doors? For some, it's the doorway of inaction. For others, it might be mindful breathing, going for a walk, talking about the situation, increasing anger by kicking an object, or calling forth a character strength. To paraphrase a popular quote: "Mindfulness can open the door, but only character strengths can keep it open."

Creating Space for Strengths

Thich Nhat Hanh explains the following in his teachings on mindfulness, peace, and the management of conflict and problems: We all need space; everybody and everything needs space; when we have space, we can feel free. This idea can be applied to plants and flowers where if they are packed closely together in the same flower pot, there will not be enough space for them to spread their roots and grow. When a wild animal is cornered or trapped, it does not have enough space, it may feel threatened, and often will lash out. When friends are overly needy or relationships/marriages are too co-dependent, problems emerge from a lack of space. Each human being needs some space to renew and replenish oneself. Our thoughts needs space in that our minds can become cluttered like a disorganized drawer; as we give time to focus on one thought or an idea, it can become like a seed that has been given room to germinate. Oftentimes our minds ruminate, over-think, and recycle the same worries over and over. In these situations, we are not giving our mind space to settle and just be. Similarly our emotions need space – when feelings are avoided or suppressed, they often fester and magnify and we feel worse. Our emotions need our compassionate attention, mindful breathing, and acceptance in the present moment.

Similarly, our strengths of character need space to develop. When space is created for strengths, our attention shifts, we see the positive, and our energy rises. There is no exact method for having a character strengths practice, instead character strengths can become part of any practice, theoretical orientation, or approach to working with people. As discussed in Chapter 2, there are important principles to keep in mind (e.g., characters strengths are dimensional; the role of context is crucial for strengths expression, etc.), tools that can work with any character strength, and interventions that can be tailored to specific strengths. Mindfulness assists by not only exploring and making room for strengths, but it brings attention to that which we value most. This opens the door to help us make a meaningful contribution to our lives and the lives of others. When the laser of our mindful attention is pointed clearly at what is best and already exists in us, the possibility of flourishing increases.

In the following subsections, I take the approach that is the reverse of the focus in Chapter 4. Here character strengths are the base and mindfulness is discussed as a mechanism or orientation for enhancing or improving the balance of strengths practice.

Signature Strengths

As discussed earlier, interventions to boost awareness and use of signature strengths are one of the most popular interventions in positive psychology (Gander et al., 2012a; Madden et al., 2011; Mitchell et al., 2009; Mongrain & Anselmo-Matthews, 2012; Rust et al., 2009; Peterson & Peterson, 2008; Seligman et al., 2005). The standard intervention with signature strengths is to help the client identify their top strengths of character and use those strengths in a new way each day. This intervention helps individuals to expand their view of themselves, to counterbalance the negative mindset, and to build a repertoire of resources in the future, theoretically similar to the role of positive emotions that broaden skills in the moment and build future resources (Fredrickson, 2001). The standard method for generating initial mindfulness of character strengths is through the online survey, the VIA Inventory of Strengths (VIA Survey; see www.viame.org). Practitioners who are mindfully attuned to their clients can also get a good sense for signature strengths through observation and discussion – looking for strengths that are most authentic, core to the client's identity, most natural and easy to express, energizing, expressed consistently across situations, and recognized most readily by informants close to the client.

When my son was two months old, he could not see far in front of him. I would position my face in front of him, and he would respond by moving his face from side to side a few times as if struggling to focus. Then, at some point, he would stop and as if he were zooming in, he would suddenly "see" me. Pausing there, he would smile. We were then connected. Similarly, when a practitioner points out and values the signature strengths of their client, they are "seeing" them. It becomes a moment of connection. Mindfulness is a mechanism to catalyze this process of zooming in to see what is best in another being.

The Virtuous Circle

Relevant to this discussion is the concept of a virtuous circle of mindfulness and character strengths (Niemiec et al., 2012). Plenty of exploration has been done on vicious circles in which negativity breeds and reinforces further negativity, as in the role of negative thinking in many psychological disorders. However, far less research has been done on the virtuous circle (or virtuous cycle). One mindfulness study informally referenced the virtuous circle to describe a qualitative analysis of a subject's experience with MBCT (Allen et al., 2009). Others have commented on the benefits of a virtuous circle with character strengths and other positive experiences (Elston & Boniwell, 2011). Similarly, when therapists undertake a priming procedure in which they focus on the patient's individual strengths (resource priming) before a therapy session, a positive feedback circuit is created that leads to strengths activation, which then connects with positive outcomes (Fluckiger & Grosse Holtforth, 2008).

Mindful strengths use creates greater mindfulness in which the individual is more tuned into the present moment – external environment, five senses, thoughts, emotions, and those best qualities (signature strengths) that reside in their internal environment. This mindfulness of strengths increases the likelihood of balanced strengths expression, thus tilting behavior/thoughts toward a virtuous circle of mutually positive effects. Likewise a strong mindfulness practice will not only encompass the actual practice of strengths and virtues, but could simultaneously elicit positive outcomes associated with character strength and an enhanced awareness of one's core identity, of which an important part is signature strengths. The virtuous circle can be broken in many ways: A general lack of strengths awareness (Linley, 2008) as well as the "taking-strengths-for-granted effect" of seeing signature strengths as ordinary rather than extraordinary (also called strengths blindness, Biswas-Diener et al., 2011) are significant obstacles impeding virtuous circles of mindfulness and character strengths.

A Meta-Strength

The attentional process of mindfulness can act as a meta-strength, a higher-order process for working with any of the 24 character strengths. In ad-

dition, some researchers have hypothesized certain character strengths might act as a master strength by which the operation and use of other strengths occurs or is filtered through. Schwartz and Sharpe (2006) propose a "practical wisdom" (i.e., the strength of social intelligence or perspective/wisdom) to serve this role, while other strengths have been suggested (e.g., self-regulation; Baumeister & Vohs, 2004, and love; Vaillant, 2008). My view is that in practice any of the 24 strengths – when operating as the individual's signature strength – has the potential to act as the "master strength" that opens up access to other strengths for a given individual. For example, a person authentically and strongly expressing their prudence or their curiosity in a balanced way fills them with joy, energy, and a sense of competence that opens them up to expressing any of the other strengths that are needed in a particular situation. Moreover, it is the attentional process of mindfulness that helps the individual to operate master strengths and other strengths. Mindfulness directs the individual's attention to what matters most in his or her life while supporting sensitivity to the context/situation the individual is in, sharpening the accuracy of the strengths use, and employing the "golden mean of character strengths" from moment to moment.

The Golden Mean of Character Strengths

Practitioners who take a strengths-based approach are well-advised to help clients understand the *golden mean of character strengths* – the right combination of strengths, used to the right degree and in the right situation. For example, the level of creativity you show at work will be expressed differently if you are supervising someone or being supervised and will be brought forth to a different degree with your spouse and with your child or friend. Those strengths you use along with creativity will vary as well – perhaps curiosity in one situation and leadership in the next. In addition, one might consider for what purpose a strength is being used and whether it is the right purpose. Of course "right" is subjective to issues of individual and group morality and the nuances of the situation. Therefore, an initial, starting point could be that a "right purpose" is beneficial for self *and* others.

Box 5.1. A Golden Mean

The Golden Mean of Character Strengths: The right combination of strengths, used to the right degree, in the right situation, for a purpose that benefits both self and others.

The concept of a golden mean comes originally from Aristotle (2000) and the entire teachings of the Buddha have been summed up as encouraging and teaching the middle way, or middle path (Kornfield & Feldman, 1996) in which one pursues balance between two extremes. The golden mean has been re-articulated by various strengths researchers (Biswas-Diener et al., 2011; Linley, 2008; Schwartz & Sharpe, 2006). There is no absolute mean in strengths expression as everything is relative to the situation/context; this aligns closely with what the *Character Strengths and Virtues* text describes as "situational themes," which nest under the character strengths which then nest under the larger virtue categories (Peterson & Seligman, 2004). Aristotle was a very practical philosopher who emphasized, above all, finding balance among life activities, such as working, learning, playing, and loving, and between excess and deficiency. This can be applied to character strengths as being overused in a particular context (excess) or underused (deficiency). For example, the overuse of bravery is recklessness while the underuse of bravery is cowardice, while at the same time, too little prudence can be cowardice and too much prudence is likely stuffiness. To find the golden mean in a given situation, the individual must be mindful of the fact that there are many strengths at play and it is very easy to overuse or overplay a strength, as well as to underuse or underplay a strength. Thus, when we speak of a golden mean, we are speaking about having a mindful awareness of ourselves, an attunement to others, and looking for a balanced expression that fits the context. A moment to moment awareness of ourselves and others in situations is the best way to monitor and therefore increase or decrease our strengths use.

Context Matters

Familiarity with the golden mean indicates the individual will be comfortable tuning into times when strengths are being overused or underused, according to the context of a given present moment. One could argue that a portion of strength underuse is due to mindlessness, complacency, and becoming lost in autopilot tendencies, unaware of potentiality and action that could be taken. Also underlying strengths underuse is a constricted view of the present moment manifested by a fixed mindset that views change in a limited way and does not look for growth opportunities. Overuse, on the other hand, can be argued, in part, as a loss of perspective in which the individual gets locked into habitual tendencies (e.g., overusing perseverance by not knowing when to quit) and has lost a mindful awareness of the big picture. Mindful awareness helps explore the nuances of strength expression, navigate the vicissitudes of life, and increase the level of discernment as individuals approach complex situations. The successful management of strengths imbalance is seen when an individual is able to maintain an authenticity with their momentum as well as not being blind to their strengths.

Chapter 12 includes a handout used in MBSP outlining overuse and underuse for each of the 24 character strengths. Becoming familiar with how each character strength can be overused or underused helps practitioners become savvy about strengths dynamics and how strengths can contribute to or even cause problems from time to time. Practitioners can help clients monitor for character strength overuse (e.g., when a client's curiosity becomes nosiness) and for character strength underuse (e.g., when a client's disinterest or apathy may mean they are using too little curiosity). As one practitioner said: "The language of overuse and underuse helps me to understand what to be on the lookout for when my clients are out of balance."

The use of mindfulness helps in exploring the nuances of context and deciphering of which strengths might be used and in what combination, and how much of a strength might be drawn back or increased incrementally. Indeed, one will use a different degree of one's love strength with a family member versus a work colleague, and the expression will look different when one is in a funeral home, a crowded restaurant, or one's home with them. While many of these decisions are automatic, mindfulness serves as a higher-order process and a resource for applying strengths contextually and finding balance. So how does one make such decisions? Research on the importance of practical wisdom – similar to the constellation of social intelligence and perspective – emphasizes that virtues and character strengths need to be balanced to prevent excess or overuse. Three issues need to be prioritized when considering the application of strengths in a particular situation (Schwartz & Sharpe, 2006):

1. *Relevance:* Does the situation require a strength?
2. *Conflict:* Which strength should I use, especially when my strengths are competing?
3. *Specificity:* What is needed to translate the strength into action?

Awareness of relevance, conflict, and specificity can assist the individual in using strengths to an optimal level that adheres to the golden mean. This is consistent with another thread of mindfulness research known as sociocognitive mindfulness (Langer, 1989; Langer et al., 2010). This slant on mindfulness emphasizes awareness of cognitive distinctions made about objects of one's mind (e.g., thoughts, feelings) and treats these as novel and emerging. This also refers to having a mindfulness of the conditionality of context and that the present experience of a situation takes precedence over previous contexts; therefore, autopilot responding needs to be broken to open the possibility of using different character strengths.

Strengths-Spotting

Strengths-spotting involves bringing consciousness to the presence of strengths in oneself and in others. This is an important aspect of learning and training in strengths. Mindful awareness of verbal and nonverbal cues is at the crux of strengths-spotting. This involves mindful listening, in which one is tuned in to the experience of the other and therefore is primed to spot strengths that arise. Mindfulness returns individuals to their senses so they can be more adept at spotting the details within or around them, such as tuning into body language,

changes in verbal fluency, word choice, and intensity. The skill of strengths-spotting assists individuals in building up a "common language" for communicating about their core qualities and discussing what is best in themselves and those around them. Becoming familiar with the character strengths, virtues, and the strength dimensions (those words in the brackets in Chapter 2, Table 2.1) of the VIA Classification is a starting point for individuals; they will then have more *strengths fluency* (Linkins, Niemiec, Mayerson, & Gillham, in press) as they will have more knowledge, depth, and understanding about strengths to be better equipped to identify strengths in oneself and others, and therefore display strengths dexterity in which they align specific strengths with tasks and apply strengths to achieve positive outcomes.

Many psychological processes are implicated in this strengths-spotting ability, such as *psychological mindedness* (awareness and understanding of psychological processes and emotional states in oneself and others), *empathic concern* (feeling sympathy and concern for others), and *perspective taking* (taking the psychological point of view of others). Researchers have described mindfulness as not only a similar construct to psychological mindedness (Horowitz, 2002), but a necessary precondition for psychological mindedness, as evidenced in moderate correlations (Beitel, Ferrer, & Cecero, 2005). Mindfulness has been found to increase empathy and perspective taking (Birnie et al., 2010; Dekeyser et al., 2008; Sweet & Johnson, 1990).

An important point to not be overlooked, especially when spotting strengths in others, is the importance of naming the strengths of others in the moment, offering a rationale for what has been spotted, and expressing the value it holds. As individuals are typically more prepared to hear negative feedback or problems, this sharing of valued qualities is a welcomed shift. See Table 5.1 for a layout of steps one can take to successfully implement strengths-spotting. Oftentimes, the recipient of strengths-spotting has never had someone point out the details of their goodness, whether that be their curiosity, their appreciation for beauty, their inherent fairness orientation, or their teamwork strength. The value potency increases when this strengths-spotting, naming, and discussing is done spontaneously.

Table 5.1
Mindful strengths-spotting: Steps for teaching oneself and clients

---

1.) *Build a language*. First, take time to build a coherent strengths language so you are priming your-self on what to look for in your client. The VIA Classification provides a great framework for buil-ding a meaningful and systematic vocabulary. Learning not only the virtue categories and strength definitions, but also the synonyms and dimensions of each character strength, will help you build a flexible repertoire for your strengths-spotting.

2.) *Fine tune your observation and listening skills*. What do strengths look like in action? The idea here is to look for a shift in your client, on both a verbal and a nonverbal level. Pay attention to changes in energy.

    a. Look for *nonverbal* cues that a strength is present by looking for improved posture, better eye contact, more smiling or laughing, increased use of hand gestures, and the expression of posi-tive emotions such as joy, excitement, and hope. In workshops around the world, after a strengths-spotting exercise, I debrief and ask participants what they noticed on a nonverbal level, and invariably someone volunteers saying they observed the phenomena of the individual's eyes "lighting up" when the person was speaking to a strength in some way.

    b. On a *verbal* level, listen for a stronger, more assertive voice, improved vocabulary and clarity of speech, and use of strength words. Some clients might be quicker and even tangential in their speech because they are excited about the topic, while others speak more slowly and are more methodical and direct with their speech when a strength is present signifying a relaxed and calm confidence.

3.) *Label character strength behaviors*. As you label strengths in yourself and in others, make note of the behavior that you are spotting that is associated with the strength or at least your rationale for how you saw the strength being expressed. If you are spotting the strength in yourself, this will help you take a stance of "owning" the strength. For example, "That enthusiasm you are sensing from me around this topic is my character strength of *zest* coming alive," or "Wow, you really dealt with that difficult colleague with a high level of *social intelligence* when you offered them different options for handling their crisis. Great job using one of your signature strengths!" In the former, you'd be simultaneously rehearsing your own internal strengths-spotting, as well as modeling for your client a way to engage in the process. In the latter, you'd be reinforcing the core essence of your client as well as giving them a positive emotional experience for them to build upon and ge-nerate resources for the future.

4.) *Build a habit by maintaining your strengths-spotting*. Repeat the above phases through practice and more practice. Similar to the development of other skills, spotting character strengths needs to become an ongoing practice for it to build. You might wish to deepen your skill of recognizing cha-racter strengths in action by keeping a log (mental or written) of behavioral expressions of charac-ter strengths.

5.) *Teach strengths-spotting to your clients (or others)*: After you feel more comfortable with your own skill of strength-spotting, reflect on how you will teach it to your client. Go through the above phases one-by-one with your client. In addition, you might share real or fictional scenarios in which character strengths are expressed and then have your client identify character strengths they see in the story. You can have your client begin to observe those close to him/her at work or in their personal life.

6.) *Express appreciation*: Many people are not practiced in giving positive feedback around strengths, or receiving it, and so working to diminish awkwardness can be helpful. Explore with your client ways to express appreciation to another to minimize discomfort and hopefully find a level of com-fort. This will often involve using curiosity and self-kindness to tolerate any initial awkwardness in practicing this new approach. Some clients may struggle with this kind of mindful strengths use and are thus invited to use their own words. For example, instead of saying "I really appreciate your prudence" it might feel more natural and genuine to say "I really appreciate the way you are careful in thinking through all the risks." But, in most cases, try to use the VIA Classification language to take advantage of the novelty and power of strengths labels.

Boosting Lower Strengths

After individuals have reviewed their rank-order of character strengths, a common phenomenon is to look toward those strengths that are lower in one's profile. Mindful awareness is needed for the individual to discern which direction to pursue in their strengths use – deploy signature strengths (referred to as "building upon" strengths) or boost lower strengths (referred to as "building up" strengths). While it is hypothesized that focusing on one's signature strengths is likely to lead to the largest benefit, another important practice consideration is to remember the principle that "all 24 character strengths matter," as each is a capacity within each individual and ultimately is important in one situation or another. Over the decades, some character strengths have developed a robust array of interventions that can be used to build them up (e.g., creativity, forgiveness, hope). For strengths with less scientific backing (e.g., prudence, humility), it is likely that awareness-building activities involving mindful reflection of past use of the strength, awareness of how others have been exemplars of the strength, and the practice of self-monitoring would each be a mindfulness-related activity to start.

In the end, it is difficult to raise any strength without cultivating a greater awareness of it. This applies to *phasic strengths* (strengths that are not signature strengths but which the individual can employ in a substantial way when the situation calls for it) and to lower strengths. Strength awareness develops through mindful practice done repeatedly. This conscious use helps to foster a mental and behavioral routine with the strength. Benjamin Franklin took this approach centuries ago (Franklin, 1962) and positive psychology scholars continue to claim its effectiveness today (Peterson, 2006).

Strength Re-Appraisals

"I love that you get cold when it's 71 degrees out. I love that it takes you an hour and a half to order a sandwich. I love that you get a little crinkle above your nose when you're looking at me like I'm nuts. I love that after I spend the day with you, I can still smell your perfume on my clothes. And I love that you are the last person I want to talk to before I go to sleep at night. And it's not because I'm lonely, and it's not because it's New Year's Eve. I came here tonight because when you realize you want to spend the rest of your life with somebody, you want the rest of your life to start as soon as possible."

Harry Burns in *When Harry Met Sally ...* (1989)

There are many ways we can approach challenges, problems, stressors, hassles, difficulties, and life issues. Often times our automatic responding kicks in, and we react in certain habitual ways. We handle these challenges by blaming, catastrophizing, worrying, isolating, yelling, over-thinking, under-thinking, etc.

Reframing offers people another angle. Sometimes reframing offers a positive perspective on something that could be seen as a negative – as in several of Harry's opening remarks when he is professing his love to Sally Albright in the film *When Harry Met Sally ...* – and in other instances reframing is less dramatic yet offers an equally compelling lens to try on. The intention of reframing is not meant to replace a diagnosis but to give the person a potential "ah-ha" moment, an insight into themselves, a positive and realistic alternative, and an approach they can take to handle their issue. Reframing requires the individual or practitioner to give pause, with mindfulness. The individual has to take notice of an experience, see the often visceral expression of strengths being overused/underused, and then consider balance. It is a moment of choice.

Consider the example of a student who has delayed for several weeks in starting the writing of a paper that is due the next day but instead is continuing to search and research the topic incessantly. A quick label on this situation would be to call it procrastination; building off this label, a menu of strategies emerges. Another interpretation would be to say the individual is underusing prudence, overusing curiosity, and underusing perseverance; this perspective moves the conversation in a different direction, introducing positive qualities that might have been forgotten or overdrawn. Which view is the student most likely to "hear"? Which is most likely to keep the student engaged in the conversation? The interpretation of overuse/underuse opens the conversation to pivotal follow-up questions about strengths use, management of overuse/underuse with strengths, and discussion of balanced strengths use. The student might speak of their passion for love of learning and curiosity to investigate topic areas in a deep way or of the use of self-regulation to temper their curious nature and a deployment of zest and enthusiasm in order to be more planful and prudent with the time remaining. Practitioners focused only on labeling procrastination are likely to miss their client's inner resources and positive potentials.

This line of questioning changes the conversation and brings the individual to view themselves from a different vantage point – a strengths perspective. In order for someone to take this perspective, the nonjudging and openness qualities of mindfulness are necessary to make the positive appraisal. In summary, here are two levels of questioning one might use in the reframing of problems using a strengths lens:

1. What character strengths might you be overusing or underusing in your avoidance of this paper project?
2. What character strengths would help you bring balance to this situation? What strengths might you use to temper your overuse or boost your underuse?

Research has found that individuals are prone to the negative and are impacted more by negative than positive events (Baumeister et al., 2001). Thus, the relevance of positive re-appraisals, or strengths re-appraisals, is of primary importance. Research suggests that mindfulness makes it easier to be positive. Mindfulness helps individuals re-appraise stressful situations in a more positive perspective; this is meaning-based coping that enables the individual to adapt successfully to challenging circumstances (Garland, Gaylord, & Park, 2009). Mindfulness has been found to decrease negative reactivity in communication (Huston, Garland, & Farb, 2011), and mindfulness is linked with positive reappraisal in that the two constructs together predicted job burnout (Gerzina & Porfeli, 2012). There appears to be a reciprocal link

of mutual enhancement between mindfulness and positive reappraisal to the degree that a positive upward spiral is generated (Garland, Gaylord, & Fredrickson, 2011).

Strength Constellations and Conflicts

It is unlikely that individuals express only one character strength in isolation. In reality, individuals express a combination of several strengths at any one time. One lecturer might be displaying a constellation of leadership with curiosity, humility, and kindness as they ask for a student's opinion on the topic being discussed, while another lecturer may use leadership with creativity, social intelligence, and teamwork as they organize a student debate around a class theme. The conscious use of character strength combinations is best viewed as an art, and the nonjudging process of mindfulness is important for discerning which strengths to call forth.

In other situations, character strengths may appear diametrically opposed. When someone witnesses an individual spout political rhetoric or biased religious views, should bravery and judgment (to challenge the individual to see other views) be used or should prudence and self-regulation (to cautiously hold back one's views for a different time and place) be employed? The answer to this will be based on the complexity of the individual's personality as it interplays with the context they are in. A mindful awareness of one's strengths, of other internal experiences (e.g., emotions being triggered), of the situation, the environment, and the potential consequences of speaking out or not are important factors to be present to. While the dyad of fairness and kindness often combine together nicely as a strengths dyad (e.g., listen to the Dalai Lama speak about anything), they can also oppose one another. If you are running late and someone cuts in front of you in line, is it more important for you to bring forth your fairness principle (e.g., everyone should wait their turn, thus this person should go to the back of the line) or your kindness strength (e.g., they must be struggling to have to cut in front of me so I'll let them be)? There are no correct answers to these scenarios and conflicts, but mindfulness can help us discern an optimal path that takes our own needs and the needs of others into consideration.

Strengths Hot Buttons/Sensitive Areas

Humans are creatures of habit and, as such, gravitate toward routine. This occurs not only in our eating, work, and sleep schedules but also in how we handle relationships. Reactivity in relationships is a manifestation of autopilot. In many instances, when we examine situations closely, our character strengths have become hot buttons – sensitive areas that are triggered. If we are in a conversation with someone new and discover 20 minutes later that we are asking all the questions, we might begin to feel frustrated that the inquiries have not been reciprocated. This may be especially triggering if the individual asking the questions is high in curiosity and is perceiving a lack of curiosity in return. Likewise, a prudent person's hot button might get pressed when others are late for a meeting, thus displaying a lack of planfulness and conscientiousness, and a kind and generous person might be triggered when they learn that a wealthy person has not offered a single donation to charity in years. Because we value our own signature strengths, it can be particularly vexing when others do not express the strengths as well.

In other instances, we might experience a hot button when we perceive someone to be overusing a character strength, such as the person high in zest expressing a bit too much energy early in the morning or the enthusiastic spiritual seeker who begins to express their spirituality by proselytizing to individuals in their community. This may trigger us regardless of where zest and spirituality fall in our own strength profile – as signature strengths, middle strengths, or lesser strengths.

Mindful strengths use is a pathway that can lead to management of such hot button issues. The next time one is triggered by another person (in any way), ask oneself which character strength(s) are being pushed in some way. Is it that we want things to be a certain way and the individual is doing something that violates this? Pausing to breathe with the tension, exploring the

strengths being used, overused, and underused, and then considering which strengths might be deployed in response, requires significant mindful awareness. Sometimes it is difficult to manage hot button issues in the heat of the moment, thus, prospectively planning for triggering situations that might arise when a particular person arrives, a specific meeting starts, or when one has to face a sensitive scenario is a useful approach.

Big Strength/Little Strength

It seems likely that each of the character strengths can be displayed in a large way that is highly impacting as well as displayed simply in everyday life. It is the latter that any of us can immediately tap into to bring about an impact on our lives or the lives of others. Researchers have examined a number of strengths in this way by describing strengths as "big" and "little." The most popular example is for creativity in which scientist Dean Simonton (2000) characterized "Big C" Creativity as typifying extreme originality and inventiveness that is immediately obvious to others, such as the great creations of famous painters, poets, and filmmakers. "Little c" creativity refers to everyday creativity or ingenuity in which a person comes up with a new way to solve a problem.

Table 5.2 offers several examples (at least one from each virtue category), showing how this conceptualization can be viewed across different character strengths. While we might not achieve or display the extremes of Big C, Big L, or some of the other Big character strengths, it is likely, if not inevitable, that we will achieve little c, little l, and other little character strengths. The name "little" is used simply as a comparison to "big," from the vantage point of comparing the impact the strengths use has on others or the enormity of the feat. This term "little" does seem a bit ironic because as we begin to examine the impact strengths can and do have on our personal lives, it is clear that there really are no "little" strengths; as noted earlier, character strengths use is quite extraordinary. Bringing mindfulness to our past and current strengths use as well as to "little" strength use is likely to assist in expanding the scope of the strength.

Table 5.2
Big and little character strength uses

Character Strength	Big use	Little use	Source
Creativity (C, c)	Creating renown works of art, music, literature	Finding a new solution to a problem	Simonton (2000)
Leadership (L, l)	Presidents, prime ministers, CEOs	Organizing a group of friends for an evening out	Peterson & Seligman (2004)
Hope/Optimism (H, h)	Having the belief: Our nation is on the verge of great things	Having the belief: I will find a good parking space today	Peterson (2000)
Love (LO, lo)	Sacrificing one's life to save one's drowning child	Expressing love on a greeting card	This volume
Forgiveness (F, f)	Forgiving a person who perpetrated a trauma	Letting go of the annoyance of being cut off in traffic	This volume
Appreciation of Beauty/ Excellence (ABE, abe)	Marveling at one of the natural wonders of the world	Appreciating the beauty of one leaf	This volume
Self-Regulation (SR, sr)	Winning a triathlon	Deciding not to go up for seconds at a buffet	This volume
Perseverance (P, p)	Surviving a concentration camp	Working hard and completing a 2-page paper for class	This volume

Putting it All Together

What follows is an example of a common, sometimes debilitating problem, while illustrating the use of mindfulness and character strengths, the importance of strengths labeling, reappraisal, and other topics mentioned in this chapter. Several years ago I worked with a middle-aged man (I'll call him "Jim") who was legally blind and suffered from social anxiety disorder (social phobia). Jim also experienced panic attacks. He wanted to learn to manage his anxiety better and to discontinue use of his anti-anxiety pills.

One day I asked Jim: "How did you make it here today?"

"The usual way – by bus," he said. "Actually, 2 buses, a little bit of biking, and a lot of walking."

"And what was that like for you to do today?"

"It was fine … I felt fine. Nothing remarkable."

"Wow, Jim … Many people would be terrified to live in the darkness that you live in as a partially blind man. Yet, you go about your day taking buses, walking down busy streets, trying to improve yourself with therapy, volunteering at local agencies … and you successfully face the challenge of riding a bike despite limited vision. What courage you have! What perseverance!"

My client was stunned. He was not accustomed to seeing himself as a person with strengths. Even more foreign to him was having actual strength labels assigned to him (he was much more familiar with his identity as a "panic disordered social phobic who drinks too much"). This was an "ah-ha moment" for Jim – not an uncommon experience for clients who experience a *strengths re-frame*.

"Jim, we've been practicing mindfulness in our last few sessions to help you learn to relate differently to yourself and to your anxiety."

"Yes."

"Take a moment to pause and bring a careful, mindful attention to your day so far," I noted, as I handed him a copy of the VIA Classification that we began discussing the previous week. "Are there any other strengths on this list that you used today?"

He studied the list of strengths. "Yeah, I used *curiosity* when I asked the person sitting next to me on the bus about her daughter. And when I noticed myself start to get anxious, like that tunnel vision feeling, I used *perspective* to step out of it and take notice of everything that was around me. Oh, and I used *fairness* because the bus driver forgot to charge me my fare and I let him know."

Jim's strengths language was opening up and becoming more fluent. He was showing an ability to view his life from fresh angles. He was now applying his mindfulness practice to strengths awareness.

We discussed strengths overuse and underuse. He observed an imbalance that was occurring internally. His underuse of bravery (i.e., not facing his anxiety, not expressing his signature strengths with confidence) and his overuse of prudence (i.e., being too cautious about each situation) were colliding to a detrimental effect. The result was one of immobilization.

"What strengths might you use to bring balance to this experience of becoming immobilized?"

"Well," Jim said, "for some reason I don't feel I can be brave. But I can be curious."

"Great, how will you do that?"

"I will look for what is new and different when I'm outside. I can ask questions when I'm sitting on the bus and around people. I'm good at asking questions."

"Any other strengths that can assist you?"

"Maybe hope – I'm not really sure how. Wisdom. Kindness. Being a more contributing team player when I'm around others."

"OK. Here's another question, Jim." I pointed to the list of character strengths: "Are there any strengths that you are using already that perhaps you had not previously been mindful to?"

"Funny that you mention that. There are. I already use the strength of judgment because I'm a thinker, always considering different views and details of situations. And I seem to always be honest about my struggles. I admit it when I'm nervous. "

"Yes, good. Those are strengths to keep in mind that you can explore further and use more consciously. I have another thought – what are you doing when you are avoiding the situations you are afraid of?"

"Typically, I'm painting. Sometimes reading a science book. Other times I go to church."

"OK, so you're using creativity or love of learning or spirituality then? Looks like several more strengths that you can bring your awareness to and re-direct or use in a new way to help you. You've described many strengths today as well as many ways you can mobilize yourself. Would you like to set up an action plan to practice using your strengths in a social situation this week?"

As Jim reflected on our sessions, there were three character strengths he ultimately found most useful in helping him move through his anxiety with mindfulness:

• *Curiosity:* Research has found that curiosity and social anxiety are incompatible (Kashdan, 2007). The research is clear that the best pathway to manage anxiety is exposure to the fear accompanied by personal skills. Curiosity is not only a skill individuals can keep with them, but it's a strength that opens one's attention in the present moment to counteract the narrowing effect of anxiety.

  – **Jim's tip:** Be curious about your anxiety. Take notice of what you are not seeing (what is your "tunnel vision" preventing you from seeing?). When anxiety arises, instead of taking an approach of, "Oh no, not again!" consider saying, "That's interesting. I wonder what's going on here?"

• *Bravery:* When you are ready to face your anxiety, you should do so with coping skills. Undoubtedly, you'll need to rally any personal courage that you'd previously been underusing. Focus on the outcome of using your bravery (Pury & Kowalski, 2007).

  – **Jim's tip:** Ask questions of oneself about the outcome of future strengths use. How will you feel about yourself after you face your anxiety? How will your behavior impact others?

- *Self-regulation:* Don't try to override panic or intense anxiety by learning relaxation techniques. These are great techniques, but there's a time and a place for their use. Research shows learning relaxation techniques for panic can actually be harmful since you cannot override your fight-or-flight response when it's fully activated in panic. Instead, train yourself to observe the moment to moment experience in your body and mind.

  - *Jim's tip:* When you practice being aware of the present moment, you are taking control of your attention. When your mind wanders to past problems or to future worries and you bring your focus back to your breath (the present moment), you are taking control of your attention (in other words, you are self-regulating your attention).

Strategies for Building an Approach of Mindful Strengths Use

Here are a few additional, practical suggestions for using mindfulness to enhance the practice of character strengths and invigorating a mindful strengths use.

Target Specific Strengths

The use of meditation techniques to target a particular character strength is not new, as leading figures in mindfulness have been teaching this approach for decades. For example, the most common character strengths to target in meditation are probably wisdom (the strength of perspective) and compassion (the strength of kindness), as these are core focus areas in Buddhist practices. Love has been a longtime focus as well, and, in particular, loving-kindness meditation has enjoyed a surge of research (see Chapter 3 for a review). Cultivating the spirituality strength has been a long-time focus of self-help and spiritual

writers and more recently of researchers (Goldstein, 2007). Forgiveness is a strength that has been targeted with mindfulness practices as well, particularly by Thich Nhat Hanh (2001), Jack Kornfield (2008), and Tara Brach (2003). For example, Brach offers a deep, three-part meditation on cultivating forgiveness that involves asking for forgiveness, forgiving oneself, and forgiving others.

Re-Envision the Strengths Paradox

Unawareness of strengths is pervasive. There is more outside of our consciousness in terms of strengths expression than what we can possibly be mindful too. Even when we are aware of our good qualities, we are highly vulnerable to the taking-strengths-for-granted effect, to seeing strengths as ordinary, and to not viewing them in a substantive way. Despite this high level of strengths blindness, when individuals are given an opportunity or reminder to consider their strengths, they typically have no difficulty doing so. This is the *strengths paradox*. A way to address the paradox is to hold a mindset that strengths work is an ongoing process of learning and growth. Every situation and experience in life is something unique to attend to in the present moment and is an opportunity for balanced strength expression. This means that strengths-spotting glasses should be worn throughout the day, at work, and when around other people; while one might take the glasses off to go to sleep, it is important they be set nearby the bed so they can be quickly put back on first thing in the morning upon awakening.

Shift From Mindless to Mindful

This exercise, used in MBSP, invites individuals to consider one activity of their regular life that they struggle with or are bothered by and which might benefit from a greater dose (i.e., frequency, intensity, or duration) of mindfulness and strengths use. Participants consider situations in which they typically display mindless behavior, such as tense discussions with a colleague, spouse, or roommate; experiences of overeating or over-drinking; or re-occurring vices, habits, or problems.

The practice involves the individual deliberately bringing mindfulness and strengths to that one activity. The target is the autopilot, mindless reactivity, and bad habits associated with that activity. When practiced regularly (e.g., each day), the individual makes shifts toward cultivating virtue, making strength use more routine, and using mindfulness to do so.

Stay Mindful of Overuse and Underuse

As each situation is unique, consistent presence to one's strengths is necessary. Mindfulness practice combats the pull of autopilot which promotes strengths underuse and challenges the loss of perspective that comes with strengths overuse. The general practices of ROAD-MAP discussed in Chapter 2 can be applied to the improvement of strengths balance relevant to this discussion. In particular, asking for feedback from others is perhaps most important. The character strengths 360 exercise focused on in MBSP (Sessions 5 and 6) is a place to start.

Make Good Use of the Adverb or Adjective

Adverbs are words that modify and give description or substance to a verb of action, while adjectives describe a noun. "Mindful" can serve as a strong adjective (e.g., mindful standing, mindful working) and "mindfully" as a wonderful adverb to virtually any action in our lives (e.g., mindfully loving). In addition, these can be used as descriptors for *any* of the 24 character strengths. To use these as adverbs or adjectives is to place a special sense of importance on the strength – to prioritize it as a focal point in one's life.

In MBSP, there is an exercise called "strengths branding" in which participants choose one of their strengths and brand themselves with that strength and its link with mindfulness. For this exercise, it's best to start with one's signature strengths as these are strengths of high value to the individual and a level of versatility already exists. Since signature strengths are part of our core identity they are likely to feel more authentic to brand to oneself than a lesser strength that is less owned by the individual.

BOX 5.2. Mindful Hope: An Example of Strengths Branding

An MBSP participant reported on the strengths branding exercise to their group:

"I brand myself with mindful hope. Hope is my highest signature strength, one that does not fail to give me energy and well-being when I need it most. When I am feeling down, I bring my attention to a glimmer of the positive within me and around me. After I feel bad about arguing with my wife, I use mindfulness to clearly see the reality of my contribution while balancing this with a view of the good in myself and my wife. I remind myself of our marriage and the possibilities that await us to discover in the future. This is idealism, I know. But that part of me is my hope coming across.

I will continue to remind myself that hope is who I am. When I notice someone smile at me at work or play I will reconnect with my hope strength in that moment. I will notice how it feels in my body – right now my hope feels like a lightness at the top of my chest and a gentle tingling in my face. I will notice hope in my thinking – right now it comes across as thoughts of excitement relating to this exercise, also as a thought relating to connecting more with others in this group outside of this session.

Sometimes, I struggle in that I become so hopeful of the things I want to accomplish that I overextend myself or over-commit. I am then unable to finish everything. My approach of mindful hope will catch this overuse early on. When I am asked to take on a new project, my mindfulness will click in and I will pause, breathe, and reflect fully on the ramifications of a yes or a no response.

In short, mindful hope means that I continue to fall back on a soft bed of being positive to others, tapping into my energy and zest, and being goal-oriented toward the future in a way that is balanced and comfortable."

Individuals brainstorm one question such as, "What does mindful prudence look like?" or "What is it like to be mindfully humble throughout my day?" This is journaled and then discussed in dyads or small groups. Box 5.2 offers an example of what mindful hope looked like to one individual practicing MBSP. Ellen Langer (2006) has observed, "If we are mindfully creative, the circumstances of the moment will tell us what to do." One might come to better understand mindful strengths use by investigating resources and materials that describe and explore one particular character strength of interest. This helps the individual to deepen their knowledge about the strength's nuances and complexities and can offer a map for one's mindful strengths use. In considering books on specific character strengths one might review the following: for mindful curiosity, read *Curious?* (Kashdan, 2009); for mindful gratitude, read *Thanks!* (Emmons, 2007); for mindful social intelligence, read *Social Intelligence* (Goleman, 2006); for mindful self-regulation, read *Willpower* (Baumeister & Tierney, 2011); for mindful bravery, read *The Courage Quotient* (Biswas-Diener, 2012); for mindful humility, read *Humility: The Quiet Virtue* (Worthington, 2007); and for mindful loving, read *Everyday Blessings* (Kabat-Zinn & Kabat-Zinn, 1997)

Set Up "Bells" of Awakening in the Environment

Thich Nhat Hanh encourages individuals to create "bells" of mindfulness to break one's habitual mindlessness and return to the present moment. Individuals might set up these external cues by using naturally occurring sounds (e.g., bells, a baby's cry) or self-created reminders (e.g., sticky notes). Whenever an individual sees a sticky note or hears the particular sound in their environment, it is a call to return to the present moment where they can re-connect with their breath and with the strengths they are wanting to develop or the strengths they might rediscover in the moment.

Other Practices

MBSP has a number of exercises that support the building of a practice that involves mindful strengths use. Review Chapters 6–14 and choose the exercises that stand out the most.

Section III: MBSP

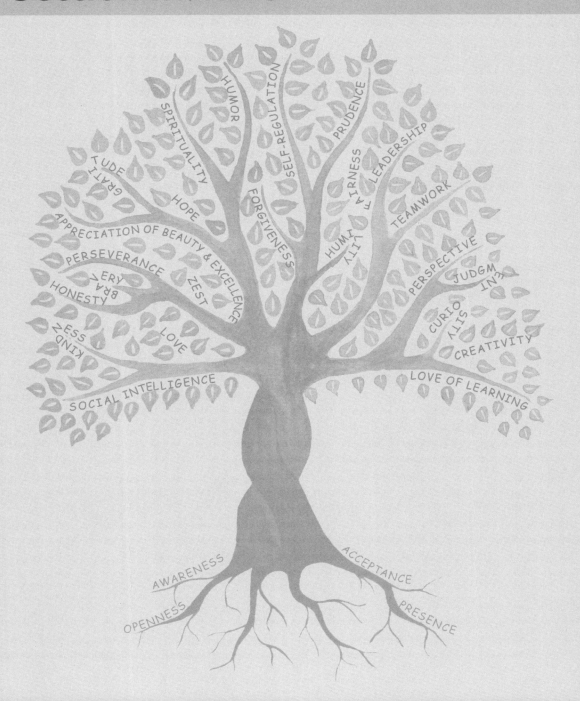

Chapter 6

Overview of MBSP

Of what avail is an open eye if the heart is blind?

Solomon ibn Gabirol

Chapter Snapshot

This chapter provides a full overview of MBSP, the first formal training program of character strengths, and serves as a precursor to the remaining chapters, which review the details of the eight MBSP sessions and possible adaptations. This overview is divided into three main sections – introductory material such as basic assumptions and comments on the change process in MBSP; important practical information for running MBSP groups such as format, timing, and key reminders; and pilot research on the MBSP program. Ultimately, what matters when it comes to running MBSP, mindfulness programs, and other group approaches is the group process and interactions that occur in the group, i.e., the relationships participants have with themselves, the relationships they form with fellow group members, and the relationship the group leader is able to establish with the members. Thus, being proficient on the points in this chapter and subsequent chapters is only part of the responsibility of the practitioner.

Opening Story[1]

A farmer came upon an eagle's egg lying on the ground. In a hurry, he picked it up and placed it in the chicken coup along with several chicken eggs. In a couple days the egg hatched and the eagle was born. Assuming he was a chicken, the eagle clucked and pecked and dug for worms. It scurried about and occasionally jumped around, flying a few feet in the air like the chickens. Over the years, the eagle grew old and tired. One day it saw a magnificent bird flying overhead with grace, skill, and profound beauty. The bird was unfettered as it glided through wind and rain across the sky.

"Who is that?" asked the eagle.

"That's the king of the birds," replied a chicken, "The bald eagle! He is one with the sky. That is his home. We are chickens – our home is on the ground."

And so the eagle lived and died a chicken, for that's what he believed he was.

---

[1] An earlier version of this story appeared in Kornfield and Feldman (1996).

Introduction to MBSP

Introduction

At its best, the integration of mindfulness and character strengths is as follows: The practice of mindfulness *is* strengths and the practice of strengths *is* mindfulness. They cannot be separated. To practice mindful breathing or walking is to exercise self-regulation. To express a curious and kindly openness to the present moment experience is to practice mindfulness. To deploy strengths in a mindful way is to strengthen mindfulness, and a strong mindfulness is a recipe for more balanced and mindful strengths use.

MBSP is the culmination and innovation of the research and practice discussed earlier, which is an outgrowth of various mindfulness programs, scientific studies, and practices, some of which date back centuries. It emerges from my personal mindfulness practice and my professional mindfulness work leading hundreds of mindfulness groups, a myriad of workshops, seminars, and retreats, and working at the intersection of the science and practice of character strengths. It is also the result of feedback from several practitioners who have piloted MBSP in different countries (spanning four continents). MBSP is an attempt to integrate the strongest practices of mindfulness and character strengths together into one program.

As one MBSP practitioner observed, MBSP brings together different energies. Mindfulness is traditionally viewed as a quieting, oftentimes a calming approach, while character strengths practices are frequently energizing and immediately engaging. With mindfulness, the attention is focused or deliberately broadened with exercises such as sitting meditation, mindful walking, etc. With the practice of character strengths, individuals share times when they are at their best and discuss the strengths they are using while spotting and encouraging the strengths in others; this tends to build energy in oneself and others. The integration of such a variety of practices and energies provides for a fascinating synergy.

There are similarities and differences between MBSP and other mindfulness programs. The majority of existing mindfulness programs have an application focus that is geared toward decreasing or managing some kind of problem (e.g.,

stress levels, pain levels, emotional imbalance, marital conflict) or preventing/managing psychopathological behavior (e.g., depression episodes, anxiety episodes, substance abuse, binge eating). It is that problem area that often attracts participants and sets an expectation or an implicit mental framework around participants wanting to "decrease" or "get rid" of something that is wrong or dysfunctional, even if the tenets of mindfulness are explained as contrary to such expectations.

MBSP offers a different focal point. It brings the focus to that which is best in individuals – that which individuals are often mindless to – their character strengths. Kabat-Zinn (1990) has explained that the purpose of mindfulness is not to point out what is wrong, but to help people find what is right. MBSP opens the door to a language for people to re-discover and uncover what is right within them.

From the vantage point of psychological treatment, some might describe MBSP as a third-wave approach. These approaches to psychological treatment – in contrast to psychodynamic or cognitive-behavior therapy approaches – directly target acceptance, mindfulness, openness to experience, and valued living (Wilson et al., 2010). Nowhere in the MBSP title are the words "therapy," "coaching," or "consulting," and while MBSP is appropriate for each of these contexts, it should not be explicitly limited to one or another. First and foremost, MBSP is a practice (hence its title). Practice connotes something to work with and improve, to develop and deepen, and to increase and explore. There is no perfection that is to be achieved, no disorder to be ameliorated. MBSP is potentially for anyone. If a person is interested in connecting more with what is good within them, in wanting to strengthen their mindfulness practice, or in becoming more aware and savvy at using their strengths, then the fit might be a good one.

The driving motivations for why people meditate are twofold – to overcome psychological/emotional problems and to expand consciousness (Sedlmeier et al., 2012). While MBSP clearly aligns with both motivations and future research might bear out the utility of MBSP for each, it is the latter motivation that is fundamental to the program. The MBSP program is rooted in the wisdom, science, and best practices that preceded it. In addition, it presents new practices, adaptations to existing practices, and the first formal integration of this material. As discussed earlier, MBSP has substantive roots in the tradition of successful, empirically based mindfulness programs, namely MBCT, MBSR, and the eminently practical, less studied mindfulness work of Thich Nhat Hanh. Compared with other mindfulness programs from the participants' perspective, the focal point of MBSP for mindfulness work (i.e., strengths, rather than depression, stress, or medical illness) differs in content and offers an explicit emphasis on increasing and balancing the good rather than overcoming what's wrong (e.g., stress, depression). That said, the reality is that most mindfulness programs start from the vantage point of helping clients focus on "what is," rather than focusing on contriving something good or plucking something out that is bad.

Throughout MBSP, lecture points and exercises are drawn from the latest research in character strengths and occasionally from the general field of positive psychology. The VIA Institute on Character is a leading authority on the education and best practices of character strengths, and this work is infused throughout MBSP. There are many other phenomena in psychology and related fields that can be found in the MBSP framework and processes, including the science around self-concordance, broaden-and-build theory, mindset, goal-setting, and meaning.

MBSP operates from several basic assumptions about human beings. These include the following:

- People can build their character strengths and mindful awareness (mindfulness and character strengths are each malleable, to some degree).
- People can use their mindfulness and character strengths to deepen their self-awareness, foster insight, build relationships, reach their goals, and build a life of meaning and purpose.
- If people focus on bringing mindfulness to who they are – namely their best core qualities – this will enable them to use their strengths in a more balanced way.
- If people consciously bring their character strengths to their mindfulness practice and to mindful living, they will find ways to become

more consistent with their practice and in turn reap the benefits of regular mindfulness practice.

The Change Process in MBSP

As one observes the interactions and experiences in MBSP groups, growth is obvious and palpable. Sometimes the result is participants feeling more comfortable to face difficulties, sometimes it is individuals clearly improving their well-being or reaching their goals. Many times individuals exclaim that they are finally "smelling the roses," acknowledging strengths for the first time, and becoming kinder to others.

The metaphor of a chick hatching from an egg is often appropriate. Each person is changing at their own pace – some are hatching as they awaken to themselves for the first time. It's not uncommon to hear the phrase – "I wish I knew this stuff 20 years ago," or even "50 years ago" as was the case of a 70-year-old woman in one MBSP group. For others, the egg has just begun to crack open as the individual is beginning to challenge previous notions and habitual thinking, perhaps battling a fair amount of internal resistance. As one man put it, "I've resisted meditation for years and I fight against coming to this group each week, but something in me says that it's important that I be here each week. I think I see wisdom beginning to bubble." And there are others who "hatched" prior to the onset of MBSP and are adding to their mindfulness and strengths-based orientation as they, like a new chick, look at life with a beginner's mind.

Change in MBSP can be subtle, substantial, or both. By subtle, I mean that the learning can come in small, incremental changes, often not readily noticeable. However, when the individual looks back six or seven weeks earlier, the change is apparent. Small shifts in thinking or slight adjustments to behavior accumulate over time. These subtleties can create substantive change. This is likened to minimalist films that typically show one character simply living his or her life and they make a small change (e.g., take a different route home) or something happens to them (e.g., a cousin from out-of-town visits for the weekend) and the viewer is then treated to very subtle shifts in the character's worldview and behavior over time. For good examples of minimalist films and character strengths and mindfulness in films, see Appendix D and Niemiec and Wedding (2014).

In contrast, change can be substantial and obvious. Most MBSP groups will have one or several members who experience a major transformation in their thinking (e.g., how they view the world), emotions (e.g., how they feel about themselves and others), and/or behavior. Later in this chapter, I refer to "centerpiece, experiential exercises" for each of the MBSP sessions; this is meant to highlight one particular exercise each week that is particularly novel and packed with potential insight and growth opportunity. The raisin exercise in Session 1 often has this effect and in Session 2, those individuals who have taken the VIA Survey for the first time and see themselves described in terms of strengths may react with pleasant surprise. It's not uncommon for individuals to have gone through life blind to many of their core, good qualities and to come across a validated test that begins to describe them as a "person of strength" is a major breakthrough for such individuals.

Running MBSP Groups

Internal Structure of MBSP Sessions

I: Opening meditation: Character Strengths Breathing Space
II: Dyads or group discussion: Review of practice with mindfulness and strengths (this is usually preceded by a brief review of the previous session and the practices being worked with)
III: Introduction to new material
IV: Experiential – mindfulness/character strengths experience
V: Debriefing or virtue circle
VI: Suggested homework exercises for next session
VII: Closing with a strengths gatha[2]

This is the standard session structure, although slight adjustments are made each week (later chapters review these details). While most facilitators will follow this format, some situations/institutions may require adjustments. This might be due to certain settings (see Chapter 15), such as the education, business, correctional, or inpatient setting. Practitioners will need to assess whether the makeup of the group's participants warrants adjustments, for example, youth populations and therapy clients. Factors that can also have an impact, though not as significant, include groups with a significant level of meditation experience (e.g., if a practitioner is leading MBSP for their sangha/community), those with extensive knowledge and practice with positive psychology (e.g., those who've undergone intensive character strengths training), the quantity of participants in the group (e.g., a makeup of 5 vs. a makeup of 15), and participants' interest/willingness to partake in discussion (self-disclosure).

Timing

Each session is typically 2 hours for each of the 8 weeks, however, adjustments can be made. Here's the breakdown of some of the costs/benefits of using different time frames.

- 1.5 hours per session is efficient, although there is less discussion and no virtue circle. It has potential to feel "rushed," so care must be taken in managing time and the leader must be very strong in managing the boundaries of each exercise.
- 2 hours is a good balance that allows for full coverage of the material, exercises, and sufficient group discussion. Virtue circles are recommended.
- 2.5 hours allows for more in-depth mindfulness practices and for longer discussion periods, Q & A, and experiential exercises.
- Note: Due to setting limitations in some schools, businesses, and clinics, 1-hour sessions may be the only option. In these instances, it is recommended the group be extended to 16 weeks where two weeks are

---

2 MBSP leaders often rotate the gathas used from those on the gatha handout, self-created, or created by group participants. The work of Thich Nhat Hanh has many gathas that could be incorporated here as well.

spent on each topic area. A similar outcome will apply to many correctional and inpatient settings for similar reasons and due to clients' decreased ability to sustain engagement for long periods of time.

Preliminary research on the length of time of mindfulness programs has found that the effectiveness of mindfulness and the number of hours was nonsignificant; this means that adaptations or abbreviated versions may be appropriate (Carmody & Baer, 2009). Indeed, the mindfulness literature has revealed a number of abbreviated, brief, and adapted mindfulness programs which have shown promising results.

Studies have shown a positive impact of brief mindfulness meditation, sometimes abbreviating MBSR or MBCT programs. For example, brief mindfulness interventions have been shown to significantly improve pain tolerance (Liu, Wang, Chang, Chen, & Si, 2012), decrease pain sensitivity (Zeidan, Gordon, Merchant, & Goolkasian, 2010), improve sexual functioning (Brotto et al., 2012), decrease psychological distress and improve life satisfaction (Harnett et al., 2010), enhance self-control (Friese et al., 2012), and improve sustained attention and decreased fatigue and anxiety (Zeidan, Johnson, Diamond, David, & Goolkasian, 2010). Before drawing quick conclusions about abbreviating mindfulness programs, it is important to closely consider the context, population being served, match of the mindfulness program, quality of trainers, and other factors.

However, as will be discussed later, clients who have participated in MBSP across several cultures and settings have overwhelmingly reported that it is very important to attend all 8 MBSP sessions.

Prerequisites

Prior to the first group, it is important participants understand the MBSP program demands. Participants are asked to make a verbal commitment to several items. In some settings, an open forum and Q & A session is utilized by the MBSP facilitator where potential participants can learn more about the program, the expectations, and ask questions. This is also an opportunity for facili-

tators to screen out individuals who might not be suitable for the program based on the setting or hoped-for group makeup. Such screenings are routinely done in clinical settings and would be less applicable in many business settings, especially those in which an entire organizational team is participating in the MBSP group.

Participants are offered several optional items that can assist in their MBSP experience. Some participants make good use of these over the weeks, others see them as useful tools for post-MBSP experiences, and some individuals find them to be a distraction from an already-full program.

Core Commitments

- Commit to attend the full 8-week program[3]
- Willingness to share with others (some of the exercises in MBSP move participants out of their "comfort zone" and then invite participants to share some of these experiences with others)
- Commit to daily engagement with homework exercises
- Attendance at an MBSP retreat (if available)[4]
- Take the VIA Survey (by Session 2)
- Maintain a journal/notebook

Optional Purchases

- VIA reports: These are in-depth reports of the participants' results on the VIA Survey (www.viapros.org)
  - VIA Me Pathways Report: A consumer-friendly report with graphs, tips, quotes, and strategies for working with one's highest character strengths.

---

[3] I am frequently asked by participants who have scheduling conflicts whether it's OK to miss sessions. My general stance is that missing one session is probably alright, but a number of factors should be weighed, such as the impact on themselves, the impact on other group members, and possible enrollment in future MBSP groups.

[4] Not every practitioner will have the resources in terms of time and setting or the interest and skill-set for leading a retreat. Thus, practitioners may decide to lead MBSP with or without a retreat. If a practitioner decides to lead a retreat then it is strongly recommended that all participants attend. MBSP retreats are conducted anytime after Session 5 and some are used as a booster session after Session 8.

- VIA Pro Report: An extensive report used to help practitioners better understand their client's strengths; reviews signature strengths, the latest research, and best practices.
- Mindfulness CDs: by Jon Kabat-Zinn (purchase Series 1 or Series 2 at www.mindfulnesstapes.com)
- Optional purchase: *Full Catastrophe Living* (Kabat-Zinn, 1990)
- MBSP materials: *Mindfulness and Character Strengths* (Niemiec, 2013) including a CD; an MBSP workbook is forthcoming.

Beginning the Group

Sessions 2–8 start with a brief meditation followed by a practice review with the questions:
- What went well (www) with your mindfulness and strengths practice this week?[5]
- What obstacles did you face? How did you face the obstacles with mindfulness and/or with character strengths use?

Materials for Practitioners to Bring to Group

- Handouts (weekly)
- Instructor agenda and other notes (as needed)
- Bell
- White board & markers
- Raisins, bowl, spoon (Session 1)
- Books, as examples (Session 1 and as needed)
- Note cards for virtue circle (Session 1, optional)
- Stone or takeaway object (Session 8)

Homework Exercises

The amount of homework in mindfulness programs is intimidating for some participants. Thus,

each session has *suggested* homework exercises participants can engage in. The basic idea is that participants will develop some kind of mindfulness practice (e.g., formal meditation, some element of mindful living, etc.) and some awareness or practice relating to character strengths (e.g., strengths journal, strengths-spotting of others, etc.). The intention is these practices offer good learning opportunities throughout the program and can serve as the foundation for the cultivation of stronger practice habits in the future.

During this course, the minimum commitment participants should expect of themselves is to do at least one of the exercises relating to mindfulness and one of the exercises relating to character strengths each week. This will help keep both domains "top of mind" and make integration more likely (i.e., integration meaning "strong mindfulness" and "mindful strengths use.")

This issue of homework in mindfulness programs has been studied but the results are inconclusive. Researchers found that out of 98 mindfulness intervention studies that they analyzed, only 24 examined the connection between homework practice and outcomes (Vettese, Toneatto, Stea, Nguyen, & Wang, 2009). Of these studies, the results were mixed as to the positive impact or lack of impact of homework on the outcomes.

Maintenance

What will the participants continue to practice following the 8-week experience? Practitioners are encouraged to reflect on this question throughout the program. This idea is mentioned at the midpoint and then explicit questions and goal-setting exercises tap into this at Session 7 and are discussed in Session 8. It is likely participants will stick with something that they enjoy and feel competent in using. Those exercises that are repeated in both the group experience and as homework will contribute to participants feeling a sense of mastery and thus assist them in keeping the practice flowing after the program.

Some MBSP groups, in collaboration with their facilitators, have decided to build in follow-up sessions, booster sessions, and/or MBSP retreats (these optional add-on features are discussed

---

[5]   What went well (www) is a common phrase used by many practitioners, often found in positive psychology, for example, Fox Eades (2008) and Yeager, Fisher, and Shearon (2011). In this context, it is used as a core question for debriefing the MBSP homework from the previous week and as a way to frame the discussion.

in Chapter 15). These are a way for participants to stay connected with one another, build upon the concepts in the program, focus on maintenance of the practices, and prevent a return to autopilot tendencies.

Virtue Circle

The virtue circle (also called strengths circle) is a core part of MBSP that offers a formal, structured way for participants to connect with one another and experiment with many of the practices. While participants practice mindful listening and speaking during the homework practice review at the beginning of MBSP groups, the virtue circle offers a very different approach and generally offers new light to practices of mindfulness (e.g., listening) and strengths (e.g., strengths valuing). This is modeled on what some secular communities have called "wisdom circle" and what many Buddhist communities call a "Dharma discussion group."

Note that an alternate title for this experience is strengths circle. Some cultures, settings, and populations will prefer this title which can be viewed as a synonymous title to virtue circle; the title does not change the intention. Practitioners working with ministers or in a religious setting (e.g., church, synagogue, mosque) are likely to use the title virtue circle, while those who are in a purely secular setting might instead choose strengths circle.

Purpose

This is a space during the MBSP session for individuals to practice mindful listening and mindful speech, as well as strengths-spotting in others and strengths valuing.

Steps

These are general guidelines. Note that each of these will *not* be applicable in all settings. For example, the approach of "bowing" might be replaced with a "talking object" (participants listen mindfully to whomever is holding the object) or simply with hand-raising.

- The interaction typically begins with the sound of the bell, followed by silence. Silence connects the sharing of the participants' and is considered the default of the virtue circle. During silence, participants enjoy their breathing and practice just being present with others.
- The facilitator reviews the purpose, the practice, and logistics of the virtue circle.
- After the facilitator bows indicating they are done speaking, there is silence.
- Anyone can begin. When an individual is ready to share something, they bow to the group to indicate their intention to speak and show respect to the group.
  - The individual practices mindful speech while sharing.
  - The individual might choose to spot strengths in another group member; they may wish to share their experience from an earlier meditation/exercise/lecture point; or they may wish to review something with the homework that they hadn't yet shared.
  - The individual indicates they're done speaking with another bow.
  - Typically, the group returns each bow.
  - Silence, until another person bows in.

Additional guidelines
- The instructor may decide to bow in at any point to let people know how much time is left; to offer their own sharing; to spot strengths; to remind people about mindful speech/listening practice; or to bring up a topic area for participants to consider.
- In most instances, before a person shares a second time, all participants would have shared one time or at least been given the space to share. The engagement of back-and-forth (i.e., cross-talk) with other participants is highly discouraged; an exception to this occurs when an individual is spotting/valuing strengths in another participant. Questions and comments are generally directed to the whole group. Participants prioritize the sharing of experiences rather than the sharing of advice.
- Content discussed in the virtue circle (what is being discussed?):
  - *Debriefing* of the most recent exercise in the group; participants share what struck them.
  - Sharing other experiences from the group, insights from the homework, progress with mindfulness/strengths practice.

- *Strengths-spotting*: naming strengths of others observed in the session.
- *Relationship valuing*: expressing appreciation for others' strengths.
- Process areas of the virtue circle (how is it discussed?):
  - *Mindful listening*: tuning in to the words being said/unsaid; body language; energy.
  - *Mindful speaking*: sharing from the heart; is also clear, direct, succinct, substantive; practicing a balance of sharing that is not too much and not too little.
  - *Strengths in motion*: the way that participants interact – with or without words – can be a display of strengths in motion. Participants will find themselves expressing the character strengths of love, kindness, social intelligence, self-regulation, perspective, fairness, forgiveness, and curiosity, among others.

Concluding the Group

For those who are implementing two-hour+ groups, it is optimal to allow the last 30 minutes (minimum) for a virtue circle. This is followed by a review of potential homework exercises for the following week and a meditation to complete the group experience. This brief closing meditation also serves as a bookend to the opening meditation of each session.

Journaling or Tracking

Both are important. Some participants will naturally gravitate toward one over another. For example, those that like to do creative writing will probably be more interested in journaling. Some individuals choose to do both but all participants should choose at least one.

Tracking sheets
The tracking sheet provided each week is a systematic way to practice self-monitoring – keeping track of your meditation behaviors, challenges, insights, strengths used, and progress. Self-monitoring is a solid, scientific tool that helps people make lasting changes in their lives. Participants

are encouraged to review these sheets periodically and look for patterns. Some questions that facilitators might ask participants include: What has stood out to you in your self-monitoring? What obstacles have been coming up in your mindfulness practices? What character strengths did you use to manage the obstacles?

Journaling
Keeping an ongoing journal (in a separate notebook, computer file, etc.) is a way to explore your experiences, feelings, and ideas in a deep way. There are no limits to where the journaling can take you. Some people take a stream-of-consciousness approach and just allow their ideas and thoughts about a particular topic to flow freely and they write down anything that comes to mind, letting go of all judgment. Research has found journaling to be an effective exercise for self-growth and for dealing with problems. While it is not necessary to re-read what has been written, it is sometimes interesting to do so. In general, participants might be asked: What have you been saying to yourself in your journal? Have you been giving yourself any important advice? What is the most important thing you have learned about yourself through journaling?

Leading Mindfulness Experiences

Before offering any guided mindfulness experience, it is important to study and practice working with the underlying ingredients of experiential exercises. The voice tone, pacing, time length, content, pauses, intentions, and structure vary significantly across types of meditations and experiential exercises. For example, a person leading a transcendental meditation will take a different approach and may sound quite different from someone leading a mindful breathing exercise.

The more that practitioners can understand about the underlying process for setting up, framing, leading, and debriefing experiential exercises, the better. Supervision and feedback from veteran practitioners is an *essential* prerequisite. Practitioners should be discouraged from simply picking up a book with meditation scripts and then reading the scripts in mindfulness sessions without previous practice and supervision.

Hypnosis scholar and master therapist, Michael Yapko (2011), offers a compelling comparison of the parallel features of guided mindfulness meditation (GMM) and hypnotherapeutic inductions. This informs practitioners about the depth and intricacy of experiential exercises. He explains there are seven similar steps between GMM and hypnosis and in his book he examines mindfulness scripts from various meditation leaders (e.g., Tara Brach) and explains how these steps unfold in the meditation experience. According to Yapko, the seven stages of experiential processes when working with a client (in the psychotherapeutic context) are as follows:

1. Prepare the client: Offer psychoeducation about the meditation and build in client expectancy of success.
2. Orient them to the experience.
3. Build a focus through hypnotic induction or mindful focusing.
4. Build a response set: Yapko refers to this as building positive momentum toward therapeutic objectives.
5. Offer suggestions for change: This refers to giving direct or indirect suggestions geared toward the client's goals.
6. Offer contextualization of new behaviors and perceptions: Draw a link between the person's current experiences and their personal life.
7. Disengage and reorient: Conclude the experience and orient them to their present moment.

These stages are not only useful for new practitioners learning to formulate and understand experiential approaches but also for seasoned practitioners to turn back toward the mindfulness exercises they are currently offering clients and ensuring these stages are accounted for. This then aids in offering a thorough, deep, and personally relevant experience for the client.

Centerpiece, Experiential Exercises in MBSP

Within the dynamics of a group process, time can easily become mismanaged. One strategy in managing time in the midst of a particular session is to recall the session's main, centerpiece exercise and to allow plenty of time for the experience and de-briefing; from there, the remaining portions of the group can be appropriately worked around that. Based on MBSP participants' feedback and MBSP leaders' observations, there is a large potential for insights and "ah-ha" moments in these exercises.

Session 1: Raisin exercise
  Why?: Shows participants that mindfulness can be brought to any experience.

Session 2: You, at your best (includes strengths-spotting)
  Why?: Shows participants they have the ability to spot strengths in oneself and others.

Session 3: Statue meditation
  Why? Allows participants to experience the application of mindfulness and strengths with fairly challenging obstacles.

Session 4: Mindful walking
  Why? Shows mindfulness is part of daily life and strengths can easily be embedded.

Session 5: Loving-kindness meditation followed by strength-exploration meditation
  Why? Shows specific strengths can be targeted with meditation and built from within.

Session 6: Character strengths 360 review *and* fresh start meditation
  Why? The perspective of others brings a new vantage point to one's strengths and the meditation brings a new vantage point to reframing/managing problems.

Session 7: Best possible self exercise
  Why? Draws a solid link between the MBSP program and future plans/goals.

Session 8: Golden nuggets exercise
  Why? Draws a connection between each participant, a key learning, and growth points.

Processes Woven in the MBSP Structure

When MBSP practitioners are studying this program, it is advisable to step back and observe the various processes that are implemented in MBSP that engender optimal flow and growth. Understanding and working with these ideas boosts the confidence of the leader and drives the focus more to the process of the work rather than getting lost in content. Becoming familiar with each of these will enable practitioners to respond more effectively to questions from participants.

- Participants apply this work to themselves (self-awareness, self-improvement) prior to focusing on relationships.
- Participants practice exercises that build from the concrete (e.g., the raisin, one's body) to the abstract (e.g., strengths, emotions, and lastly thoughts).
- Participants explore and experiment with experiences before having them explained in detail (usually).
- Participants practice with both direct (i.e., guided mindfulness meditation) and purist (i.e., open-ended) mindfulness experiences each week to highlight the value of each and reach the personal interests of a wider range of individuals.
- Practitioners and participants employ a growth mindset in the practice of exploring and seeing opportunities and strength at challenging times.
- Practitioners take an "hourglass approach" in terms of session content in most groups by going from general to specific to general. For example, an overview and review; specific new content; summary and ideas for moving forward.
- Practitioners facilitate a particular strengths process for participants: aware, then explore, then apply (see Chapter 2 and Chapter 13).
  - Aware: Helping individuals to better *access* themselves.
  - Explore: Helping individuals to *explore* their previous/current strengths use.
  - Apply: Helping individuals to *align* their strengths with what they are doing to create their best life.

Key Reminders

In each session, the following underlying themes are useful to give priority to:

- *When there is doubt or particular emotionality, consider asking a question or allowing for silence for the group to be with the experience.* The former means to unleash your curiosity, the latter means to use your self-regulation (controlling the impulse to have to say something).
- *Emphasize discussions over Q & A.* While creating opportunities to ask questions is important, this does shift the focus toward one individual's needs and away from the group dynamic, therefore pros and cons must always be weighed. The group itself is a mindfulness community thus finding ways to catalyze this maintains the community's authenticity.
- *Emphasize experiences and practices.* Practitioners offer insights and principles to lead participants to greater self-knowledge, but it's the live practice that usually has the biggest impact. A group session that does not have a healthy couple of doses of practice/experience is less likely to have an impact.
- *Strike a balance of dyad homework reviews and large group reviews.* The former allows for every participant to share while the latter allows every participant to hear how others are doing.
- *Prioritize stories, personal examples, and metaphors.*
- *Give participants space.* As discussed in Chapters 5 and 15, participants need space to share their experiences. In some instances, I've allowed the homework practice review and debriefing to take up over half of an entire session. The leader's inclination might be to share more knowledge – and this is a treasured part of MBSP – however, individuals will likely learn more through discussions that help to solidify applications. Individuals may spontaneously create or discover inspiring material and show interest in sharing stories, quotes, sacred readings, poems, movie examples, and handcrafts. For example, one woman rallied her creativity to make special quilts for her grandchildren and effort was made to allow for group time to share this.
- *Integrate a bell.* When possible, allow the bell to do the "talking." Bells can begin and end meditations, begin and end strength exercises, serve as a cue to return to the present moment, and can offer a simulation of present moment awareness that participants can repeat outside of the group.
- *Maintain a consciousness of integration areas (strong mindfulness and mindful strengths*

use). The following two questions can go through the facilitator's mind while leading groups:

- As participants practice mindful sitting, walking, eating, talking, and listening, do they seem to be aware of those strengths they are naturally using?
- As participants discuss strengths, might a mindful pause or inquiry help to harness mindfulness to explore the strengths further?

- *Relationships are a focal point.* In discussions, examples, lectures, and responses to questions, emphasize the focus as bringing benefit to both one's relationship with *oneself* AND one's relationship with *others*. This is also evidenced in the weekly meditations and the virtue circle. In this way, relationships are a meta-theme of MBSP.

Overlapping and Opposing Phenomena

MBSP facilitators should be aware that there are many tensions present in mindfulness and strengths processes. Each of these dynamics exists when working with mindfulness and character strengths and each dynamic has both similarities and contrasts. While care must be taken in teaching or addressing the differences, each can become an important teaching point. Some are more process-related, some more content-related, and others are directly related to the approach of the practitioner. Many of these can be addressed in discussions or in Q & A periods.

- *Changing vs. accepting.* Change and acceptance are often two sides of the same coin in which one automatically affects or creates the other. They often appear to be in opposition, such as when an individual wants to change something about themselves or their present moment and the task at hand is to move toward greater acceptance of how things are in the moment.
- *Mindfulness vs. relaxation.* Mindfulness practice sometimes leads to greater physiological relaxation and a serene mind and relaxation approaches sometimes lead to greater mindfulness. However, it's important to explain to par-

ticipants that the purpose of mindfulness is to create greater awareness not to intentionally bring about relaxation.

- *Being vs. doing.* Connecting with what "is" in the present moment, allowing oneself to be as one is, being present to the raw essence of a sound or with one's movement – these are examples of being. Doing is the mode of action, of work, and of multi-asking.
- *Reacting vs. responding.* Reacting is automatic and habitual, it is often an immediate impulse, while responding is an action that is conscious, deliberate, and skillful.
- *Having thoughts vs. metacognition.* Metacognition refers to thinking about one's thinking, being aware of one's thoughts, beliefs, and mental processes.
- *Relationship with oneself vs. relationship with others.* How we connect with and respond to our mind and behaviors forms the way that we relate to ourselves.
- *Character strength vs. talents, skills, and interests.* Character strengths are who we are at our core and are different from other types of strength. Talents are what we do well, skills are what we have gained proficiency to do, and interests are passions that engage us.
- *The teacher/leader in front of the room vs. the teacher/leader within.* The former is an approach focused on lecturing and imparting knowledge, and presents a distance between expert and student. The latter approach is more collaborative and emphasizes the student as expert with the answers within, and the approach is to create opportunities for the student to access and unleash insights.
- *Mindfulness and character strengths vs. other areas of positive psychology.* Mindfulness and character strengths have a natural integration, harmony, and mutual benefit, and while other areas commonly studied in positive psychology may not be the focal point of the sessions, many emerge as a result of this work such as positive emotions, resilience, and flow.
- *Mindful eating vs. savoring.* Savoring involves intentionally staying with the positive and relishing in it. Mindful eating is to observe and notice the changing present moment experience of eating which may or may not be pleasant.

- *Mindful listening/speaking vs. active-con-structive responding (ACR).* ACR is a particular way of responding in a positive, genuine and encouraging way to someone who shares good news. The former is the larger construct that includes ACR and can be used as an approach whether the news is good, bad, or neutral.
- *Bare attention vs. focusing on strengths.* The former refers to a raw, pure focus on the breath or present moment. It is the clear seeing of something without its label, such as being present to a sound without naming who or what is producing it. A focus on strengths in a meditation experience is not bare attention to whatever is present, but instead is deliberately bringing something to the mind, followed by mindful observation. Sometimes this is called guided mindfulness meditation.

Managing Challenges in MBSP Groups

The following are typical issues that can emerge when teaching MBSP, and are common in most mindfulness intervention programs that are longer than a couple weeks. Some of these are issues that emerge from participants and others are issues that occur within the practitioner. This is not an exhaustive list; however, understanding these ideas may serve to generalize to other issues that may emerge.

Issue: Practitioner feels overwhelmed or confused as to what action to take.

Potential adjustment: The first step is to pause and check in with oneself. Take a "10-second breathing space." Ask yourself: Is inaction what is needed right now? Often individuals need to remind themselves not to "do" anything, but instead to just "be present" to the experience happening in them and around them. The practitioner should also remind themselves of one of the purposes of the A-E-A model, that the model serves as a lighthouse offering a guiding ray of light as to what might be a next step for the client. Does the individual need further *awareness* of their strengths, deeper *exploration* of their strengths, or are they ready to *apply* some step to move forward with their goals or life plans?

Issue: Participant feels overwhelmed noting there is too much material.

Potential adjustment: The participant should be asked whether they are finding time to build practices relating to strengths and relating to mindfulness each week, even if they aren't practicing daily. You can clarify with them that the main task in terms of homework practice is to do "something" with mindfulness and "something" with character strengths each week rather than to feel they must do every assignment each week perfectly. They can also be reminded that by making it to the group each week they are showing a good commitment to the practices and to the others in the group. This consistency and success can be built upon.

Issue: Participant says they are frustrated with the MBSP experience.

Potential adjustment: If the facilitator suspects that this might be a common experience among several other members then some time might be allotted to discuss the frustration openly. This can be accompanied with a mutual practice of mindful breathing, mindful communication, and character strengths expression.

Issue: Practitioner does not feel ready to lead a group; may feel a lack of confidence.

Potential adjustment: These individuals are encouraged to consider applying MBSP first in a one-on-one situation. This helps practitioners become more comfortable with the material, handling logistics and handouts, and applying it to others' needs. For many practitioners, a 1-on-1 situation is less intimidating than a group situation. Years ago, I took this approach with MBCT. While I had been leading a weekly mindfulness group experience for years, I wanted to fine tune the material and some of the meditations before implementing the more formal structure with a group. I discussed this possibility with two or three individual clients suffering from recurrent depression. Upon hearing their interest and collaboratively integrating mindfulness into this treatment plans, I adjusted the MBCT to fit with this individual work. This made the transition to the group setting several months later more seamless.

Issue: Individuals present a question and the leader does not know how to respond.

Potential adjustment: Depending on the question, it might be important to respond with "I don't know," "I will investigate that," "Let's investigate this together," or use it as a growth opportunity by inviting the individual to take action in some way and report back to the group. Here are some examples that have occurred in MBSP groups and challenges that can be posed directly to the individual in the group setting:

- After several group sessions a woman exclaims: I just don't understand what mindfulness is. I just don't get it.
  - *Challenge:* Use your love of learning to read a mindfulness passage or article and listen to one mindfulness CD track. Report back to the group explaining what mindfulness is and your experience of it.
- A woman noting she doesn't agree with the VIA Survey results, noting two strengths among her top five that should not be there.
  - *Challenge:* Describe these two strengths and why you think they are important qualities in human beings. Why have the great philosophers, world religions, and other thinkers valued these two strengths throughout time? Please re-evaluate yourself from the context of these descriptions. We'll check in on this challenge in a couple of weeks.
- A man explaining he doesn't think he'll benefit from using his signature strengths more.
  - *Challenge:* This might be true if you continue to use your signature strengths in the same way and the only thing that changes is frequency. Instead, consider how you can widen the way you use your signature strengths. Reflect on how you can be mindful of the potential of strength overuse while simultaneously consider situations and scenarios in your life in which you are underusing these strengths.

MBSP for the Practitioner

Your Presence
Since those who lead MBSP groups practice character strengths use and mindfulness meditation on a regular basis, the ability to maintain a connectedness to oneself during MBSP sessions is likely to come naturally. Practitioners use their mindfulness and strengths consciously and deliberately during groups. Mindful speech, listening, breathing, and strengths expression are modeled in each session. In short, MBSP practitioners "walk the talk" by practicing and integrating mindfulness and character strengths regularly.

Practitioners can turn to their signature strengths when they are confused, concerned, elated, or content. Practitioners are encouraged to share their signature strengths and examples of their use, overuse, and development over the weeks with the group. For example, those high in curiosity can turn to posing questions to the group, those high in gratitude might express this heartfelt feeling to the group, those high in teamwork might pose a query as to how the group can connect together to address a particular topic, and those high in perspective/wisdom might spontaneously offer an inspirational quote.

Mindful practitioners know when to "hold the moment" for participants by being present to difficulties, joys, and moments of insight. Several books have discussed this role of the mindful practitioner such as *The Mindful Therapist* (Siegel, 2010) and *Therapeutic Presence: A Mindful Approach to Effective Therapy* (Geller & Greenberg, 2012). In the latter, therapeutic presence is the state of bringing one's whole self to the encounter with a client by being completely in the moment – physically, emotionally, cognitively, and spiritually. This is explained as involving a philosophical commitment to be present and engaging in a personal mindfulness practice to cultivate this.

A foundational aspect of mindfulness practices is the practitioner's personal warmth and compassion for others, which practitioners cultivate in their own mindfulness practice. MBSP practitioners exude this friendliness and kindness in their interaction and leadership of MBSP sessions. As described by Segal, Williams, and Teasdale (2013), kindness and compassion are the ground from which mindfulness is practiced, taught, and cultivated.

One MBSP leader was struggling to find balance in managing the often uplifting effect of character strengths exercises and the often calming effect of mindfulness exercises. At times during groups, these shifts in energy led her to feel as if something was wrong in the group or that she was not taking the optimal approach. She began to place greater emphasis on her "presence" to the group. In addition, she brought greater mindfulness to this internal experience. She realized she would have to deepen her bravery strength in leading the group as well as increase her curious questioning. For the remainder of the MBSP sessions, she built in additional personal mindfulness practice immediately prior to each group experience and made deliberate effort to be present to herself, the energy of the content, and the group's energy. This had a remarkable impact on her feeling more centered in the group and more connected to its shifting energy from moment-to-moment.

The Value of Priming

Strengths priming serves the function of getting oneself ready to use a strength in action and it brings the strength into consciousness. Research has found that priming either mindfulness or strengths prior to a session has good benefits.

- Priming with strengths (thinking or talking about a client's strengths for 5 minutes prior to a session) led to greater strengths activation as rated by independent observers, fostered mastery experiences, improved the therapeutic relationship, and enhanced therapy outcome (Fluckiger & Grosse Holtforth, 2008).
- Priming with mindfulness (practicing mindfulness for five minutes prior to a therapy session) led to therapists perceiving themselves as being more present in sessions; while clients thought therapists were present whether or not they did the exercise, clients did perceive therapists to be more effective when they primed with mindfulness (Dunn, Callahan, Swift, & Ivanovic, 2012).

Prior to some MBSP groups, I would prime myself to a particular character strength I wanted to be sure to express. I did not want the group members to perceive me in a higher light of some kind. And, I knew that I could easily slip into an expert-mode, a "telling" approach, and spending too much time reporting facts and figures (e.g., research tidbits). This is alright at times but my sense was this should not be the emphasis, therefore, shortly before particular sessions

I primed myself to humility – sometimes I would reflect on humble thoughts, image a humble person, and remind myself of the real reasons I was there. I reminded myself that my positive psychology and mindfulness colleagues and I are each standing on the shoulders of many great thinkers and leaders that preceded us, who also were standing on the shoulders of earlier great thinkers. The strength of humility also helps to build the perspective that MBSP work is really about the individuals in the group (not the facilitator), and what matters most is helping participants learn, experience, and get the most out of each week.

Before starting an MBSP program, and prior to a given group, consider what strength(s) you would like to bring forth in the group. Also, consider implementing a personal practice of mindfulness prior to each session.

Research on MBSP

As with any new program, research is needed to evaluate the program's structure, populations of benefit, change mechanisms, and overall effectiveness. Research on MBSP is underway and ongoing. Initial pilot data on MBSP has been conducted and reveals promising results. The data and findings are provided in this section.

Qualified Practitioners

Practitioners implementing MBSP should be knowledgeable *and* experienced with both mindfulness and character strengths, and supervision and/or co-leadership of the sessions should be implemented where appropriate.

In preparation for this book, I piloted MBSP groups with different populations. In addition, a handful of specially qualified practitioners from around the world piloted the program with different populations and offered me feedback and critiques to improve MBSP, to enhance cross-cultural viability, and to boost ideas in adapting MBSP to special populations (Chapter 15). Many of these suggestions have made it into this book;

some have been integrated into MBSP as formal and optional features of the program.

Here are the rigorous criteria used to select the MBSP practitioners to lead pilot programs (note: the majority of individuals who showed interest in leading an MBSP group did not meet these criteria):

- Maintenance of a regular, personal mindfulness meditation practice of some kind (ideally the individual would have regular participation with a local sangha/community of mindfulness/meditation).
- Personal practice regularly paying attention to, deploying, and/or increasing one's own character strengths.
- Experience applying mindfulness to individuals of the same demographics and problems one is intending to implement MBSP with (e.g., clinical clients; general population; students; business professionals).
- Good knowledge of VIA character strengths – background, benefits, interventions, exploratory questions; has experience using the VIA Survey; uses a strength-based approach that includes strengths discussions with clients/employees/students.
- First-hand experimentation or at least has read recent articles exploring the integration of mindfulness and character strengths.
- Familiarity with the MBSP program (Chapters 6–15).
- Willingness to offer feedback (e.g., discussing critiques, strengths, ideas, adjustments of MBSP group) before, during, and after the 8-week pilot experience.
- Willingness to receive feedback and discuss (by Skype) the experiences of the MBSP group, including adjustment strategies for improving as the leader from session to session.
- Willingness to collaboratively make adjustments to best fit the culture and setting. Practitioners found that very minimal changes were needed in this vein (see Chapter 15 for a discussion).

These criteria directly express that those who lead MBSP, mindfulness meditation groups, or related mindfulness experiences should be engaged in a practice of mindfulness themselves. Kabat-Zinn (2003) relates this necessity to authenticity, explaining that mindfulness cannot be taught in an authentic way if the instructor is not practicing in their own life.

The first and second criteria in relation to a personal practice are the most crucial and form the basis for one's work in the group. In addition to one's own conscious self-growth process, practitioners should have experience applying the concepts with their particular client population and be psychologically flexible as they apply the material. Those practitioners who meet these criteria are more likely to be comfortable with the material and be more adept at handling resistance, questions, or struggles that may emerge in the group experience.

MBSP – Initial Pilot Research

In 2011, I conducted a small pilot study with an experimental group (8 individuals completed MBSP) and a control group (7 individuals who received no intervention). The experimental group consisted mostly of experienced meditators who were part of a local sangha/mindfulness community, while the control group was a mix of meditators and nonmeditators. Groups completed a set of pre- and post-intervention measures. The measures completed were:

- Mindfulness: The Five Factor Mindfulness Questionnaire (Baer, Smith, Hopkins, Krietemeyer, & Toney, 2006): 39 questions with subscale measures including observe, describe, act with awareness, nonjudging, nonreacting; results also reveal a total score for mindfulness.
- Signature strengths use: four questions courtesy of the VIA Institute that address identity and signature strengths expression.
  - Signature strengths/flourishing link ("My greatest fulfillments in life occur when I express those parts of myself that are core to who I am").
  - Signature strengths – work ("My work is an expression of who I am at my core, not just something I do well").
  - Signature strengths – relationships ("My personal relationships give me the opportunity to express the best parts of myself").

- Signature strengths – community ("My activities in my community are vehicles by which I express my best self").
- Depression: the 2-question depression screen assessing sadness and anhedonia.
- Happiness: the 5-question Satisfaction with Life Scale (Diener, Emmons, Larsen, & Griffin, 1985).
- Flourishing: the 8-question Flourishing Scale (Diener et al., 2009).
- Meaning: one question from the Flourishing Scale taps meaning.
- Engagement: the Positive Psychotherapy Questionnaire, courtesy of Tayyab Rashid (2008), also called the Orientations to Happiness Questionnaire, includes several questions on engagement. These 7 questions were extracted and used to elicit a total score for engagement, including knowledge; activities; problem-solving; concentration; flow; management; accomplishment.

Findings

I calculated the means of several variables for the experimental group and the control group. The experimental group (MBSP) *increased* substantially from pre- to post-test on the following:
- Flourishing
- Engagement
- Signature strengths/flourishing link
- Signature strengths – work
- Signature strengths – relationships
- Signature strengths – community

In the Experimental group (MBSP) there was *no changes* or negligible changes on the following variables:
- Depression (2 questions)
- Meaning (1 question)
- Mindfulness overall

Those variables in which the experimental group was *substantially* higher than the control group include:
- Flourishing
- Engagement
- Signature strengths – work
- Signature strengths – relationships
- Signature strengths – community

Limitations

In addition to the small sample size, the groups were not randomized (but were self-selected) and were not equivocal on all demographics, as evidenced by the experimental group having greater levels of previous meditation experience than the control group. In addition, this pilot group represented one of the early versions of MBSP which has since been revised and improved.

Summary

The experimental group had what appeared to be five meaningful differences over the control group, namely in flourishing, engagement, and use of signature strengths in important domains of life. There were no changes in mindfulness, which is not surprising since the experimental group consisted of long-time meditators who practiced weekly in a mindfulness community together (e.g., ceiling effect). There were no changes in depression; however, this was not a clinical group (it was a healthy group from the community), so this, too, is unremarkable. Future studies will need to include more in-depth measures of meaning and purpose.

This initial pilot evidence that MBSP might lead to improvements in certain areas of well-being, particularly among meditators, should be viewed with caution until further research validates and extends these findings.

MBSP – Qualitative Feedback

Eight initial MBSP pilot groups ranging from 3–13 individuals from six countries (United States, Denmark, Hong Kong/China, France, Portugal, and Australia) were conducted. The perception of individuals was unilaterally positive. Without exception, every participant completing MBSP reported experiencing an increase in their overall well-being at the end of the program. Nearly every person also reported an improvement in their stress management. There have been no reports of worsening well-being or stress management to date. No negative "side effects" of MBSP have been reported to date.

In early 2013, I reviewed the (confidentially submitted) qualitative reports of individuals completing MBSP from these eight groups. Strong positive effects were demonstrated on *all* of the following (with the strongest reported first):

- Overall well-being
- Sense of who you are (identity)
- Meaning in life
- Sense of purpose
- Engagement with life tasks
- Management of stress
- Quality of relationships
- Sense of accomplishment
- Management of problems

When asked what participants feel they are able to do as a result of completing MBSP, a number of areas were highlighted. The most common included:

- Aware of my signature strengths
- Deepened my mindfulness practice
- Used strengths to deal with my problems/difficulties
- Spotted strengths in others more frequently
- Used mindfulness to face my problems/difficulties
- Started a new mindfulness practice
- Verbally appreciated strengths more in others
- Used my strengths more often
- Overcame more obstacles in my mindfulness practice

Across the MBSP groups, which varied in time length (1.5 hour sessions and 2-hour sessions) and population, the following qualitative feedback was reported: Participants strongly preferred or expressed interest in 2-hour sessions and found that this was "just right" in terms of the amount of time in a session. In general, participants found that eight sessions was the right number of weeks. A moderate percentage of participants preferred additional sessions, while an interest in fewer sessions was not reported. The interest in having additional sessions might be managed by adding the optional features discussed in Chapter 15, such as the MBSP Retreat and MBSP booster sessions.

Within a given MBSP group, the majority of participants wanted large group discussions to be about ⅓ of the time of the group experience, with very few wanting more or less time. The majority of participants found that having about ⅓ of the

group time spent practicing with strengths or a mindfulness meditation to be optimal; about one-quarter of participants wanted more time spent on these practices and no one reported wanting less time. In terms of benefit to one's learning and growth, participants ranked the lecture/input periods and the whole-group discussions as most important; this tended to be followed by group meditations, then homework exercises/practices, then one-on-one activities with group sessions. Despite being ranked the lowest, participants tended to report appreciating having time for dyadic experiences, which are part of several MBSP sessions.

During mindfulness practices, the three most significant obstacles that emerged for individuals were:

- Not enough time/too busy
- Forgot to practice
- Mind wandered too much

Regarding homework offered in MBSP, the majority of participants reported that the right amount of homework was being suggested each week, with a handful of people saying it was too much. That finding notwithstanding, it is interesting to note that when asked about how much of the homework participants completed on average (from 0%–100%), most participants did not report completing 90–100%. Nearly ⅔ of participants reported completing 50% or more and about ⅓ of people reported completing between 10–40% of the homework. In terms of which homework exercises people practiced routinely, the following were the most frequently endorsed:

- Mindfulness meditation
- Reflection on past use of strengths
- Observing others' strengths
- Tracking strengths use
- Appreciating others' strengths
- Working with using strengths

In terms of attendance at all 8 sessions (i.e., not missing any sessions), the vast majority of people believe it is "extremely important" to attend all 8 sessions.

There are a variety of mindfulness and strengths practices that participants report as their favorite practice in MBSP. The two most beloved mindfulness practices were the character strengths breathing space exercise and the loving-kindness meditation. The two most beloved strengths practices were the character strengths 360 exercise and the strengths interview.

When asked about the benefits of the virtue circle that is part of the MBSP 2-hour sessions, several benefits/comments have been reported:

- I see it like a sacred space where respect, awareness, reflection and recognition take place. This gives great value to the group.
- Mindful listening practice; getting comfortable with silence helped me.
- The process was very enabling; we all had a chance to easily make comments.
- Being verbal in our appreciation of others was a good benefit.
- I found it helpful to recognize that things could just come up naturally during silence. It was a revelation to me … also, hearing how others in the group were impressed with my strengths.
- We got to know each other and felt closer. It gave reassurance to my personal experience (i.e., that I was in line with others). New aspects of the experience of the workshop for me were integrated.
- Someone said something positive about me that really surprised me.
- It gave me time to explain what is on my mind without others interrupting; it catalyzed mindful listening.
- I really enjoyed listening to others' thoughts, experiences, and their personal journey.
- Others' comments increased my awareness of character strengths.

When queried about the impact of MBSP on one of their relationships, the vast majority of participants stated MBSP has had a positive impact and they were able to name a specific instance. Here are a few examples:

- At about the time this group began I got a call from my son. I had not heard from him for 6 years. I am using mindfulness and character strengths in my dialog with him.
- It opened a channel of communication with my husband.
- This has affected my relationship with myself – I have more confidence.
- In my relationships, I have slowed down my thought processes, and learned to recognize

my strengths and the strengths in others. I am a calmer, happier, more joyous person who is not afraid of facing life's obstacles. In fact, now I welcome them.

- I've been able to take several of my relationships to a deeper level. My acceptance of "what is" has improved considerably. The way I relate to challenges posed to me by others has improved considerably.
- MBSP allows me to take a few steps back and to realize that my strengths might be different from the strengths of others.
- I am more mindful of others. I don't react as impulsively. I reflect on what is happening around me.
- It has most certainly had a positive effect on my relation to my family – more presence, joy, and positivity. When I give more, I get more back! I have really felt that.
- I noticed an increased attention/closeness to my immediate family and friends. I'm taking more of a beginner's mind, not responding to my own thoughts but instead I'm listening and pausing – I'm often in "being mode" now.
- More of the time I can reframe my close relationships in positive ways and use mindfulness when I get irritated and anxious. I feel I have more tools.
- It has helped a lot with my dealing with my business partner relationship. I'm able to use mindfulness while communicating and responding to her, and with positive tones, recognizing the rough emotions and thoughts I still get, but not to be too affected by them. It has been effective and I was able to get better results and more positive responses from my partner. I also feel a lot more at peace in my heart.
- My relationship with my staff improved because I focused more on their strengths and they were very happy and worked harder as a result.

Final comments

These quantitative and qualitative findings suggest MBSP may be able to have an impact in a number of ways on individuals. Due to the research limitations discussed, no definitive conclusions can be drawn about the program as a whole, how it compares to other mindfulness or positive psychology programs, or who will benefit most from the program. Therefore, researchers are encouraged to study MBSP and practitioners are encouraged to study, understand, and wisely implement the program with appropriate caveats.

MBSP – Most Common Q & A

What's the biggest focus of MBSP?
It is certainly both mindfulness and character strengths. Each is the priority and each can be the basis to serve the other. An easy way to think of it is breaking the integration down into 2 parts:
1. Adding character strengths to your mindfulness practice (strong mindfulness): When one doesn't want to meditate, call forth perseverance. When one is struggling with mindful eating, call forth curiosity about the food or self-regulation with the pace of eating. Such an approach helps to make mindfulness stronger.
2. Adding mindfulness to your character strengths practice (mindful strengths use): When one is engaged in a strengths practice such as using signature strengths in new ways, call forth mindful awareness to remember to do it each day, but also to pay attention to the thoughts and feelings involved in using one's strengths. Another part of character strengths work involves finding the balance to not overuse or underuse one's strengths and to be sensitive to the context one is in. Therefore, maintaining a curious and open mindfulness approach will help the individual be aware of how one is using one's strengths and whether one is coming across too strongly in a given situation.

It is artificial to say one is more important than the other. They are interconnected. MBSP helps people learn about mindfulness and about character strengths. Both are taught, both are discussed, both are experienced live, and both are practiced, but it is ultimately the integration that is the focus.

How is MBSP similar to other mindfulness-based programs?
MBSP is similar to other mindfulness-based programs, such as MBSR and MBCT, in that there is a solid 8-week structure that includes a variety of learning modalities and practices. The intention of these mindfulness programs is that participants will learn approaches they can use the rest of their lives. Each of these three mindfulness programs uses the raisin exercise, body scans, walking meditations, and sitting meditations as ways to help participants deepen their experience of the present moment.

How is MBSP different from other mindfulness-based programs?
MBSP differs in that it focuses mindfulness on character strengths. It explicitly trains participants on both mindfulness practices and character strengths practices, and, in turn, how each enhances the other. This synergy can then be used to create one's best life or to manage problems.

In addition to content differences in each of the eight sessions, another difference occurs in how practitioners and clients perceive the programs. A mindfulness program designed to help someone overcome overeating or manage suicidality is going to create certain expectations among participants in regard to overcoming problems and fixing one's deficits. Regardless of the approach taken by the facilitator, this perception of using mindfulness as a technique to fix oneself may become a lingering issue. The focus of MBSP is explicitly on exploring what is good and strong in individuals and then finding ways to harness this in one's life with mindfulness.

More specifically, many mindfulness-based programs were created with particular populations in mind, for example, individuals with chronic pain, stress, or medical illness (MBSR), recurrent depression (MBCT), borderline personality (DBT), and substance abuse (MBRP). However, most of these programs have found a broader audience can benefit from the program. MBSP was created to be intentionally broad and wide-reaching in terms of nonclinical/clinical populations and use in various settings.

Do most other mindfulness-based programs focus solely on the negative or dealing with deficits?
Absolutely not. Mindfulness involves paying attention to one's experience in the present moment, which might be positive, negative, neutral,

or somewhere in between. Mindfulness programs focus on enhancing the quality of this attentiveness to oneself. In addition, the tone and atmosphere of the majority of mindfulness programs is intended to be a positive and accepting one (e.g., consider the engaging debriefing of exercises and sharing of personal experiences that occurs in MBSR groups).

Mindfulness naturally engenders positive emotions and a meta-analysis on MBSR among healthy subjects found the program had a strong effect on improving psychological well-being (Eberth & Sedlmeier, 2012). In addition, a randomized trial of MBCT found an increase in positive affect and pleasantness of daily life experiences compared with a control group (Geschwind, Peeters, Huibers, van Os, & Wichers, 2012). While many mindfulness programs do measure positive outcomes (e.g., positive mood, vitality), this is still an emerging part of research protocols.

Prior to MBSP, there has been a lack of mindfulness programs that focus explicitly on building awareness, exploration, and enhancement of positive phenomena as the main approach and intention, and there are none that focus directly on core character strengths.

To be clear, just as MBSR, MBCT, and other mindfulness programs do not negate or avoid focusing on positive elements in the human experience (e.g., the "pleasant events calendar" used in MBCT, values clarification in ACT, and healthy communication practice in MBRE), those who participate in MBSP do not avoid focusing on negative or afflictive elements of experience. Some aspects of MBSP focus explicitly on problems or struggles (e.g., Session 6), and participants report an improvement in managing problems and stress as a result of the MBSP program.

If mindfulness and character strengths are each constructs associated with well-being by themselves, why bother integrating them? Is this overkill?

As noted in Section 1, these two areas share benefits as well as seem to offer unique pathways to well-being. It is suggested that their integration brings forth unique dynamics (e.g., virtuous circle) that an explicit focus on either one may not readily elicit or may not elicit as strongly as the two together. In addition, the combination may

assist individuals in maintaining changes longer over time. Similar to any change process, individuals engage in practices to grow and improve oneself, as well as to come to know oneself in a deeper way. Mindfulness offers a lens for seeing oneself and others with clarity, and character strengths present a language for understanding one's potential and the good that can be expressed to others.

If mindful attention is essentially a bare attention that focuses solely on "what is," is it contradictory to deliberately focus on something else, like character strengths?

MBSP teaches both bare attention and attentiveness to areas to which we are often blind to (e.g., character strengths). Just as other mindfulness programs help participants bring their attention to "something" (e.g., relapse triggers, painful emotions), MBSP does the same but brings the focus to strengths.

MBSP does not teach participants that they *should* be high on a particular strength, instead it encourages participants to be mindful of themselves to discover (or re-discover) their strengths.

There is indeed a risk that when a person purposefully brings mindfulness to something specific – the person can get lost in that specific "thing." As an example, consider mindful walking where the practice is to be mindful of the body, its movement, the environment, the mind (e.g., observing thoughts of "I'm afraid to walk" or an emotion of excitement). Why not also be aware of the character strengths being used in the moment (e.g., zest, appreciation of beauty)? Why not observe these strengths rise and fall as they are employed by the walker? Strengths are simply part of our consciousness like anything else.

In addition, the intention here is that this strengths awareness will deepen and strengthen the mindfulness (e.g., participants believing that they can use their strengths to pull themselves back to the present moment when their mind wanders). This also may increase the enjoyment of the experience because the person is aware that they are using their strengths, which tends to lead people to feel good about themselves. Consider the person being aware that as they practice mindful walking they find they are closely aware and connected to the beauty of nature around them or that they are using curiosity as they explore their environment.

Other MBSP exercises involve deliberate thinking about and reflection on strengths (mindful reflection or reflective thought; Amaro, 2010). The challenge here is that the reflection is mindful in that one allows the mind to explore and investigate the strength and when the mind strays too far from the strength exploration, one "catches" the mind and guides it back to the task at hand. This is mindfulness.

Finally, all the mindfulness work – and all mindfulness programs – are really a springboard and a lead-in to something else: to greater awareness in daily life and daily interactions. Thus, the hope is that integrating consciousness about strengths while practicing mindfulness will do just that.

Mindfulness-Based Strengths Practice (MBSP)

Session 1:
Mindfulness and Autopilot

Session 2:
Your Signature Strengths

Session 3:
Obstacles are Opportunities

Session 4:
Strengthening Mindfulness in Everyday Life (Strong Mindfulness)

Session 5:
Valuing Your Relationships

Session 6:
Mindfulness of the Golden Mean (Mindful Strengths Use)

Session 7:
Authenticity and Goodness

Session 8:
Your Engagement with Life

Chapter 7

Mindfulness-Based Strengths Practice

Session 1: Mindfulness and Autopilot

The unexamined life is not worth living

Plato

Opening Story[1]

There once was an old woman who spent much of her day sitting at the edge of her town. She encountered various travelers passing through who were interested in the town in which she had lived for so many years. One day a man approaching the town asked her a question:

"What are the people like in this town?"

"What are they like in your hometown?" replied the old woman.

"Oh, the people are difficult, mean-spirited, and selfish. Don't get me started!" he exclaimed. "They are not people you can trust! I was happy to leave."

"I think you'll find the people here to be the same," noted the old woman.

The man went on his way. The next day a second traveler approached the town and asked the woman the same question.

"What are they like in your hometown?" she asked in return.

"Well, they are generally quite kind and very thoughtful," he observed. "They work hard, are fair and honest, and are accepting of one another. I was disappointed to leave."

"I think you'll find the people here to be the same," replied the old woman.

Structure for Session 1[2]

I   Welcome and Positive Introductions [30 min]
II   Raisin Exercise and Debriefing [25 min]
III   Mindfulness and Autopilot [20 min]
IV   Body Mindfulness Meditation (Body Scan) and Debriefing [20 min]
V   Virtue Circle – [20 min]
VI   Suggested Homework Exercises [5 min]
VII   Closing: Brief Meditation [1 min]

Note. If possible, arrange the participants in a circle of chairs so that each participant can view one another. The times noted are approximate and set for a 2-hour session; for a 1.5-hour session, it's advisable to eliminate the virtue circle and limit the raisin exercise to 20 minutes.

---

[1] An earlier version of this story can be found in Roger Walsh's (1999) book *Essential Spirituality*.
[2] Practitioners might consider using the opening stories at some point during MBSP group sessions.

I   Welcome and Positive Introductions

The opening words of any new group or program are important as they contribute to the impressions and expectations individuals are forming about the practitioner and the program as a whole. There are a number of core points to get across in the introduction. Most relate to the creation of a good group experience:

- Offer gratitude to the individuals or institutions involved in the logistics that made the group experience a reality; introduction to the group facilitator; novelty of the program – comment that this is a special opportunity.
- The group experience emphasizes *growth* (a mindset that looks for opportunities to learn at every turn), *education* (building knowledge), and *experiences* (live practice of tools that can be readily applied in daily life):
  - Therapeutic vs. therapy: Those MBSP groups that are not set up as therapy groups might explain that the group is intended to be "therapeutic," meaning beneficial and supportive of one's personal growth, learning, and development.
  - Many learning opportunities will be utilized, including meditations, large group discussions, dyad exercises, didactic input, Q & A, group experiential exercises, and homework practices. An approach promoted throughout the program is that the group participants learn not only from themselves and the facilitator but from one another and the wisdom of the group-as-a-whole.
  - Hopes (of the facilitator):
    - "Stretch" oneself: See this group as a laboratory to explore and discover new ideas about oneself and others. Allow oneself to by challenged, to be wrong, to struggle, and to find well-being along the way.
    - Commitment to the group: Set a plan and intention to stick with the entire program through the challenges and positives. It is highly recommended individuals attend all 8 meetings. Part of

this involves a commitment to the other group members who begin to count on seeing one another and learning from one another each week.
  - Confidentiality is encouraged in the group (note: therapy groups will need to discuss this in greater depth including the limits of confidentiality as well as cover relevant institutional policies).
  - Group norms are relayed and discussed: timing, set-up, and structure of MBSP; internal structure of a given group session, group breaks (if any); other policies.
- Positive introductions: In addition to sharing one's name and what they do during a typical day, it's important for the group to get to know one other in a deeper way. One way to do this is to offer a question that elicits substantive sharing but is not personal in an uncomfortable way. The question "What matters most to you?" allows individuals to share briefly (e.g., "My relationship with my children") or go deeply into examples, whichever they feel comfortable with. An alternative approach is: "Share something good that happened to you recently" or "Share one positive quality about yourself."
- About MBSP (refer to Handout 1.1): This course will help you develop mindfulness and character strengths. This first session will focus only on mindfulness and next week we'll focus mostly on character strengths. Then, at Session 3 and onward, we will discuss and practice bringing mindfulness and strengths together. In each group, we will practice exercises that will build upon one another from week to week and that you'll be able to apply in your home practice. There are many positive outcomes, such as greater happiness, less depression, and higher meaning and engagement in life, that have been connected with mindfulness and character strengths use. Therefore, mindfulness and character strengths can become pathways to what we want most out of life. This program, MBSP, is about building a strong base for our lives, about delving deeper into self-awareness, reaching and expressing our inherent goodness, and connecting more with others.

II Raisin Exercise

Main Teaching Points

- Introduction: Little to no introduction is typically offered, instead participants are invited to engage in a practical experience in which they approach "the object" (raisin) being handed out as if they are encountering it for the first time (beginner's mind). See Box 7.1 to read the meditation and Chapter 4 for additional details.
- Key reminders when leading the exercise:
  - Incorporate all 5 senses.
  - Pause 5–10 seconds in between statements/sentences.
  - Participate in the experience while leading it.
  - Refer to being watchful of the wandering mind and the task to return to the present experience.
- Debriefing: Allow space for participants to discuss their experiences. Consider using a white-board to track what participants observed. Some questions include:
  - What did you notice during the experience?
  - Is this how you typically eat raisins?
  - What did you notice about the raisin that you hadn't noticed before?
  - What did you notice about your attention?
  - Why do you think we did this exercise?
  - Might what we did with the raisin be applicable to other areas of our lives?
- Participants are encouraged to take this approach of beginner's mind with the entire MBSP experience. Some participants might

---

Box 7.1. Raisin exercise[3]

Take the object in the palm of your hand or between a finger and thumb and pay attention to seeing it … Seeing the object as if you've never seen such a thing before. Looking at it carefully, turning it over. Observing the highlights, folds, and where the light hits and where it doesn't.

Lifting the object up to the nose and with each in-breath, carefully seeing what smells you detect. You might take notice of any differences in smells from your right nostril and your left nostril. You might bring the object toward one of your ears and between a finger and thumb press gently on the object. See if you detect any sounds coming from the object. And then take another look at it.

And if, while we're doing this exercise, you notice yourself having certain thoughts like, "What a weird thing this is" or "I don't like this" or thoughts about your day, then simply note those as thoughts you are having and return your attention back to the object … Back to experiencing the object as if for the first time.

Begin to slowly lift the object up toward the mouth, noticing how your arm seems to know exactly how to do that. Roll the object along your upper and lower lip and notice the sensations this creates. Placing the object in your mouth, and without biting it, notice how it is received. Be present to simply having the object in your mouth.

When you're ready, positioning the object between your upper and lower teeth, noticing how your tongue automatically helps out. Pressing down on the object one time and noticing the tastes that are released and the change in the object. Pressing down on the object a second time and continuing that process of chewing … Noticing the change in consistency of the object and the tastes of the object.

Before swallowing the object, notice your intention to swallow it … Bring to your awareness how you position the object toward the back of the throat and the role of your tongue and saliva. When you're ready, swallow the object … Following it down your throat and sensing it moving down through your body.

Taking notice of any lingering pieces of the object in your mouth and any taste that remains … And sensing or knowing that your body is now one raisin heavier.

---

3 This exercise was initiated and pioneered by Jon Kabat-Zinn and the many subsequent leaders of MBSR (Kabat-Zinn, 1990). Many versions have appeared as this exercise has become a staple element of most mindfulness programs. A similar version can also be found in Segal et al. (2002).

view this as putting on their "beginner's hats"; the leader also takes this approach in many respects.

III   Mindfulness and Autopilot

Main Teaching Points

- Make a connection between the raisin exercise just experienced and autopilot and everyday mindlessness.
- Draw or describe the continuum of awareness: on one end is autopilot, mindlessness, and everyday distraction and the other end is mindfulness, presence, and here and now (see Chapter 1 for model and discussion).
  - Offer examples of autopilot when driving, working, reading, eating, etc.
  - Mindfulness is viewed as keeping one's attention alive in the present moment (Nhat Hanh, 1979) and paying attention on purpose, in the present moment, without judgment (Kabat-Zinn, 1994).
    - Emphasize the normalcy of autopilot (that it is not good or bad) and that it can be adaptive but also can lead us to miss many opportunities in life.
  - The paradox of mindfulness: it's simultaneously one of the easiest approaches (we can drop into mindfulness at any moment, during any activity) and one of the most difficult (e.g., facing pain or emotional turmoil directly)
  - Our first task is to understand how pervasive autopilot is: "Catch AP-ASAP" ("catch auto-pilot, as soon as possible") becomes a key phrase to remember and a key idea that can be highlighted each week.

IV   Body Mindfulness Meditation

- Listen to Track 2 of the attached CD for the body mindfulness meditation.
- Introduction: The body mindfulness exercise (also known as, and referred to interchangeably, with body scan) is another classic mindfulness exercise made popular in MBSR and MBCT. This involves bringing a careful, open and ac-

cepting awareness to our body in the present moment. The purpose of this exercise is not relaxation – although that might happen for you – but the main purpose is simply awareness. We will practice being open and curious to our bodies in order to tune in more closely. See Box 7.2 to read an abridged version and Chapter 4 for other details. The exercise is commonly done sitting or lying down; the version discussed in MBSP is usually done sitting ina chair (this promotes the application of mindful sitting throughout the day – in meetings, when at a computer, while eating, etc. whereas lying down is often synonymous with sleep).
- Note: In terms of time management, this exercise is quite malleable and can be adjusted to fit shorter time periods or as long as 45 minutes.
- Key reminders when leading the exercise:
  - Ideally use a bell to open and conclude the experience.
  - Focus on a couple of lower body regions, upper body regions, face, top of head.
    - Use the breath to "breathe into" each body region.
    - Encourage curiosity, openness, and acceptance of each area – exploration and investigation, then letting go.
  - As a conclusion, bring attention to the body-as-a-whole, experience a sense of oneness.

Debriefing

Participants drive the debriefing of this novel exercise. Depending on the size of the group, it might be possible to hear what the experience was like for each individual. Here are some questions to get the discussion going:

- What struck you during this experience? – What did you notice?
- How did you handle your autopilot mind during this experience?
- What was it like to practice being open and curious to your body?
- What does relaxation or peace mean in terms of body sensations?
- How do you typically approach your body?
- Why do you think we practiced this exercise today?

Box 7.2. Body Meditation (Abridged)

Take a moment to get comfortable in your seat. See about taking on a posture of strength in which your back is straight yet comfortable and your feet are firm on the floor. Take notice of the present moment around you – what you see, the sounds and smells you take in, and the contact your body makes with the chair and floor.

Take a moment to re-discover your breathing. Allow yourself to connect with your breathing. Notice the sensations involved with each in-breath. Perhaps you can feel the tiny sensations in your nostrils as you breathe in. Do you notice the sensations in your chest and stomach with each in-breath? As you breathe out, take notice of the sensations throughout your body.

Let's practice bringing this open and curious approach to the rest of the body. Bring your attention to your left foot. As you breathe in and out, explore your left foot. What sensations do you notice? Perhaps you can feel the contact of your sock or shoe with your foot? Maybe you notice other sensations such as a lightness or heaviness in the foot? Maybe a sensation related to temperature such as a warming or cooling or a sense of moisture – wetness or dryness in the foot? Whatever you notice, practice accepting that sensation as part of your experience in this present moment. Allow it to be as it is. Breathe with the sensations. Breathe with the left foot. If your mind wanders away from focusing on your foot, simply bring it back – back to exploring your foot fully. Continue to explore the whole foot – the toes, the top and bottom of the foot, the ankle, right down into the muscles and bones of the foot. Practice taking that gentle approach with your left foot – open and curious to what you'll discover. Then, when you're ready, on an out-breath, let go of the left foot. Simply releasing it, letting it dissolve away.

Move the spotlight of your attention up your body to your lower left leg.

[Parts of the preceding language are then used to help individuals explore the rest of their body going through their legs, arms, hands, torso, chest/stomach, back, shoulders, neck, face, and up to the top of the head]

Now that you have brought a greater awareness to the various parts of your body in the present moment, allow yourself to connect with your whole body. As you breathe slowly and deeply, notice your wholeness and how your body is far greater than just a collection of muscles, organs, bones, and joints. Feel that wholeness … Body and mind connected as one. Breathe with your body-as-a-whole. (Longer pause).

In a moment, we'll bring our attention visually back to the room. Notice how you feel as you prepare to do so … Taking notice of your body in the chair and the realization that there are people around you. Bring an awareness to your eyelids, a part of our body we often pay very little attention to. Take conscious control of the muscles in your eyelids and open your eyes just about 10% of the way. Notice the effect of bringing in just a little bit of light. Slowly, under your conscious control, lift them 25% and then 50%, bringing in more light and color. Notice the changes and how you begin to orient to the room – to the light, the colors, and the people around you. Continue lifting your eyelids until you're fully alert and present in the room and to the people around you.

Summing Up the Session

- When we slow down, we start to see what our minds are actually doing!
- Mindfulness practices tell us something about our minds and how we handle things. For example, are we being judgmental? Reactive?

Too quick to accept? It's not just about eating a raisin or listening to our bodies, it's about everything we do. Mindfulness is thus about our everyday life.

- The raisin exercise and the body mindfulness meditation can serve as *microcosms* for how we might live our life – with awareness. Why not approach every task with greater mindfulness? What would happen if we did?

- Handout 1.5 offers a summation of key points on mindfulness.

V   Virtue Circle

- See detailed discussion in Chapter 6 which reviews the purpose, process, and guidelines for the virtue circle as well as information that helps practitioners to introduce this aspect of MBSP to participants.

VI   Suggested Homework Exercises

- Bring your VIA Survey results next week (take the VIA Survey at www.viame.org). This refers to the free results that rank-order one's character strengths from 1–24. The purchase of in-depth reports (VIA Me Report or VIA Pro Report) is optional; those that do purchase the optional reports are encouraged to bring them to the group.
- Body mindfulness meditation, 1 ×/day.
- Practice mindfulness with one routine activity each day.
- Track your experiences on Handout 1.2 and/ or in your journal.
- Reflect on a "You, at your best" experience. Participants do not have to write this down but should be ready to share their story at the beginning of next week's class.

Review of Suggested Homework Exercises

- Highlight the importance of the suggested homework exercises each week. This serves as the connective tissue between sessions; it is important for deepening the work and it maximizes personal benefits and well-being.
- A common question emerges at this point: How long should the body mindfulness meditation be practiced each day? My preference is not to set an exact time or to require participants to listen to a particular mindfulness meditation CD (however, a large number of people do decide to listen to CD meditations each day). What is most important is setting up a regular routine. MBSP work is long-term, so why set oneself up with a sense of frustration or failure at the onset? I believe it's much more important for someone to do 5–10 minutes every day than 45 minutes twice a week. Once a routine is set, it can be built upon over the coming weeks and months. Thus, I encourage people to listen to their body/mind and their personal needs, set up a routine, and monitor their experiences and progress.
- Routine activity: Individuals are asked to consider one activity in their daily life that they typically do on autopilot (e.g., brushing their teeth, feeding their dog/cat, washing their hair, helping their child get dressed, cooking breakfast) and do the activity *every day* this week with mindfulness. Just like individuals ate the raisin, the practice is to tune into and even savor their routine with their senses. If there is time, it increases accountability to go around the circle hearing which routine activity each person will focus on. It's OK if more than one person picks the same activity.
- Distinction between journaling and self-monitoring. People often prefer one or the other but it's perfectly fine to do both. The former is more for self-exploration and creative reflection, while the latter is more for tracking tasks, behaviors, and keeping accountable to the practice each week (see Handout 1.2).

Handouts

- Handout 1.1: Overview of Mindfulness-Based Strengths Practice (MBSP) (2 pages)
- Handout 1.2: Tracking & Suggested Exercises (1 page)
- Handout 1.3: VIA Classification (1 page)
- Handout 1.4: You at Your Best (1 page)
- Handout 1.5: Mindfulness – General Description (2 pages)

VII Brief Meditation

- Conclude with a 1-minute meditation that invites participants to bring their attention to their body in the present moment, followed by a focus on their in-breath and out-breath.

Additional Considerations

Virtue Circle Tip

- In this session, participants begin to understand and involve themselves in the virtue circle. To facilitate this learning, consider handing each individual a 3 × 5 card at this session or Session 2. You might explain the main ideas practiced in the virtue circle each week and individuals could jot these down and refer to the card as needed in future sessions. For example, one participant might write the following to serve as a list of reminders: mindful listening; mindful speaking; strengths-spotting; strengths valuing; strengths use.

More Questions to Consider

- What are you resonating with at this moment?
- What brought you to want to take this course?
- What do you hope to get out of this course?
- Have you had experience with mindfulness or meditation in the past?
- Have you spent time studying your strengths of character?

Practice Trap

The topic of homework and to what level it is "required" may come up. This question should be handled with care. A balanced response is one that encourages participants to work through the majority of the homework but also conveys that participants should be kind toward themselves and to what is realistic in their present day life.

Ultimately, what do practitioners hope for? That the participants will make strides in their mindfulness practice and their character strengths practice each week. Therefore, participants who complete a homework assignment/practice in each area are likely to be on the right track.

Participants can be reminded to do as much as they can so they can benefit more from the program. For some participants, less is more; some dig in deeply in one practice (e.g., one man established a steady 1-hour body mindfulness practice each day and did no other homework the first two weeks). This is something to celebrate and the effect this had on his life should be explored. A general motto is to fit MBSP into your naturally flowing life and "try your best to put forth your best effort and that is *good enough*."

Lesson learned: Encourage wide use and experimentation but also self-kindness and self-understanding; don't set participants up with negative feelings of discouragement or overwhelm at the onset of the program.

MBSP Handout 1.1

Session 1:

Overview of Mindfulness-Based Strengths Practice (MBSP)

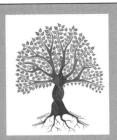

Overview

MBSP is an 8-session program that brings the practice of mindfulness and the practice of character strengths together. It includes discussions, meditations, strengths practices, lecture/input, and homework exercises. There are two general categories of integration:
1. Strong mindfulness: improving mindfulness practices by weaving in character strengths.
2. Mindful strengths use: improving character strength use by weaving in mindfulness.

Description

This 8-week workshop/program is about engaging more deeply with life. The crux is self-awareness and self-discovery. It combines two powerful and popular approaches that are being used in schools, clinics, universities, scientific labs, and businesses worldwide: mindfulness meditation and character strengths. Emphasis is placed on exercises that are discussed and practiced each week. This course teaches the basics of mindfulness and of character strengths, and offers more advanced, practical ways to integrate the two. It presents a unique angle to living one's best life, re-discovering happiness, achieving goals, finding deeper meaning and life engagement, and coping with problems.

Mindfulness Practices

Participants practice mindful breathing, listening, speaking, eating, walking, mindfulness of problems, loving-kindness meditation, brief mindfulness, and many other practices.

Character Strength Practices

Participants practice strengths-spotting, use of signature strengths, character strengths 360, strengths branding, strengths interview, valuing strengths in others, best possible self, strengths goal-setting, strengths-activity mapping, strengths gathas, and many others.

Core Topics

The following are the eight core themes by session:

Session 1: Mindfulness and Autopilot
• Autopilot is pervasive; everything starts with awareness

Session 2: Your Signature Strengths
• Identify what is best in you; this can unlock potential to engage more in work and relationships and reach higher personal potential.

Session 3: Obstacles are Opportunities
- The practice of mindfulness and of strengths exploration leads immediately to two things – obstacles/barriers to the practice and a deeper awareness of the little things in life.

Session 4: Strengthening Mindfulness in Everyday Life (Strong Mindfulness)
- Mindfulness helps us attend to and nourish the best, innermost qualities in ourselves and others; conscious use of strengths can help us deepen and maintain a mindfulness practice.

Session 5: Valuing Your Relationships
- How we relate to ourselves is an important element of self-growth. This has an immediate impact on how we connect with others.

Session 6: Mindfulness of the Golden Mean (Mindful Strengths Use)
- Mindfulness helps to focus on problems directly and character strengths help to reframe and find different perspectives not immediately apparent.

Session 7: Authenticity and Goodness
- It takes character (e.g., courage) to be a more authentic "you" and it takes character (e.g., hope) to create a strong future that benefits both oneself and others.

Session 8: Your Engagement with Life
- Stick with those practices that have been working well and watch for the mind's tendency to revert back to automatic habits that are deficit-based, unproductive, or that prioritize what's wrong in you and others. Engage in an approach that fosters awareness and celebration of what is strongest in you and others.

Benefits

- Builds deeper knowledge of the best qualities in people.
- Cultivates strengths awareness and strengths use.
- Boosts mindfulness as an always-available approach to use in life.
- Offers several concrete practices to boost happiness and manage stress and difficulties.
- Previous participants have experienced increases in happiness, flourishing, engagement, meaning, purpose, better relationships, and improved stress and problem management.

Purposes of MBSP

- Despite the many benefits of mindfulness, most people who start a mindfulness practice do not keep it up. Character strengths offer ways for individuals to better deal with obstacles and barriers that naturally emerge.
- Character strengths work offers a common language to capture positive qualities individuals can learn and bring their mindful attention more closely to.
- Mindfulness and character strengths are interdependent and can create a virtuous circle of mutual benefit.
- Mindfulness facilitates increased self-awareness and potential for change activation by bringing one's character strengths more clearly into view.
- Offers a path for individuals to use their best strengths more, and be more attuned to a balanced expression that is sensitive to the situation and to potential overuse/underuse.

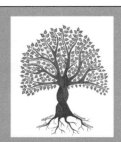

MBSP Handout 1.2

Session 1: Mindfulness and Autopilot

Tracking and Suggested Exercises

Suggested Exercises/Homework This Week:

- Bring VIA Survey results next week (www.viame.org)
- Body mindfulness meditation, 1 ×/day
- Practice mindfulness with one routine activity each day
- Track your experiences here and in your journal
- Reflect on a "You, at our best" experience (see Handout 1.4)

Day/Date	Type of Practice & Time Length	Strengths Used	Observations/Comments
Wednesday Date:			
Thursday Date:			
Friday Date:			
Saturday Date:			
Sunday Date:			
Monday Date:			
Tuesday Date:			
Wednesday Date:			

MBSP Handout 1.3

Session 1:

The VIA Classification of Character Strengths

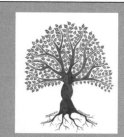

WISDOM

Creativity: Originality; adaptive; ingenuity
Curiosity: Interest; novelty-seeking; exploration; openness to experience
Judgment: Critical thinking; thinking things through; open-minded
Love of Learning: Mastering new skills & topics; systematically adding to knowledge
Perspective: Wisdom; providing wise counsel; taking the big picture view

COURAGE

Bravery: Valor; not shrinking from fear; speaking up for what's right
Perseverance: Persistence; industry; finishing what one starts
Honesty: Authenticity; integrity; telling the truth
Zest: Vitality; enthusiasm; vigor; energy; feeling alive and activated

HUMANITY

Love: Both loving and being loved; valuing close relations with others
Kindness: Generosity; nurturance; care; compassion; altruism; "niceness"
Social Intelligence: Aware of the motives/feelings of self/others

JUSTICE

Teamwork: Citizenship; social responsibility; loyalty
Fairness: Just; not letting feelings bias decisions about others
Leadership: Organizing group activities; encouraging a group to get things done

TEMPERANCE

Forgiveness: Mercy; accepting others' shortcomings; giving people a second chance
Humility: Modesty; letting one's accomplishments speak for themselves
Prudence: Careful; cautious; not taking undue risks
Self-Regulation: Self-control; disciplined; managing impulses & emotions

TRANSCENDENCE

Appreciation of Beauty and Excellence: Awe; wonder; elevation; admiration
Gratitude: Thankful for the good; expressing thanks; feeling blessed
Hope: Optimism; future-mindedness; future orientation
Humor: Playfulness; bringing smiles to others; lighthearted
Spirituality: Religiousness; faith; purpose; meaning

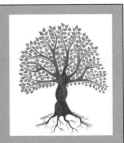

MBSP Handout 1.4

Session 1:

You at Your Best

Think of a specific time, recently or awhile back, when you were at *your* best. You were really feeling and acting at a high level. Perhaps you felt you were really engaged in what you were doing? Perhaps you felt like the experience you were part of was a very successful one? Most likely you felt like you were your authentic self, being who you are. It may be a specific experience in a relationship, in a work/school environment, or while socializing. Or, a specific time period might come to your mind. Reflect on this "story." See if you can frame your experience with a beginning, middle, and end. **Be sure to consider the character strengths that you used in that experience.** You might take the approach of replaying and reliving the positive experience just as if you were watching a movie of it. If you are sharing the story with someone, brainstorm the character strengths that each of you observe in it; if you are only reflecting on the story, be sure to consciously name how each strength was expressed.

Goal

Re-experiencing and savoring moments like this in your mind can lead to greater happiness and a greater chance that you will savor future moments as they happen in the present moment. Research has shown that this type of savoring (mindful reflecting) is beneficial, even if you do not write anything down.

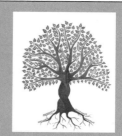

MBSP Handout 1.5

Session 1:

Mindfulness – General Description

What Is Mindfulness?

Mindfulness means paying attention to the present moment without judgment. Much of our life is spent in "autopilot" or in states of mindlessness in which we are going through the motions of life, barely present. This leads to distraction, forgetfulness, and suffering. When we are mindful, we are "tuned in" to our present experience; we are "alive." This is also referred to as "being" mode rather than "doing" mode.

What Is the Scientific Definition of Mindfulness?

Mindfulness is (1) the *self-regulation* of attention to immediate experience, with (2) an orientation of *curiosity*, openness, and acceptance. This means that when we are being mindful we are taking control of what we focus on – we are controlling our attention. As we attend to our present moment – whether this be to an emotion, a thought, a belief, an impulse, a sensation, or to something in our surrounding environment – we need to approach that "thing" with a curious, open, and accepting attitude.

What Is the Purpose of Mindfulness?

The purpose is NOT relaxation, inner oneness, or relief of symptoms, although these are all possible "side effects" of mindfulness practice. The purpose of mindfulness is *awareness* of the "here and now" and the changing moment-to-moment experience of our minds and bodies. This is how mindfulness is different from many other types of meditations and mind-body therapies that seek to produce a specific outcome.

Why Is Mindfulness Important?

When we are "mindless" (in auto pilot) and caught up in our thinking, we are less aware of what is going on in our internal and external environment. Two things often result: (1) we miss the details (often positives) of life and (2) we miss opportunities to grow or challenge ourselves. Mindfulness opens the door of opportunity to these potentials. In addition, mindfulness practice has been associated with a large number of benefits ranging from greater well-being, better management of medical and psychological problems, and increases in particular character strengths.

How Is Mindfulness Practiced?

Anytime you bring your attention to the present moment with curiosity, openness, and/or acceptance, you are practicing mindfulness. This can occur "any" time, whether you bring your attention to how you are sitting, your movement as you walk, your breathing as you work, the road and landscape while you are driving, the food you are eating, the smile on the person's face you are talking with, etc. Here are three ways to practice:

Formal

Some people practice mindfulness meditation for a certain amount of time each day. It is a "formal" practice when you carve out part of your daily living to practice mindfulness, for example, 2×/day for 10–15 minutes each or every morning from 9:00–9:30 a.m. The most common form is concentrating on following your breathing while you sit.

Informal

Informal practice means to "use it when you need it." When you are feeling stressed, anxious, depressed, overwhelmed, or helpless, take a moment to slow down, pause, and "just be." Breathe. Become aware of your body, your thoughts, your emotions (feelings), your behavior, and your environment. What is your body saying to you right now? What are you thinking about? What emotions are you present to right now? What do you need? What would "self-care" look like for you in this moment?

In-the-Moment

1. Practice returning to the present moment whenever your mind wanders off.
2. Whenever possible, do one thing at a time (multi-tasking can lead to mindlessness).
3. Pay full attention (all five senses, when possible) to what you are doing right now.
4. Practice "being" while you are … eating, driving, talking, listening, working, praying.

Mindfulness Resources

Books

Mindfulness and Character Strengths: A Practical Guide to Flourishing by Ryan Niemiec (2013)
The Miracle of Mindfulness by Thich Nhat Hanh (1979)
Full Catastrophe Living; and *Wherever You Go, There You Are;* and *Coming to Our Senses* by Jon Kabat-Zinn (1990; 1994; 2005)
The Mindful Way Through Depression by Williams, Teasdale, Segal, & Kabat-Zinn (2007)
Mindfulness; and *The Power of Mindful Learning* by Ellen Langer (1989; 1997)
Eating Mindfully by Susan Albers (2003)
Mindless Eating: Why We Eat More Than We Think by Brian Wansink (2006)
The Mindful Brain: Reflection and Attunement in the Cultivation of Wellbeing by Daniel Siegel (2007)
Loving-kindness: The revolutionary art of happiness by Sharon Salzberg (1995)

Websites

www.viacharacter.org/mindfulness (Mindfulness-Based Strengths Practice; MBSP)
www.mindfulnesstapes.com or www.umassmed.edu/CFM/index.aspx (Jon Kabat-Zinn)
www.iamhome.org (Thich Nhat Hanh & The Mindfulness Bell)
www.tcme.org or www.savorthebook.com (Mindful eating)
www.mbct.com (for depression)

Chapter 8
Mindfulness-Based Strengths Practice
Session 2: Your Signature Strengths

Character and personal force are the only investments that are worth anything.

Walt Whitman

 Opening Story

"Like watching flowers opening and blossoming." This was the observation of one MBSP leader in reference to the changes she was observing session-to-session in the participants. She described one participant, Kara, who was a very cynical person. Kara scowled a lot, was quick to point out the flaws of situations, and struggled to connect with others in the group. Kara's profession was a business manager who got things done through power and control. While not completely unpleasant, she was quick to become demanding, negative, and critical of her employees. As a result, her employees tried to avoid Kara whenever possible.

During the strengths-spotting exercise in this session, Kara found it easy to offer a fellow group member positive feedback about the strengths they were expressing. Even more significant to Kara was the observation that this activity, and her actions, led the other group member to experience a big lift in energy and positivity. Simply giving this member feedback led to a pleasant, comfortable, and uplifting exchange.

Kara worked hard to develop the skill of strengths-spotting in each MBSP session and a few group sessions later, she made an announcement to the group: "My whole leadership approach is going to change because of this and it all stemmed from that first strengths-spotting exercise we did. I will become a better leader because of this."

Structure for Session 2

I	Opening Meditation: Brief Body Mindfulness Meditation [10 min]
II	Practice Review [15 min]
III	You at Your Best with Strengths-Spotting [35 min]
IV	Your Signature Strengths [25 min]
V	Body Mindfulness or Mindful Breathing Exercise [10 minutes – Time permitting]
VI	Virtue Circle [25 min]
VII	Suggested Homework Exercises [5 min]
VIII	Closing: Character Strengths Breathing Space [5 min]

Note. Times are approximates. This is for a 2-hour session; for a 1.5-hour session, it's advisable to eliminate the virtue circle and body mindfulness while shortening each section accordingly; the body could then be emphasized in the other brief meditations.

I   Opening Meditation

- Brief body mindfulness meditation: Starting with the body mindfulness creates a good flow from Session 1 to Session 2 and reinforces the importance of this practice.

II   Practice Review

- For some newly formed groups, the openness promoted by mindfulness in the first session carries into this session and the participants are ready to share experiences and open up to the group. For some groups, this takes more time as individuals become more trusting and comfortable with the structure, the group norms, and the practices.
- Debriefing the homework exercises for this session is usually guided by questions relating to two strands:
  - The mindfulness practices – the body scan practice and mindfulness of a routine activity. What went well (www) this week? What surprised you? What challenges did you face?
  - VIA Survey results: What was your reaction to the VIA Survey?
    - o It's important for participants to share their initial impression to their results, which often emerges as an emotional response (e.g., surprise, joy, disappointment). Group facilitators can normalize the various reactions that emerge. Some curiosities and inquiries by participants about the VIA Survey at this point are best held off to later in the group or at a future session because the you-at-your-best exercise should precede didactic and Q & A about strengths.

III   You at Your Best
With Strengths-Spotting

- Listen to Track 3 of the attached CD for the you at your best exercise with strengths-spotting in oneself.

- Set-up: Arrange individuals into dyads. Offer a personal or professional example of a time when the facilitator was "at their best."
- Instructions: Per the homework suggested for this week (see Handout 1.4), this exercise involves one person telling the story of a time when they were at their best (the storyteller) and the other person listens carefully to the story and practices spotting the character strengths present (the strengths spotter). When the story concludes, they discuss the strengths in the story. It is important for each person to have a turn so after about 10–15 minutes, switch roles.
- During these and other dyad/small group exercises, the facilitator might choose to walk around the room and "listen in" to each interaction and be available to answer questions if some individuals are "stuck."
- Important strengths-spotting tip to share with participants:
  - For each strength that is spotted, go beyond the strength label. Offer the rationale for what you saw.
- Debriefing:
  - As the listener, how easy was it to spot character strengths? As the speaker, did you notice character strengths while you were talking?
  - What did you learn about yourself?
  - Did you notice yourself naturally using some character strengths while listening?
  - What is it like trying to learn a new language?

IV   Your Signature Strengths

Main Teaching Points

- We have now begun the practice of strengths-spotting. We can think of strengths-spotting as occurring on two levels, which we will practice throughout MBSP:
  - Character strengths in others
  - Character strengths in oneself
- We need a "common language" in order to take either path.
- Offer background/history of positive psychology and the VIA Classification of universal

strengths and virtues (see Handout 2.2 and discussion in Chapter 2). This discussion includes commentary on what is meant by "VIA." It is a Latin word that stands on its own and means "the way" or "the path." For the purposes here, VIA refers to three things: a classification, a survey, and a nonprofit organization that educates practitioners, organizations, and the public about strengths research and practice.

- Signature strengths – *what they are* (highest strengths that we self-endorse, are energizing, natural to use, core to who we are, nominated by family/friends, and used across settings), *why they are important* (pathways to life goals, outcomes we want), and *research findings* (link between signature strength expression and happiness, engagement, meaning, less depression).
  - Specific research has found that using one signature strength in a new way each day for one week has been linked with increases in happiness and decreases in depression for 6 months!
    - ○ Give personal example of signature strengths use.
  - Other research on signature strengths might be offered at this point. Practitioners can stay updated by checking in on the latest research summaries on the VIA website here: www.viacharacter.org/www/en-us/research/summaries.aspx
  - Two parallel ideas: All 24 strengths matter; signature strengths seem to matter most.
    - ○ When these are posed as questions, they might look something like:
      - · Do you express who you are across settings and situations?
      - · Get to know the full language – use it, post it, practice it, discuss it. Do you value all 24 character strengths and understand the importance of each in your daily life and communications?
- Last week we discussed how common autopilot is in our life. Equally pervasive is strengths blindness. Probably all individuals can benefit from greater strengths awareness. Some research has found that only about one-third of people have a meaningful awareness of their strengths, while other research finds that less than 20% of people are flourishing. These data indicate that there is more we can do to express our full potential.

- Comment on a strengths process model that will be discussed in future sessions – the aware-explore-apply (A-E-A) model which involves individuals first becoming aware of their strengths (Sessions 1 & 2), exploring their strengths (Sessions 3–6), and applying/maintaining their strengths use (Sessions 7–8).
- *Brief group exercise:* Challenge the group with this: Choose a signature strength people in the group might not know about you (a less obvious one). In one sentence, share a behavior (without mentioning the word) in the last day or two that is associated with this strength. Other participants will guess the strength.

V   Body Mindfulness Meditation or Mindful Breathing Meditation (time permitting)

- To save a bit of group-time, practitioners can offer a "taste" of the body mindfulness meditation that infuses a few explicit character strengths.
- Begin to weave in strengths words, especially curiosity, perspective, and kindness (e.g., offering the metaphor of kindness droplets spreading throughout the body).
- A formal debrief can then be done, or the conclusion of the body scan can flow seamlessly into the virtue circle.

VI   Virtue Circle

The practitioner might transition immediately from the meditation into the virtue circle, noting that when the participants open their eyes they will be in the virtue circle. Participants may choose to share their experiences with the body scan, or turn to other key aspects of the virtue circle, such as strengths-spotting/valuing. Concluding the body scan in this way can help participants sharpen their mindful listening and speech because they'll have just emerged from meditation.

VII Suggested Homework Exercises

- Body mindfulness meditation (with self-regulation, curiosity, kindness), 1 ×/day)
- Character strengths breathing space exercise, 1 ×/day
- Tracking/journaling (see Handout 2.1)
- Use one of your signature strengths in a new way each day
- Practice mindfulness with a different routine activity each day
- *Bonus:* Select a current book you are reading, a TV show you watch, or recent movie/play you saw and write about the strengths you spot in the main character(s).

Homework Exercises Review

- When explaining the mindfulness of a routine activity assignment, it should be noted that participants should choose an activity different from the previous week and then focus on that routine activity on each day of the coming week.
- For the "signature strengths in new ways" exercise, practitioners might consider printing and handing out the following blog article that reviews two examples for each of the 24 character strengths: http://blogs.psychcentral.com/character-strengths/2012/04/new-ways-to-happiness-with-strengths/ (also found in Chapter 2).
- Handout 2.3 presents an opportunity for participants to really dig in and begin exploring their character strengths in a deep way. Participants could explore one or more of these questions in their journal, discuss them with family or friends, and monitor changes in their thoughts about them. In addition, these become useful questions for MBSP practitioners to know well and query at different points in the MBSP course as needed.
- For the bonus exercise, if a participant prefers suggestions for exploration, they can review Handout 2.5 for a list of various movies with positive psychology themes.

Handouts

- Handout 2.1: Tracking & Suggested Exercises (1 page)
- Handout 2.2: VIA Fact-Sheet (2 pages)
- Handout 2.3: Exploring Strengths (1 page)
- Handout 2.4: Character Strengths Breathing Space (1 page)
- Handout 2.5: Positive Psychology Movies (1 page)

VIII Closing meditation

- Introduce the character strengths breathing space exercise as a way to "frame in" the onset and conclusion of sessions (see handout 2.4). Explain that it is a three-minute meditation that is three steps, each about one minute long. It has been adapted from MBCT (Segal et al., 2002) in a way that keeps the integrity of the mindfulness focus while highlighting the character strengths involved. Track 4 of the attached CD is the character strengths breathing space.

Additional considerations

Group Observations

Participants are eager in this session to discuss their VIA Survey results and to begin spotting strengths in one another during the exercises. Facilitators do well to encourage strengths-spotting by modelling it for the group and offering queries about strengths. Participants will bring up new insights about their strengths that take many forms. One woman who was brand new to mindfulness and strengths practiced the body scan exercise each day before Session 2. After getting her rank-order of character strengths and learning that one of her top strengths was appreciation of beauty and excellence, she immediately understood why she was eager to practice the body scan each day outside. She previously had not made the connection between mindfulness and her strengths.

An older man who was very quiet in regard to sharing and offering comments took his turn to offer an "at your best" story. Honesty, authenticity, and psychological bravery were strikingly clear in the story as evidenced not only in the truthfulness offered but in the examples of how he faced difficulties within himself, refusing to run from challenges or make excuses. When the strengths spotter pointed out this poignant honesty, he seemed pleased. It was as if the strength-spotter saw the true essence of who this man was. This was quite validating for him and opened him up to become more comfortable and talkative in the group.

When participants are practicing mindful listening, probably any given signature strength can be deployed. Those high in appreciation of beauty have noted that they tune in closely to the beauty of what is being said; those high in judgment/critical thinking begin to form alternate views but stay open to the view being shared in the moment; and those high in love convey a sense of warmth and care with their body language and nonverbal attentiveness.

During the strengths-spotting activity, practitioners might encourage one or both individuals to close their eyes for part of the time. This approach of shutting off one of the senses frequently enhances mindful listening and can help individuals to speak clearly, directly, and from the heart. There may be some initial discomfort that emerges from the novelty of the exercise and individuals should be encouraged to face the tension with mindfulness.

More Questions to Consider

- What was your reaction to the VIA Survey results?

- It is useful to periodically query the group about their character strengths, e.g., who here is high in self-regulation? In curiosity? Such questions might be used as a springboard to discuss the particular strength or to help participants get to know one another better.

- Question to ask oneself: What did I do well as the practitioner in today's session? It will always seem more pressing to look for what went wrong and notice how things did not go as planned. There is a place for that too. But it's more likely the "What went well?" question will get lost in the shuffle, and the practitioner will have lost the opportunity to build off successes and strengths.

Practice Trap

It's important to evaluate early on in MBSP how hard you, the facilitator, are working. The facilitator should not be working harder than the group. In past groups, I would occasionally feel extra tired or tense; these were indications I was working too hard, "trying my heart out" to get individuals to understand the concepts, be inspired by the ideas, or I was simply trying to impart too much knowledge. In essence, I was overdoing it. Change happens within the individual and it is often the individual's practice work and discussion insights that keep them coming back. It's more likely that a question back to the individual, silence/pauses to sit with a key point, and exercises designed to keep individuals focused on the work themselves, will elicit change than the practitioner imparting one more interesting factoid.

Lesson learned: When in doubt, turn to a group exercise, meditation, or inquiry.

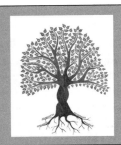

MBSP Handout 2.1

Session 2: Your Signature Strengths
Tracking and Suggested Exercises

Suggested Exercises/Homework This Week:

- Body mindfulness meditation (with self-regulation, curiosity, kindness), 1×/day
- Character strengths breathing space exercise (Handout 2.4)
- Track your experiences here or in your journal
- Use one of your signature strengths in a new way each day (Handout 2.3)
- Practice mindfulness with 1 routine activity each day
- **Bonus:** Select a current book you're reading, a TV show you watch, or recent movie/play you saw and write about the strengths you spot in the main character(s).

Day/Date	Type of Practice & Time Length	Strengths Used	Observations/Comments
Wednesday Date:			
Thursday Date:			
Friday Date:			
Saturday Date:			
Sunday Date:			
Monday Date:			
Tuesday Date:			
Wednesday Date:			

MBSP Handout 2.2

Session 2:

VIA Fact-Sheet

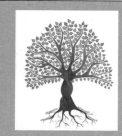

VIA Institute (www.viacharacter.org)

- The VIA Institute on Character (once called the Values in Action Institute) was created in 2000 by Dr. Neal Mayerson, under direction and collaboration with Dr. Martin Seligman, founder of positive psychology.

- The VIA Institute was initially and has continued to be supported generously by the Manuel D. and Rhoda Mayerson Foundation, a private family philanthropy.

- The VIA Institute on Character is a global, *nonprofit* organization located in Cincinnati, Ohio.

VIA Classification

- The VIA Classification is the result of a three-year project reviewing the best thinking on virtue and positive human qualities in philosophy, virtue ethics, moral education, psychology, and theology over the past 2,500 years (e.g., from the works of Aristotle and Benjamin Franklin to King Charlemagne and the tenets of the major world religions).
  - Involved extensive historical review and analysis using specific strength criteria.
  - The work was conducted under the auspices of the VIA Institute, Seligman, 55 scientists/ scholars, and directed by professor/researcher Dr. Chris Peterson.

- Six core themes emerged – wisdom, courage, humanity, justice, temperance, and transcendence – found across religions, cultures, nations, and belief systems.

- Applying various criteria, these "virtues" were subdivided into 24 universal character strengths that represent the pathways to the virtues.

- This work is discussed at length in the scholarly text *Character Strengths and Virtues: A Handbook and Classification* (2004), authored by Peterson and Seligman and published by Oxford University Press and the American Psychological Association.

VIA Surveys (www.viame.org)

- The VIA Survey (VIA-IS) measures the 24 character strengths.

- The VIA Survey has been taken by 2 million people in every single country around the globe. It gives the user immediate feedback on their top strengths of character. It is the only strengths survey in the world that is free, online, and psychometrically valid.
  - It has been found to have good, acceptable levels of reliability and validity.
  - Results moderately correlate with reports by the respondent's friends and family.

- The VIA Youth Survey is a validated measure of the 24 character strengths in youth between the ages of 10–17. Youth receive free results, and have the option to purchase a detailed youth report.

- As of 2013, both surveys are validated and available as briefer surveys, only at www.viame. org. Users now can complete the surveys in half the time. Other versions are available for researchers to study or use with students, employees, subjects, or other groups.

VIA Reports (www.viapros.org)

- *Free report:* After anyone takes the free VIA Survey, they are offered immediate results including their profile of character strengths, ranked from 1 to 24. Cost: Free.
- *VIA Me Pathways Report:* A consumer-friendly report with graphs, tips, quotes, and strategies for working with one's highest character strengths. Cost: $20.
- *VIA Pro Report:* An extensive report used to help practitioners better understand their client's signature strengths, overuse/underuse, the latest research, and best practices. Cost: $40.
- *VIA Pro TEAM Report:* An extensive report used by consultants and leaders in the business world to capitalize and leverage team strengths. Cost: $15 per team member.

Character

- *Definition:* Character strengths are stable, universal personality traits that manifest through thinking (cognition), feeling (affect), willingness (volition), and action (behavior).
  - When expressed in balance, character strengths are morally valued and beneficial to oneself and others. These positive psychological characteristics are considered to be the basic building blocks of human goodness, authenticity, and flourishing.

Signature Strengths

- Character strengths can be developed. It is likely that most people can enhance their capacity for expressing each of the 24 character strengths.
- Studies have shown that using one's signature strengths in a new and unique way is an effective intervention: it increased happiness and decreased depression for 6 months. The use of signature strengths has been found to be beneficial in different settings including work and education.
- Deploying one's signature strengths at work is linked with greater work satisfaction, greater well-being, and higher meaning in life. Expressing 4 or more signature strengths at work is linked with more positive work experiences and meaningful work.
- Two of the most important predictors of employee retention and satisfaction are: Reporting you use your top strengths at work and reporting that your immediate supervisor recognizes your top strengths.
- Research has found there is a strong connection between well-being and the use of signature strengths because signature strengths help us make progress on our goals, allow us to express our true passion and meet our basic needs for autonomy, relationship, and competence.
- Practitioners who focus on a client's strengths immediately prior to a session increase strength activation, improve outcomes, foster a sense of mastery for the client, and strengthen the practitioner-client relationship.
- Character strengths buffer people from vulnerabilities (e.g., perfectionism and need for approval) which can play an important role in managing depression and anxiety.

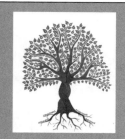

MBSP Handout 2.3

Session 2:

Exploring Strengths

Take the VIA Survey online and review your resulting list of strengths from 1–24. Explore your reaction to these results. **Read the following questions and circle those that stand out to you.** It might be helpful to ask "Why?" or "How?" after many of the questions:

- Do the top strengths seem like the "real you" – the core of who you are?
- When you use your top strengths, does it feel authentic?
- What is your gut reaction to the results?
- What surprises you most about the results?
- Which strengths seem to make you feel happy when you use them?
- Which strengths are you most interested in learning more about?
- What are your signature strengths? In other words, which strengths are most authentically you, come natural to you, and give you energy when you practice them?
- Which of your signature strengths are you most mindless to (not tuned into when you are using them)?
- Which strengths do you feel a sense of yearning in which you would like to use them more?
- When you think about a time when you were functioning at your best, which strengths did you use? Write this out as a story. Share it with someone.
- Which strengths give you a sense of excitement and enthusiasm as you think about using them? In other words, which strengths make you feel happy?
- When you think of a time when you were anxious, depressed, or highly stressed, which strengths did you use to move forward?
- Consider your past or current mentors (or personal role models, living or dead). What strengths did they embody? How did they express them? What strengths did they see in you?
- Which of the higher strengths are you most interested in building upon and expanding?
- Which of your lower strengths are you interested in building up?
- Which strengths are best for you to use in your family/relationship life, in your work life, and in your social life? Note that in each domain the combination of strengths you use might be very different.
- Which strengths might you use in order to reach your goals and/or to create a better future for yourself?
- Which strengths do you practice regularly and which just seem to come naturally where you do not even think about them until you are already using them?
- Which strength might you ask a friend or family member for encouragement and support as you attempt to bring greater mindfulness to it?

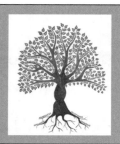

MBSP Handout 2.4

Session 2:

Character Strengths Breathing Space

While this exercise can be expanded to much longer time frames or contracted to briefer periods, the intention is that it provides a meaningful brief "space" to generate an awareness of the present moment and a connection with the breath while using character strengths. This brief mindfulness meditation builds directly from the 3-minute breathing space exercise used in MBCT (Segal, Williams, & Teasdale, 2002).

Participants may view the following three categories as three steps that flow together. Take about one minute for each step.

Awareness [Curiosity]

Take notice of your present moment. Open yourself to it. Observe the details. Take an interest in this moment. Notice what you can sense right now – aware of sounds rising and falling, the contact your body makes with your seat. Allow your curiosity to explore the moment fully. Practice being curious about your thoughts and feelings, interested in whatever is in your presence right now. Simply notice these happenings in your present moment and let each one go. If you find yourself getting caught up in one sensation or feeling, simply say, "What else? What else is happening in my present moment? What else is there to be curious about and take an interest in?"

Concentration [Self-Regulation]

Allow your attention to narrow to just one thing – your breath. This is the concentration phase of the breathing space, where the idea is to let go of all the happenings in your present moment with the exception of your breathing. Allow yourself to feel the fullness of your in-breath and the fullness of your out-breath. Feel the sensation of your breathing in your body. Concentrate just on the breath. When your mind wanders away from your breath, simply bring it back to the breath. Over and over – bring your focus back to your breath. Each time you bring your attention back to your breath, you are practicing self-regulation. This means you are "taking control" of your attention. Always back to your breath.

Expanded Awareness [Perspective]

While you continue to focus on your in-breath and out-breath, you can also allow your attention to expand to your body-as-a-whole. As you breathe, notice your wholeness, the oneness of your body and mind. Allow yourself to feel a sense of completeness or oneness. This can be viewed as using your strength of perspective – stepping back to see the wider view of your body/mind and your place in this present moment. This allows you to see and breathe with the bigger picture.

MBSP Handout 2.5

Session 2:

Positive Psychology Movies
Adapted from Peterson and Seligman (2004) and
Niemiec and Wedding (2014)

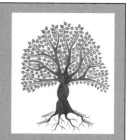

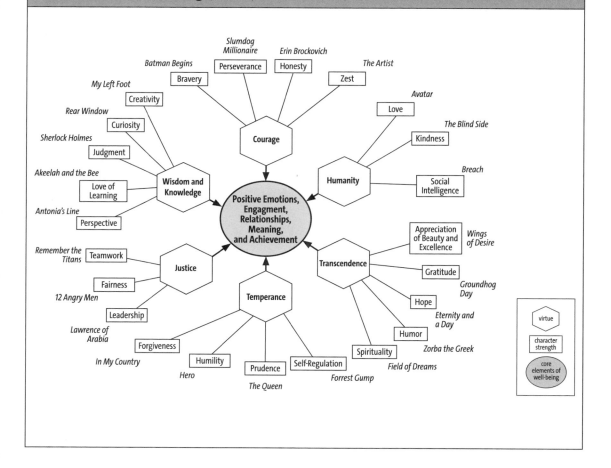

Chapter 9

Mindfulness-Based Strengths Practice

Session 3: Obstacles are Opportunities

Knowing is not enough; we must apply. Willing is not enough; we must do.

Goethe

Opening Story

In ancient India, a common sport had been for men to fight barehanded against tigers. One sturdy fellow, the world champion of his day, could vanquish even the largest, most vicious tigers, with little hurt to himself. One day a Hindu sage remarked to him, "It is a great challenge you have met, to be able to master tigers. However, it is a greater challenge to be able to master yourself. Conquer the beasts within. That is the more difficult task." (Marvin Levine, 2009, p. 40).

Structure for Session 3

I   Opening Meditation: Character Strengths Breathing Space [3 min]
II   Practice Review [20 min]
III   Strengths and Positive Outcomes and Managing Obstacles [10 min]
IV   Statue Meditation [20–30 min]
V   Debriefing the Statue Meditation [20 min]
VI   Virtue Circle [20–30 min]
VII   Suggested Homework Exercises [5 min]
VIII Closing: Brief Body Mindfulness Meditation or Leaf Meditation [2–10 min]

Note. Times are approximates. This is for a 2-hour session; for a 1.5-hour session, it's advisable to eliminate the virtue circle and shorten each section accordingly.

I   Opening Meditation

- Character strengths breathing space
  - The previous session concluded with this meditation so starting with this meditation in Session 3 offers nice continuity and flow for the participants.

II   Practice Review

- What went well (www) this week? Particularly important focus areas include: setting up and becoming more regular with a mindfulness practice, using one signature strength in a new way, and mindfulness with a routine activity.

- Debriefing: Participants will begin to make more frequent connections between mindfulness practices and their use of character strengths. For example, in discussing bringing mindfulness to a routine activity, one woman practiced making her bed each morning with mindfulness. While doing the activity, she became aware of how her signature strengths were a natural part of the experience, including appreciation of beauty in that she slowed down to notice the details of the soft, high thread count of her bed-sheets and appreciation of excellence as she naturally smoothed out each wrinkle on the bedspread to make a very precise and clean look. She also used prudence as she carefully tucked in all corners and aligned the bedspread, and creativity as she arranged several ornamental pillows in a pattern on the bed.
  - For this woman (and the group), this was an example of a simple, mundane task, easily taken for granted, in which her signature strengths were at play to some degree in the experience. Mindfulness helped her slow down and pay attention to notice them in the first place. These strengths were then top-of-mind for her as she went about her day at work and faced the challenges and stressors of her day.

III   Strengths and Positive Outcomes

Draw the connection between some of the homework on character strengths and the reaching of valued outcomes. Consider setting up an interchange like the following:

- Query the group: What matters most to you? What do you want most out of life?
  - Write down responses on the board.
  - Typical responses include: happiness, financial security, good relationships, peace, health, happy children, greater spiritual consciousness.
- Then ask: How can you reach any of these outcomes without using your character strengths (both your signature strengths and other strengths too)?

- Allow for responses and brief conversation
- Character strengths can serve as the pathways to reaching each of these positive areas. It is unlikely one can experience these valued outcomes without significant character strengths use.

Offer the metaphor of two trees to serve as a big picture view of the integration of mindfulness and character strengths:

- Picture this: Two, tall trees growing side by side as they branch out toward the limitless sky. With solid trunks that twist around each other, each tree has an extensive root system spreading several yards long and wide. Some of their roots intertwine and begin to depend on one another as they nourish one another becoming one in the same; other roots go their separate ways, extending deeper and deeper. The trees are of similar height and are so close to one another that their branches interconnect. As time goes on, the branches from each tree weave in and around one another. This occurs so seamlessly that when the passerby gazes up at the trees, their tops have become one.
- Mindfulness and character strengths are like these two great trees, separate but connected, independent yet interconnected, synergistic and mutually supportive. Their expression in the world is often viewed as though they are unique entities, yet there is a potential in each person to bring them together in a harmonious way that benefits oneself *and* others. Each has a deep root system; some roots are shared and others distinct. Those who practice mindfulness and character strengths taste a unique fruit that positively impacts their health and well-being, and brings great benefit to those around them.

Managing Obstacles

In mindfulness practice, individuals inevitably begin to confront challenges and struggles. These can be seen as barriers on an obstacles course, coming in all shapes and sizes from physical to mental to emotional to environmental (see Handout 3.2). The open, curious, and accepting attitude of mindfulness helps individuals see the obstacles more clearly and to face them. It also helps individuals become *aware* that they have strengths and to better *access* them. Mindfulness helps individuals become more in touch with reality and what "is" – especially what "is" when it comes to the interior life. Often negative thoughts and beliefs cloud the picture and one's self-perception. MBSP is about accessing what is there as well as exploring what is possible.

The core exercise practiced in this session gives participants the opportunity to directly face obstacles by consciously using mindfulness and character strengths.

Take note of any obstacles or challenges that emerge. See these as opportunities … opportunities for you to use your mindful breathing and your strengths. What strengths are you turning to right now? Which strengths will you deploy to help you? Focus on your in-breath and out-breath. (Repeat these themes over and over for a few minutes. Use your best judgment to find the balance of not doing this exercise too long or too short. The intention is that the participants experience some obstacles, and have the opportunity to face them with mindfulness and strengths).

IV The Statue Meditation

Refer to Box 9.1 for a description of this meditation.

Each individual will vary significantly in terms of their response to this exercise, the degree of discomfort, and the timing of when obstacles become challenging. Practitioners should make note that nowhere in the script are there phrases like "Keep your arms up," "Try to do this as long as you can," "You might feel some pain but keep it up," or "Don't put your arms down." Such phrases should never be used. Instead, you'll see that other than the first sentence there is no referencing to what they *should* do with their arms, there are only three reminders:
1. Make note of the obstacles that emerge
2. Turn to mindfulness
3. Turn to character strengths.

That's it. Over and over.

Disclaimer: To date there have been no issues with an individual becoming upset or complain-

---

Box 9.1. Statue Meditation

Let's take a moment to do an experiment. Let's start by taking a moment to practice standing meditation. Allow yourself to take on a posture of strength as you stand. Find a good place of balance for your body. Typically this means to set your feet shoulder-width apart and align your whole body as if there's a straight line from the top of your head and down your neck, spine, through your legs, out the bottom of your feet. Allow your body to be strong and steady but comfortable. Do not lock any of your joints. Your knees can be ever so slightly bent. Check your elbows and your jaw to make sure they are unlocked. Allow your chin to be level and eyes just gazing comfortably yet focused in front of you.

Find your breath (pause). Connect your attention to your breath for the in-breath and the out-breath (pause). Allow your breath to be an anchor, connecting you solidly to the present moment. With each breath you can find yourself more aware and strong in the present moment. (Repeat as needed allowing a couple minutes for participants to connect with their breath and establish their breath as an anchor).

Now, with this next part, pay attention and listen to your body. When you're ready, extend your arms in front of you and curve them a bit as if you were hugging a large ball (demonstrate as you lead this). Continue to follow your breathing. Feel the fullness of your in-breath and the fullness of your out-breath (pause). Take a moment to consider – what character strengths could you use right now? Choose any of the 24 strengths … and use one or more. Practice mindful standing, aware of your balance and steadiness, aware of your breath anchor helping you stay connected with the present moment experience.

---

ing that a physical problem worsened because of the exercise; however, the group facilitator bears some responsibility for the participants so one's best judgment and any disclaimers should be used. Several individuals have completed this exercise and later shared that they once had shoulder surgery, back surgery, and other body-related issues, and many of them do indeed note the "obstacle" of discomfort during the experience; however, each seemed to enjoy the challenge and the new "coping skill" of using strengths and mindfulness in the moment. It makes the practice come alive for them. The fruits of the practice become immediately clear.

V   Debriefing the Statue Meditation

The debriefing of this exercise is as crucial as the exercise itself. Here are some strategies to assist in the debriefing. Draw two columns on the board: one labeled "Obstacles" and the other labeled "Character Strengths Used." Ask the group what they experienced in general. Also, move into the specifics writing down the obstacles/challenges/difficulties they faced as well as any of the 24 strengths (and qualities of mindfulness) they used to deal with them.

- Jot down obstacles of the body (e.g., discomfort in arms, tension in shoulders, imbalance in standing) and the mind (e.g., how long will this go on?; I am frustrated with the facilitator for making us do this; I want to give up; I can't be the first one to quit; am I doing this right?).
- Jot down all the strengths that are mentioned. Query for specific strengths you are curious about and suspect they used (e.g., perseverance and, self-regulation had to be used). A few previous examples from MBSP participants include:
  - I used teamwork by looking at everyone around me doing the same thing. Everyone had their arms up. We were all a team working together. Knowing this helped me.
  - Bravery because I faced my discomfort directly. I didn't give up when I felt a struggle.
  - I felt grateful. It seems weird but I had had surgery in my left shoulder and even though I felt some tension there I felt grateful that it is so much better than it had been. And as the exercise continued I was filled with awe and gratitude at how well my shoulder was doing.
  - My arms were just too sore so I put them down. I was exercising judgment/critical

thinking by considering an alternate approach and I was using kindness toward myself because I was listening to my body's needs and responding with care.
  - I felt really connected in the moment. This was a sacred experience. This filled me with greater energy. I could have gone on for an hour. So, I was using my spirituality strength.
- Emphasize that they already had the strengths within them, they just had to remember to turn to them.
  - Note that every single one of the 24 strengths was at their disposal and possible for them to have used.
- Emphasize that they directed mindfulness to their strengths, to their body, and to their breath anchor. Ask participants about how they used mindfulness during the activity. What role did mindful breathing and mindfulness of the body have?
- Potentially, if it comes up, make note that they used a diversity of strengths, some are more mind-oriented (judgment), some more heart-oriented (gratitude), some more interpersonal (teamwork), and some more intrapersonal (curiosity).

While processing participants' experiences, highlight the core themes of today's session:
- Obstacles are opportunities for growth, for learning, for strengths use, and to deepen mindfulness practice. This is a growth mindset approach rather than a fixed mindset of rigidity where we are locked into processing and handling problems in only one way.
- As we continue to practice mindfulness and strengths use, obstacles will emerge. They will come up in our mind and our body. A big part of mindfulness is about how we deal with the obstacles. When we bring strengths to the practice to help us, this is called strong mindfulness because we are making our mindfulness practice more solid, secure, and strong.
  - Remind participants that they have now successfully used mindfulness and strengths to deal with many obstacles so they can certainly use both mindfulness and strengths when obstacles come up in their life and in their daily practice.

- Another thing that happens as we practice mindfulness, is we begin to notice the little things. We begin to smell the roses, to notice the smiles on the faces of our loved ones, and to see ourselves and our strengths more clearly. These little things are important. They really matter.
  - It is possible to see each of the character strengths in terms of big and little. It is the view of the little that matters most in MBSP. It takes mindfulness to bring our attention to these smaller, everyday displays of character strength. See Chapter 5 for examples and discussion.

VI Virtue Circle

- Conduct the virtue circle consistent with previous sessions.

VII Suggested Homework Exercises

- Body mindfulness meditation, 1×/day
- Character strengths breathing space exercise (1×/day formal practice; also informal practice as needed)
- Tracking/journaling (including tracking obstacles in your meditation practice and how you handled them, see Handout 3.1)
- Speak up! Strength spot, then appreciate – tell two people this week about your appreciation of their strengths in action
- Strengths-Activity Mapping (see Handout 3.3)

Homework Exercises Review

- Invite participants to be sure to use the character strengths breathing space exercise with some kind of regularity, scheduling it into daily life. Sometimes it is useful to pair it with other routines – before/after meals, before bedtime, first thing done while still lying in bed, etc. In addition, participants are encouraged to use it informally, which means to begin to

turn to it when they are feeling stressed or upset.
- For the speak up! exercise, encourage participants to be spontaneous with their strengths-spotting and strengths valuing; another approach is to plot out what might be said before approaching the person. Individuals can choose whomever they wish – someone in their personal life, or a random stranger such as a store clerk.
- Review the strengths-activity mapping handout. Describe the purposes of this exercise: to increase mindfulness of daily activities and the impact this has on our lives and to draw connections between activities and our strengths of character. Participants are free to choose either of the two options – whichever interests them more. One is more reflective, the other is more prospective and action-oriented. This activity ties in closely with the theme of noticing the "little," everyday use of character strengths.

Handouts

- Handout 3.1: Tracking & Suggested Exercises (1 page)
- Handout 3.2: Growing from Obstacles (1 page)
- Handout 3.3: Strengths-Activity Mapping (1 page)

VIII Closing Meditation: Leaf Meditation

- Time permitting, conclude the group with a brief meditation that allows people to walk away with the realization that little thing matter. This is an insight that tends to emerge as individuals practice mindfulness. This can be done with strong effect by meditating on one leaf. If this is not possible, then conclude with an abridged body mindfulness meditation emphasizing appreciation for one's body.
- Leaf meditation: Individuals practice applying beginner's mind to one leaf, taking in the

details, scent, texture, and wider perspective. Individuals notice the connection of the leaf with the larger whole (e.g., tree), seeing it as a living organism. These latter themes are present in many of the meditations and teachings of Thich Nhat Hanh (1998; 2009). See Box 9.2 for details.

Box 9.2. Leaf Meditation

Let's take a moment to look at this leaf closely. This is an object that is very easy to pass over and take for granted. Let's take a different approach to it. Using your breath to help you anchor into the present moment, observe the leaf. Turn the leaf over and explore it with some of your senses. Look at it deeply. Take a moment to "be" with it. Notice the colors, shapes, and texture of the leaf. Perhaps there's a sound you can notice. Maybe you can detect a scent from the leaf? (Long pause).

Can you see the life within the leaf? Maybe you can see the "veins" of the leaf that served to sustain its life. Can you see how the leaf is connected to all of nature? Perhaps you can see the tree in it, the sky, the cloud, and the sun? Without these elements, there would be no tree and therefore no leaf. Bring your mindful attention to your feelings from moment to moment as you experience this leaf. Take note of any thoughts or feelings related to the preciousness of this one object. Might we give such mindful attention to other things in our life? Our loved ones … our work … our day-to-day activities … our breath?

This leaf is one of the little things in life. And little things matter.

Additional Considerations

More Questions to Consider

- Looking at previous life experiences, how have you used mindfulness or character strengths to handle difficulties and life obstacles?
- How have you used your strengths to "bounce back" in your life?

- Think of something (or someone) you have given attention to that others typically have passed over. Name that "little thing" and describe the mindful attention you gave it?

Observations

The diversity of experiences and discussions that emerge in any particular session is striking. As the leader, one can take a quick snapshot at some point during the experience. Here's a sample of what was going on during one random moment of a group session. This is what I observed around me during the homework review of one MBSP group's Session 2:

- One man was showing his dyad partner a sheet of his top signature strengths and discussing how he uses them in his daily life
- One woman was speaking to her partner about the character strengths she observed in the characters of *The Hunger Games*.
- One woman was speaking to her two partners about the importance of savoring food as opposed to swallowing it whole.
- One woman was speaking to the role of acceptance with a challenge in her life and how she told herself "it's OK, I can face this. I can handle this. It's OK."
- One man was using the dyad experience to brainstorm about how he might use his character strengths to handle a particular situation in his life.
- One dyad was beginning to discuss character strengths combination as one man described bringing curiosity and kindness together in a more conscious way in his life; rather than being a passive observer, he decided he would take an approach of kind listening and curious questioning of people he encountered during the day such as the grocery store clerk, the drive-through window attendant, and his work colleagues. He reported an increase in energy from taking this approach.

Look for the positive contagion effect where one positive experience boosts another which opens individuals up to further positive emotions and exchanges. This is often evidenced in spontaneous strengths-spotting that participants offer to one another. This brings more quiet individuals into the fold and tends to direct individuals to reflect on previous strength-based exercises while intensifying an appreciation for the present moment. This virtuous circle naturally arises in the group and outside the group. One MBSP participant shared that she practiced mindful listening to her husband (who is not in MBSP) by being totally present and attentive to his words and compassionate and understanding of his stories. The next day, for the first time in years, he began taking the same approach as he listened to her.

Taking the Signature Strength "Pill"

One MBSP participant who suffered from depression explained her observations of the "signature strengths in new ways" exercise this way: "I have begun to practice mindfully using one of my signature strengths every day, usually in a new way," she said. "This has become my anti-depressant. I feel worse when I don't take this 'pill' and I feel better when I take it."

This participant's finding is aligned with empirical data that has shown this exercise can lower depression over long periods of time (Gander et al., 2012a; Seligman et al., 2005). MBSP practitioners need to be cautious to not suggest participants do an exercise such as this one as a replacement of other depression treatment (e.g., medications). It is, however, a wonderful and important adjunct.

Integrating Mindfulness and Character Strengths

As this is the first session in which mindfulness and character strengths are more explicitly integrated, it is useful to look for opportunities to draw connections. A common scenario at this stage is the individual who is attempting to become routinized with their mindfulness practice. One strategy is to inquire about the individual's signature strengths and ask them whether these strengths could be employed. A group brainstorm around the topic is also a good idea. Here are some examples for making good use of character strengths to assist in becoming regular with mindfulness practice each day:

- Practice mindfulness outside (or in front of a window) with my eyes open (if I'm high in *appreciation of beauty/excellence*).
- Merge it with meditative reading (if I'm high in *love of learning* or *perspective*).
- Merge it with mindful walking (if I'm high in *zest*).
- Practice mindfulness regularly with another person or as part of a spiritual community (if I'm high in *teamwork* or *spirituality/religiousness*).
- Infuse the practice with a blessing component at the beginning and end of the practice (if I'm high in *gratitude*).

Practice Trap

Be sure to take notice as to whether character strengths pull the person away from the present moment. For example, during the statue meditation exercise, one participant noted they used creativity to come up with many different ways to distract from the arm fatigue and shoulder tension; they played numbers games in their mind, focused on a nearby fan, and planned out the activities of the rest of their day. While this can be celebrated as a use of creativity in managing a stressor (i.e., developing multiple pathways to manage a problem) it should also be identified as an avoidance of the present moment. This individual was doing everything they could to shift away from the present moment rather than facing it, particularly because it was uncomfortable. While this dynamic may or may not be pointed out directly, the facilitator should not forget that this participant was indeed using a character strength at a difficult time and that this might be a resource in the future for the individual.

> **Lesson learned:** Strengths can have different effects – contributing to and enhancing present moment awareness or distracting the person from it.

MBSP Handout 3.1

Session 3: Obstacles are Opportunities

Tracking and Suggested Exercises

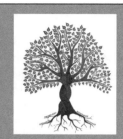

Suggested Exercises/Homework This Week:

- Body mindfulness meditation, 1×/day (track the obstacles to your practice and strengths you use)
- Character strengths breathing space (same time each day; and use it to face challenges)
- Track your meditation obstacles and experiences here and in your journal (see Handout 3.2)
- Speak up! Tell 2 people about your appreciation of their strengths in action
- Strengths-activity mapping (see Handout 3.3)

Day/Date	Type of Practice & Time Length	Obstacles to My Practice	Strengths Used	Observations/Comments
Tuesday Date:				
Wednesday Date:				
Thursday Date:				
Friday Date:				
Saturday Date:				
Sunday Date:				
Monday Date:				
Tuesday Date:				

MBSP Handout 3.2

Session 3:

Growing from Obstacles

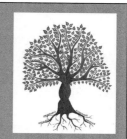

There are a multitude of barriers that can block the path of mindfulness practice and mindful living. The first step is to "catch" the obstacle as soon as possible, whether the obstacle appears to be internal (body sensations, thoughts, emotions) or external (environment, current situation). To "catch" the obstacle means to notice it and face it directly. Rather than avoiding it or directly trying to change it, consider the following two general approaches:

1.) *Take a "growth mindset" approach:* How might you view the obstacle, stressor, difficulty, or challenge as an opportunity for growth and learning? This approach involves viewing yourself as a person who is growing and improving and as someone who welcomes obstacles because they are "learning opportunities" for growth.

2.) *Use your signature strengths:* How you might use your best qualities – your signature strengths – to help you address the obstacle? A person high in curiosity might take an interest in the wandering mind while a person high in forgiveness might remind themselves that they are adept at "letting go" and can use this to manage thoughts.

Common Mindfulness Obstacles

Wandering mind: My mind didn't sit still:
- Judging mind
- Planning mind
- Wanting/craving mind
- Storytelling mind

Tiredness: I fell asleep. I'm too fatigued.

Pain or discomfort: My body tension and discomfort increased when I slowed down.

Excessive self-talk: My mind is negative. I have bad memories. I cannot stop worrying.

Irritation: I'm frustrated. I'm too upset.

Perfectionism: Am I doing it right? Am I good enough? Am I enlightened yet?

Expectations: Nothing is happening. I'm not making any progress. My mind keeps wandering so what's the point?

Schedule challenges: I don't have time to practice meditation. I've got too many things to do. Now is not the best time. I forgot to practice.

The conditions aren't right: It is too hot/cold here. There is too much noise here. I'm too hungry or full.

Feeling obligated: I have to meditate. I have no choice in the matter. I'm doing this to please someone else.

Boredom or lack of pleasure: I don't like this. What's the point? Is it almost over?

Strengths as obstacles: My curiosity is making my mind wander. My kindness (or humility) is driving me to focus only on others. My self-regulation is driving me to control everything. My prudence is holding me back. My creativity won't keep still.

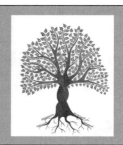

MBSP Handout 3.3

Session 3:

Strengths-Activity Mapping

As we go about our day we might not be paying much attention to the character strengths we are using in the moment. Our signature strengths come naturally to us but that doesn't mean we are always using them mindfully. Often, we are missing opportunities. We might be missing a chance to develop a strength, to attend more closely to an important interaction, or a chance for greater self-awareness.

Choose *one* of the following two activities:

Version 1 (Reflecting on your day)

Jot down your responses to the following questions:
- Consider an activity you do that's a routine. What strengths are you using to do it?
- Consider a regular activity that involves connecting with someone. What strengths do you use in the interaction? Explain.
- Consider an activity that involves some kind of work. What strengths are using? Explain.

Version 2 (Self-monitoring)

Bring your laser of mindfulness to one part of your day such as the morning, the afternoon, or the evening (e.g., a four-hour period). Commit to mindfully observe yourself as you go about your activities. Set an alarm on your watch or phone for every 15 minutes. Each time the alarm sounds, write down your response to these questions:
- What are you doing?
- What character strengths are you using? Explain how you are using each strength.
- How strong, on a scale of 1–10, are you using each strength (where a 10 is the highest degree possible)?

Chapter 10

Mindfulness-Based Strengths Practice

Session 4: Strengthening Mindfulness in Everyday Life (Strong Mindfulness)

Make the most of yourself, for that is all there is of you.

Ralph Waldo Emerson

Practicing mindfulness and strengths together is like having a second world open up to me.

MBSP participant

 Opening Story

A while back I was struggling to turn out of a downtown parking garage. Growing impatient, I forced my car into the rush-hour traffic so I could get on with my day. In doing so, I cut off another driver and I became the recipient of a short barrage of honks.

The other driver and I met up at the next traffic light. Simultaneously, we rolled down our windows and my heart began to race. I, the initial guilty party, decided to wait to see the approach she would take. Although I felt tensions rise, I also experienced flashes of curiosity, wondering what she would say.

How would she attack me? Would it be full of inflammation and obscenity? Would it be polite and gentle?

She dove head-first into yelling and blaming. I decided to argue in return. And back and forth we went. As we argued, I thought to myself how silly I must look since I was the one at fault. Eventually, we hit a stalemate and the light turned green. I drove off feeling worse.

I found myself wishing I would have admitted I was in error. I thought about how things might have been different for her if I had apologized and given her an opportunity of forgiveness. Instead, I took a nonskillful, mindless approach and I fueled her anger with further arguments. I was struck by how my mindless driving slipped into mindless listening and mindless speech.

I will never know the degree to which this situation impacted the rest of her day — did it cause a negative ripple effect in some way? When she tells the story to others, will she be digging into internal negativity? Will it cause her additional suffering?

As I drove off, my mind meandered around these questions and my lack of character strengths use — it was an underuse of kindness, judgment, and perspective for sure. In that moment, I became determined to use greater mindfulness the next time a similar situation emerged. Ten minutes later after picking up my wife, I saw a homeless woman at the corner asking for money. I'd previously driven passed this woman several times but this time I felt compelled to give her money and a packaged granola bar. So I did. She thanked me and I drove off.

When I was giving the woman money and food, I was drawing no conscious connection between the "bad" and the "good" incident. It was only a few minutes later that I realized there was perhaps a redemptive quality to my act of kindness. In a flash, my lapse in mindfulness had shifted back to mindful living.

Did my awareness of my flawed behavior coupled with my *intention* "to be better next time" spur an attitude toward strength use? Did training in mindfulness and character strengths create a stronger framework where mindlessness can only fester so long because other resources are nearby? I had committed a small tear in the web of human interconnectedness, and I then somehow sought to repair that tear as soon as possible through character strength expression. We might call this *strengths redemption*.

 Structure for Session 4

I   Opening Meditation: Character Strengths Breathing Space Exercise [3 min]
II   Practice Review [20 min]
III   Signature Strengths in a Flash Exercise [20 min]
IV   Walking Meditation [30 min]
V   Mindful Living [5 min]
VI   Virtue Circle [30 min]
VII   Suggested Homework Exercises [10 min]
VIII Closing Meditation: Strengths Gatha [2 min]

Note. Times are approximates. This is for a 2-hour session; for a 1.5-hour session, it's advisable to eliminate the virtue circle and shorten each section accordingly.

I   Opening Meditation

- Character strengths breathing space exercise: allowing for more silence and less guidance at each phase.

II   Practice Review

- Before beginning the homework review, reiterate and really emphasize how MBSP is all about "practice" when it comes to mindfulness work, mindful living, and character strengths work. We improve each of these through practice, practice, practice. It's noteworthy to think of "practice" as both a noun and a verb, i.e., "I have a strengths practice" and "I am practicing my mindfulness." Homework is, of course, one type of practice.
- Kabat-Zinn (2003) has commented about what is meant by the practice of meditation and he

explains that rather than a rehearsal for performance, practice is the actual engagement in the discipline that can be best understood as a way of being that is embodied and grows over time. Indeed, we are the result of our practice and we are the practice itself.

- Dyads or small group discussion of homework: Prioritize a review of the management of obstacles in the participants' meditation practice, the speak up! exercise, and the strengths-activity mapping.
  - When debriefing, the facilitator should emphasize the use of strengths to handle obstacles; how naming obstacles turns something that's typically vague and semi-conscious and gets in our way, into something that's much more *concrete*; the reframing that obstacles are opportunities for growth; and that we are already using our strengths but typically are not mindful of this.
  - The metaphor of a wall can be used. Some obstacles seem intimidating and insur-

mountable like a large wall. Rather than a futile struggle to hurdle the wall/obstacle in one big jump, it might be best to divide the wall into several "smaller obstacles" that one can manage and approach with strength.

- If dyads are implemented, consider having one person in each dyad introduce the other person to the larger group by sharing the insights/ideas they heard the other person describe.

III   Signature Strengths in a Flash Exercise

- Signature strengths in a flash exercise: Each person shares one example of how they used one of their signature strengths this week. However, the challenge is to use mindful speech that is brief, clear, specific, and from the heart. In a friendly way, the facilitator may impose a 30-second limit (using a timer). The facilitator, of course, should model an example using mindful speech.
- Group strengths: The signature strengths in a flash exercise can be a good lead-in to discussing the strengths of the group. Participants have discussed and begun to explore their individual strengths as well as observe and spot strengths in others. Another level is to consider the character strengths of the group-as-a-whole. This might simply be the strengths that were highest on the VIA Survey for most members or the strengths most frequently spotted at this point in the MBSP program. Or, it could be viewed as a general characteristic the group takes on, for example, some groups are always laughing and telling jokes (humor), others are highly supportive and empathic (kindness), while others are very enthusiastic and energized (zest). Of course, there may be several strengths that characterize the group; several strengths may combine to create new strengths (e.g., judgment, self-regulation, and perseverance seem to characterize "patience"). This inquiry and discussion of group strengths is repeated at least one other time in Session 8.

- The concept of strong mindfulness is explained (it might be noted that the participants explicitly practiced strong mindfulness last week when they practiced bringing character strengths to their experience of holding their arms out). See Chapter 4 to learn more about strong mindfulness.
  - This concept refers to bringing character strengths to our mindfulness:
    - To make our mindfulness practices stronger because strengths help us overcome obstacles and difficulties with the practice.
    - To deepen our experiences of mindful living.
    - To supercharge and reinvigorate any mindfulness practice.

IV   Walking Meditation

- Start with a brief standing meditation (just as they did last week), then after a few minutes, share some of the features of walking meditation and the way that it will be practiced.
- It's usually best to invite participants to follow along one-by-one. Everyone is invited to walk in silence, slowly, with open attention to their bodies, minds, and external surroundings. The primary intention is to practice walking with mindfulness and secondarily, to consider the character strengths one is deploying in the walk.
- Periodically, the facilitator may offer reminders, questions, and cues (to help break participants' autopilot tendencies) with comments such as the following:
  - I wonder if you are taking notice of your posture as you walk.
  - Are you aware of how you place each foot down? What part of your foot touches the ground first?
  - Have you stayed connected with your breathing as you move?
  - Are you striking a balance of external and internal mindfulness? Taking in the visuals, sounds, and external elements, as well as noticing your body and feelings, moment-to-moment as you walk?

– What character strengths are you aware of as you walk? What strengths are you naturally using? (See discussion and examples in Chapter 4 that describe ways in which each of the 24 character strengths are part of or might enhance mindful walking.)

○ Here is an important part of the experience: About mid-way through the exercise, it's typically useful to invite participants to share aloud the strengths they are using as they continue to walk. They're encouraged to name the strength and give a brief (one-sentence) rationale of how they are using it.

· "I'm noticing zest because I'm feeling more energized and enthused as I continue this exercise."

· "Prudence – I'm watching every step I make and it's as though I'm being very careful to not step on a single bug."

· "Appreciation of beauty because I'm taking notice of details I had never seen before. They are quite striking and beautiful."

• Some practitioners will feel more comfortable processing strengths use following the walk due to concern that naming strengths during the meditation might pull the individual out of the present moment experience. This is an important concern for practitioners to be sensitive to. At the same time, however, it is typically much easier for participants to identify strengths in the moment while they are being deployed than reflecting back on the experience and attempting to recall subtle strengths use with accuracy. Practitioners can strike a balance with this dynamic by allowing a period of time for walking in silence, followed by monitoring and expressing strengths aloud as they are noticed, and then concluding with further mindful walking in silence.

V Mindful Living

• As this session is about "strong mindfulness," the leader should look for other opportunities to draw the participants' connection to using

strengths to promote mindful living (see Chapter 4). If this can be done through experiences happening in the group already that is ideal. Walking is just one example of an aspect of daily living that is done in the session. Examples may come elsewhere such as while participants are listening or speaking, query the character strengths they are using in the moment; ask them which strengths they could use to strengthen their mindful speech and mindful listening.

• Practitioners also might ask participants certain questions that elicit discussion and insights relating to mindful living.

– What does "mindful living" mean to you?

– How might you deploy your signature strengths to live with greater mindfulness?

– What area of mindful living (e.g., eating, driving, consuming, etc.) is in most need of your mindful attention and character strengths use?

VI Virtue Circle

VII Suggested Homework Exercises

• Walking meditation, 1×/day.
• Character strengths breathing space exercise.
• Track mindfulness practices, including mindful walking, eating, driving, etc (see Handout 4.1).
• Conduct a strengths interview with a family member, friend, or colleague (see Handout 4.2).
• Create a gatha that reflects or inspires your mindful strengths use or strong mindfulness (see Handout 4.3).

Homework Exercises Review

• Encourage participants to engage in a new meditation practice this week – the walking meditation.

– For those that have a steady, wonderful body scan or sitting meditation practice going and don't want to give it up, tell them they don't have to give it up! Invite them to consider adding in walking meditation at the beginning or ending of their regular practice. Another option is to do what some mindfulness communities do which is to weave walking meditation in the middle of sitting meditation where mindful walking becomes the centerpiece of the whole meditation experience.

- For those that are not steady with a regular meditation practice, the walking meditation provides a new and fresh opportunity to engage. For many, it is a novel practice and being mindfulness-in-motion, it allows participants to be active, burning excess mental energy while practicing.

• Tracking/journaling: The facilitator might give mention to pay particular attention this week to the various aspects of mindful living and the character strengths used to engage fully in each, e.g., prudence and kindness while driving, self-regulation and curiosity while eating, etc.

• Strengths interview: For this exercise, ask participants to identify one person in their life that they'd like to interview about their strengths (if there's time, you might query the participants as to who comes to mind that they would like to interview). Participants are welcome to follow the questions and structure on the handout verbatim, to be spontaneous with their own strength-based questions, or a hybrid of these two approaches.

- This strengths interview is done prior to the exercise covered next week, the character strengths 360 exercise, in order to first allow individuals to become accustomed to talking with people in their life about strengths, starting with someone they probably know well and are already comfortable with.

• Gatha: This will be a new concept to the majority of participants. A gatha is a Sanskrit word meaning short verse, poem, or song. Take a moment to explain the handout, noting what a gatha is, how it's different from a mantra (in which individuals repeat a word or sound with the intention of creating a relaxed or oneness state), and emphasize that the gatha practice helps to create an experience both in the mo-

ment *and* for the immediate future based on the gatha's contents. Said another way, the gatha is a catalyst for mindfulness and an intention for the immediate future.

- Encourage participants to tap into their creativity strength and note that they will be welcome to share their gathas with the group in a future session or keep them private, whichever they prefer. I have found the first gatha by Thich Nhat Hanh described in Handout 4.3 to be very powerful over the years. It has helped me prepare my body and mind for difficult meetings, shift my worries to a simple focus on the present moment, and boost my confidence at times when I felt lost.

- Sometimes the reaction individuals have to this exercise is "I can't" or "I'm not creative." The idea is to bring mindfulness and character strengths to the task and simply put pen to paper. I'll never forget one woman whose reaction initially was "What is Ryan talking about with this exercise? I cannot do that." But, she started to write a strengths gatha and the words flowed out. That week ended up being a particularly challenging week for her because she was almost fired at work, her chronic pain flared up, and she was "stood up" by a new date. She turned to her gatha all week long. She called it her "saving grace."

- What follows is an example of a strengths gatha, accompanied by explanations of each line in brackets:

  ○ Breathing in, I see my strengths ["seeing" is likened to a turning inward to look and to re-discover]

  ○ Breathing out, I value my strengths ["valuing" involves appreciating the strengths one "sees" in oneself]

  ○ Dwelling now in my strengths ["dwelling" involves "being present" to one's inherent goodness]

  ○ I express myself fully ["expressing" is likened to "doing" and taking action for the good with one's strengths. Since this is the final line of the final exercise for Session 4, it can serve as a lingering, positive energy as individuals move forward with their day]

Handouts

- Handout 4.1: Tracking & Suggested Exercises (1 page)
- Handout 4.2: Strengths Interview (1 page)
- Handout 4.3: Strengths Gathas (1 page)

VIII Closing Meditation: Strengths Gatha

- Conclude the session with a strengths gatha (one of those that focus on strengths on the handout or even better, one you have personally created). This is important and timely since you'll have just explained this exercise and because the participants will be expected to create a gatha as homework. Track 5 of the attached CD offers an example of a strengths gatha.

Additional considerations

Applying the Adverb or Adjective

"Mindful" and "mindfully" can be used as modifiers to describe the action or inaction in our life. There is always an opportunity to be mindful. Mindful describes our approach as one that is attentive, curious, and connected. This can be applied to aspects of mindful living as discussed in today's session – walking, driving, eating, seeing, working, playing, etc.

Mindless Walking Practice

Many times, the best way to learn about a new practice is to practice its opposite. On some occasions in Session 4, I precede the walking meditation practice with a practice of "mindless walking." The group and I act as if we are running late for an appointment and we walk very fast as if we are stressed, preoccupied, and/or upset. Then, the shift to mindful walking becomes even more dramatic. Participants typically relate to mindless walking because it is a big part of their lives

and they can readily observe the "tunnel vision" or unitary focus that emerges in which everything is blocked off except for getting to the appointment. This fun, often humorous practice elevates the importance of mindful walking as well as the strengths use therein.

Practice Trap

It's around this time that participants are really digging in and exploring their strengths more deeply and beginning to ask questions about the overuse of strengths, the problems strengths can cause, and the dark side of strengths. These focus areas are purposefully included later in the program in Session 6. Practitioners are also typically attracted to these issues and readily want to address them. This is a trap for the practitioner (and participant) because the more crucial exploration material of strength use, strengths fluency, and strengths application – all of which are rich for cultivation – can get lost. The overall process is that participants build competence in their strengths use and mindfulness for several sessions which leads into issues of overuse, hot buttons, and the handling of problems.

People are fascinated by overuse but this can come at the expense of not having adequately explored their strengths. One example is found in a human resources manager who had the strength of prudence in her top 5 rankings of strengths. She wanted to be coached by me because she said she was overusing her prudence strength. When I asked her to tell me first about how she uses her prudence, she was silent. I encouraged her to tell me about the good of her prudence, how she used it in different settings, and how others might describe it in her, and she had nothing substantive to say. Therefore, this woman had minimal mindfulness of her strength yet was eager to begin figuring out how she overused it and could decrease the use. She was glossing over a core part of herself, a quality that had helped her accomplish so much over the years.

> **Lesson learned:** Becoming mindful that strengths use precedes delving into strengths overuse.

Group Snapshot

Every group of individuals that gathers for an MBSP experience is different, as is each particular session. No two are ever the same. However, insights can be gleaned by practitioners from studying previous participants' responses. What follows are the main points shared by each individual during the homework review of one MBSP group's Session 4 (names have been changed to protect confidentiality):

- Margaret opened the discussion. She shared how she has become more aware of how we all have such different filters or lenses by which we view the world. She realizes she has used her love of learning strength her whole life and that this is what fills her and ignites her passion; she becomes triggered by anti-intellectualism of individuals and the culture as a whole. Her lens, which she notes can be narrow at times, is through love of learning. Up to this point in MBSP, she explains her focus has been more on the practice of mindful eating and on using two of her signature strengths in new ways. She is struck by the finding that she can use mindfulness to ignite her senses and is particularly excited to tap this in an upcoming drawing class she is taking.

- Evan went next. He explained he is resonating closely with mindfulness of activities of daily life. He sometimes forgets the other homework exercises and has stuck with this one consistently. He has practiced mindfulness for years but previously had not engaged in any mindfulness of daily life activity. There was something about this focus in the homework that served as a catalyst for him to jump in with it. Consequently, he has noticed a boost in a few of his strengths that are outside of his top 5, namely bravery and gratitude. In a recent social activity that was of little interest to him, he used these strengths – bravery to attend the event and gratitude as a mechanism for connecting with others socially. He was surprised by the amount of enjoyment he experienced. He noted he also appreciates having his three humanity signature strengths "on queue" to use as needed in social situations.

- Sally then explained that she feels she is selfish at times when she guards her time closely and insists on keeping to a plan and schedule. Thus she has been challenged by the homework exercises. She then explained that she particularly appreciates the character strengths breathing space exercise and doing it in three-minute increments. She discussed her use of mindfulness with a routine activity (making her bed) and linked her strength of gratitude with this, in that she felt grateful that she had the ability to make her bed, and to move her muscles and body in a way to make the bed. She told a story of how she used her signature strengths in her relationship when she went away for the weekend and "unselfishly" placed the attention and focus on her partner for the weekend. This was different for her and it felt good; she used her humanity and "other-oriented" strengths to do so.

- Martina noted she has been working with the body scan practice. She has incorporated this in her prayer life. She has practiced using her strength of gratitude in a new way each day, finding new blessings to count and people to thank in her life. She explained that brushing her teeth mindfully each day has served as a good reminder for her to expand mindfulness to other activities.

- Jim explained that the key word for him in the discussion so far was the word "expand." He said this taps into how he is approaching his development and learnings in regard to both mindfulness and character strengths. He notices this expansion during the perspective phase of the character strengths breathing space exercise, as well as in the exercise using signature strengths in new ways ("expanding" the use). He stated he is attempting to memorize the VIA Classification "language" so that he can more readily spot character strengths in others and in his daily activities.

- Merle explained that this group marks the first time in her life that she has taken the time to focus on strengths (she's a woman in her late 60 s). This newness is a breath of fresh air for her. She has also become aware of a deeper sense of trust that has emerged strongly as she develops her signature strengths, namely a deeper trust in herself. She recalled examples of how others brought forth a strength that is one of her signature strengths and how it felt like an affront to her because they were using too much of the strength or in a way she did not like. Her thought was – "I don't want anyone to mess with my identity" (my top signature strengths). But, when this occurs, she stated she was able to notice it quickly and come back to reality (the present moment) and re-adjust.

- Ava noted she has leaned more toward the mindfulness practice than the character strengths practice this week. While she was eating one day, she suddenly awoke from autopilot and began to eat mindfully. She was aware of this and labeled it, which, in turn, was positively reinforcing for her. She gave an example in which she returned to the office after being gone for a week and discovered she had 1,100 e-mails to catch up on. She felt deluged and stressed by this and was working hard on de-cluttering her e-mails when her flow was suddenly interrupted by a colleague walking into her office to ask her a question. She didn't react abruptly. Instead she consciously paused, breathed, and shifted her focus to the person telling herself, "be here now." Ava was really pleased that she responded mindfully instead of reacting habitually and felt energized by this small example that showed potential for creating more meaningful interactions with others.

- Ted shared that he was challenged by a recent vacation which disrupted his mindfulness routine and his strengths practice. He "let go" of this disruption and the imperfect homework practice he had and regrouped. He noted he is working on one of his lower strengths – self-regulation – by setting a schedule to practice mindfulness at two particular times during the day. He noted this had worked well prior to his vacation and that he was struck by how the self-discipline had carried over into other domains of his life.

MBSP Handout 4.1

Session 4: Strengthening Mindfulness in Everyday Life

Tracking and Suggested Exercises

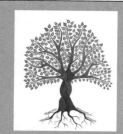

Suggested Exercises/Homework This Week:

- Walking meditation, 1×/day
- Character strengths breathing space exercise
- Track all mindfulness practices, including mindful walking, eating, driving, etc. below
- Conduct a strengths interview with a family member/friend/colleague (Handout 4.2)
- Create a gatha that reflects or inspires your practice with mindfulness and strengths (Handout 4.3)

Day/Date	Type of Practice & Time Length	Obstacles to My Practice	Strengths Used	Observations/Comments
Tuesday Date:				
Wednesday Date:				
Thursday Date:				
Friday Date:				
Saturday Date:				
Sunday Date:				
Monday Date:				
Tuesday Date:				

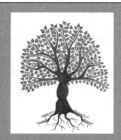

MBSP Handout 4.2

Session 4:

Strengths Interview

Instructions

Invite someone in your life (family member, friend, acquaintance, neighbor, co-worker) to allow you to interview them about their strengths. You might explain it this way:

> "I am spending more time focusing on what is *strongest* in myself and in the people around me. I would like to learn about your strengths and how they connect with who you are, as well as with your past successes. Thank you for your willingness to explore this with me."

Tips

- Approach the interview with a beginner's mind – listening to the responses as if for the first time, with a sense of newness and freshness, fully tuned in.
- Allow the interview to take a life of its own. Remember this is someone you have a relationship with; we cannot control relationships, so just *allow* the interaction to unfold.
- Keep the focus on the other person. You can make time to share your own story and feedback, if you wish, following the interview.
- During the interview, which of your signature strengths will you be mindfully using?
- Are there other strengths you will practice using (e.g., curiosity)?
- Practice mindful listening. When your mind wanders or you lose track of what to ask, trust in yourself (return to your breath, return to your strengths).
- If the person shifts to speaking of the negative, dwelling on what went wrong, or becomes tangential, shift the focus back to strengths.
- Use these questions below as a starting point; you might wish to map out these and other questions before you meet with the person.

Questions (see also Handout 2.3 Exploring Strengths)

What was one of the best experiences of your professional (or personal) life – a time when you felt most alive, engaged, and proud of your work? I'm wondering about a time when you felt you were *at your best*, perhaps it was when you were most successful, most happy, most connected with people, or all of the above. After the story, together, practice spotting strengths.

What are you *highest* strengths? (Feel free to hand the person the VIA Classification as a cue)

How have you used your strengths to *overcome* adversity and stress in your life?

During a typical day, when do you feel most *energetic* and *alive*? What are the *little things* in life that matter most to you? Which of your strengths contribute to these?

What *engages* you most – or connects you most with the present moment? What activities give you the most *pleasure*? What gives you a sense of *meaning* and purpose? How often do you tap into that experience of meaning? How might your strengths help you to search for or discover meaning?

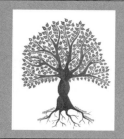

MBSP Handout 4.3

Session 4:

Strengths Gathas

Gathas are short verses that help us practice mindfulness in our daily activities. Some are rhythmic and metered. A gatha may be a poem, a song, and/or a guided meditation. Thich Nhat Hanh describes them this way: "A gatha can open and deepen our experience of simple acts which we often take for granted. When we focus our mind on a gatha, we return to ourselves and become more aware of each action. When the gatha ends, we continue our activity with heightened awareness." See Thich Nhat Hanh's website on this topic: http://www.plumvillage.org/

Examples from Thich Nhat Hanh

From *The Miracle of Mindfulness* (Thich Nhat Hanh)

Breathing in, I calm my body,
Breathing out, I smile,
Dwelling in this present moment
I know this is a wonderful moment

From *Present Moment, Wonderful Moment* (Thich Nhat Hanh on "mindful driving")

Before starting the car
I know where I am going.
The car and I are one.
If the car goes fast, I go fast.
If the car goes slowly, I go slowly.

Mindfulness and Character Strengths (Ryan Niemiec)

Breathing in, I see my strengths,
Breathing out, I value my strengths,
(inhaling) Dwelling now in my strengths,
(exhaling) I express myself fully.

Breathing in, I see my potential,
Breathing out, I see my forgiveness and humility,
Remembering and using my strengths,
I grow and deepen.

Chapter 11

Mindfulness-Based Strengths Practice

Session 5: Valuing Your Relationships

In this life we cannot do great things. We can only do small things with great love.

Mother Teresa

The source of love is deep in us and we can help others realize a lot of happiness. One word, one action, one thought can reduce another person's suffering and bring that person joy.

Thich Nhat Hanh

 Opening Stories

A Tibetan monk, released by the Chinese after years of imprisonment, was received by the Dalai Lama. When this worthy asked, "Were you ever in danger?" the monk replied, "A few times I was in danger of losing my sense of compassion for the guards." (Marvin Levine, 2009, p. 50).

This second story comes from Kornfield and Feldman (1996) who describe a young woman beginning to practice loving-kindness meditation on a daily basis. She filled her heart with love and directed it toward herself and toward others. Each day when she went to the market she encountered a shopkeeper who subjected her to unwelcomed caresses.

One day she could stand no more and began to chase the shopkeeper down the road with her upraised umbrella. To her mortification she passed her meditation master standing on the side of the road observing this spectacle. Shame-faced she went to stand before him expecting to be rebuked for her anger.

"What you should do," her master kindly advised her, "is to fill your heart with loving-kindness, and with as much mindfulness as you can muster, hit this unruly fellow over the head with your umbrella." (p. 274–275).

 Structure for Session 5

I   Opening Meditation: Strengths Gatha [3 min]
II Practice Review [30 min]
III Valuing Your Relationships [30 min]
IV Meditation: Loving-Kindness Meditation and Strength-Exploration Meditation [30 min]
V   Virtue Circle [20 min]

VI   Suggested Homework Exercises [6 min]
VII   Closing: Strengths Gatha [1 min]

Note. Times are approximates. This is for a 2-hour session; for a 1.5-hour session, it's advisable to eliminate the virtue circle and shorten each section accordingly.

I   Opening Meditation: Strengths Gatha

- Part of the homework for this session was to create a strengths gatha. See if there is a participant who would like to share their gatha; ask them to read it slowly two times. The leader can still invite and close the gatha meditation with the bell. If no one volunteers, use the strengths gatha on the handout.

II   Practice Review

- What went well in the practice of mindfulness and strengths this week?
- If possible, create dyads based on individuals' preferences for the activity they would like to discuss the most – the strengths interview, the strengths gatha, or mindful walking/daily practice. This self-selection approach is a way of going with the energy of each individual, boosting motivation, and covering all the topics.
- It's fascinating to hear the responses to each of these exercises. There are often one or more participants who conduct the strengths interview with their spouse. It's enlivening to witness their excitement and surprise as to how different it was to communicate with their partner in this way. These are individuals with decades of marriage under their belt but, like all marriages, fall into certain routines; often these routines do not involve the use of curiosity, exploration, and direct and explicit questioning around what is best in the other.

III   Valuing Your Relationships

On Valuing

- To value is to give something our attention and therefore place our energy on it. Our relationships are one of the areas most important for our well-being and happiness. Thus, learning to place attention and value on relationships is important.
- For many of us, valuing and placing attention on something (like relationships) is not enough. It's the putting of these "values" into action that ends up mattering and having the impact. This putting of values into action is what is known as *character*. Participants did this explicitly with the strengths interview this week, during the strengths-spotting/valuing within the group over the last 4 weeks, and with the mindful listening/speaking practices.
- We can approach this topic of exploring the value of our relationships and how they matter from at least two angles – our relationships with other people and our relationship with ourselves. Let's consider examples and the science.

Relationship With Others

- In the science of positive psychology, one of the most striking findings comes from what is referred to as the positivity ratio. Through complex, mathematical formulas, scientists (Barbara Fredrickson & Marcial Losada, 2005) devised a ratio for optimal well-being or flourishing. They found that a ratio of three positive emotions/sentiments expressed for every one negative emotion/sentiment expressed is a good recipe for flourishing. This is useful because research finds that less than 20% of people are flourishing (Keyes, 2002). It's also useful because research repeatedly finds that "bad is stronger than good," e.g., bad feedback is stronger than good feedback, bad health has a bigger impact on us than good health, bad relationships impact us more than good relationships, people are motivated to avoid bad self-definitions than to pursue good ones, and so on (Baumeister et al., 2001). We are wired to focus on what is wrong. Thus, we need the positivity ratio to find balance and to function at a high level.

- This ratio becomes more steep (and one could say, more pertinent) for couples/marriages (Gottman, 1994) and teams (Losada, 1999; Losada & Heaphy, 2004). For a marriage or team to flourish, the positivity ratio extends to 5 : 1.

- Now, apply this positivity ratio of emotions to character strengths. Might a good marker for marriages, teams, and other relationships be to strengths-spot/strengths-value at 5 for every 1 critique/negative comment? This is not a research finding but is a potential marker for a strong strengths-spotting ratio that creates a virtuous circle of positivity to improve relationships and strengths awareness/knowledge and could change the culture of a team or relationship.

- One could then apply this same thinking to oneself for the 3 : 1 ratio. Oftentimes, our mind is occupied with self-criticism, self-doubt, self-disappointment, worry, etc. What if an individual kept those thoughts, but was able to observe them as they occur and balance them by reflecting on their character strengths and other good qualities three times as much?

- The positivity ratio thus helps create further rationale for the importance of strengths mindfulness and strengths-spotting in relationships.

Relationship With Ourselves

- We each have a mind that suffers at times. It is interesting to view our mind in this way – as an entity that suffers. This helps us understand the importance of empathy for ourselves and the need to show compassion for that suffering "entity." Sometimes our mind is struggling because it's not getting what it wants, it was hurt, or various other reasons. We can notice this and treat that part of ourselves with care. This is part of creating a good relationship with oneself.

- This concept of "relationship with oneself" is less obvious because many people do not think of relating to themselves. But, consider this: How do you approach yourself when things go wrong? How do you treat yourself? If you examine your self-talk (your thinking), how do you typically approach yourself? Some people approach themselves with heavy criticism and self-judgment while others might approach themselves as perfect entities never doing something wrong. If you observe what you are saying to yourself, would you ever say those things to other people? Probably not. We are usually much harder on ourselves.

- It's important to come to know *how* we are relating to ourselves and not simply becoming familiar with the content of what we are saying. Mindfulness approaches do not try to change the content of thinking per se, rather they help participants to shift in how they relate to themselves. Mindfulness and character strengths help individuals to relate to themselves in a compassionate, open, curious, and accepting way. Entire programs that train people on how to build self-compassion exist. In this session, participants will engage in one practice from these kinds of programs.

- Leaders in the field of self-compassion and loving-kindness offer the following observations:
  - The popular mindfulness teacher Tara Brach (2003) explains that there are two wings of awareness – mindfulness and

compassion – and without both wings one will not be able to fly. Individuals need both as they encounter life and grow in their consciousness.

- Sharon Salzberg (2011) has described loving-kindness as a quality of the heart that recognizes how connected humans are and is a form of inclusiveness and caring for others.

- Acceptance is an important part of our relationship with ourselves. One form of acceptance is self-compassion. As Christopher Germer (2009) describes: "acceptance usually refers to what's happening to us – accepting a feeling or a thought – self-compassion is acceptance of the person to whom it's happening. It's acceptance of ourselves while we're in pain" (p. 33).

- Kristin Neff (2003a) explains that self-compassion involves self-kindness rather than self-judgment; perceiving one's experiences as part of the larger human experience rather than viewing experiences as isolated from others; and facing difficult thoughts/feelings with mindful awareness rather than over-identifying with them as truths or facts about oneself.

• Let's consider an example offered by one luminary (I'll call her "Joan") in the area of loving-kindness meditation, which is a practice that helps individuals foster a different way of relating to themselves. Before embarking on loving-kindness practice, Joan cites an example of how she frequently critiqued herself, calling herself "clumsy" and other names. When she'd trip over a table in her house and spill the glass of milk she was carrying, she would immediately berate herself: "You clumsy fool!" Joan would say. Over time she began to practice loving-kindness every day, for months. One day she noticed an important shift that had taken place in how she related to herself. She was walking across her room, tripped over her table and spilling milk on the floor, she said, "Joan, you're so clumsy, but I love you anyway." An automatic shift had occurred in Joan. She had learned to relate to herself in a new way, applying a more compassionate and accepting approach to herself.

• Subtle changes in how we approach ourselves can have a significant impact. We can use mindful awareness of our moment-to-moment experience to better understand how we relate to ourselves. We can use character strengths as a language that offers a major shift in that relationship. When we are looking for strengths in ourselves, we are more curious, open, and exploratory; we probably see ourselves in a more positive, balanced, and accepting way.

IV   Meditation: Loving-Kindness Meditation and Strength-Exploration Meditation

1. *Preparation and background for the facilitator to consider.* For the sake of time and reasons explained later, I usually merge two meditations. One of these is a guided mindfulness meditation (GMM) that is more leader-controlled as the leader guides the participants through a process focused on one particular character strength (love). The second meditation is open-ended, more participant-controlled, where each individual chooses a strength they'd like to focus on. It's generally a good idea to explain both meditations before starting; noting that one is mostly guided and the other is mostly open-ended; and noting that each involves the participants selecting something that will help in the meditation. For the loving-kindness meditation, participants will need to image an experience in which they felt loved by someone; for the strength-exploration meditation, participants select the strength ahead of time that they would like to focus on. How do participants select the strength for the second part? Offer these questions:

- Do you have a particular emotion/feeling about one of the 24 strengths that you are trying to better understand?

- When you think of your signature strengths, do you feel a lack of energy, excitement, or confidence about one in particular?

- Is there a signature strength that you don't agree with, that you don't accept, are unsure of, or that you don't want?
- Is there a particular character strength that you are curious to learn more about?

2. *Introduction to the meditations.* We can build our relationship with ourselves through a practice of mindfulness, as well as with a focus on specific character strengths. The first meditation on loving-kindness is centuries old. It involves first imaging a time when you felt deeply and genuinely loved, imaging the person who was offering you this love, feeling this in your body in the present moment, and then stating four meditation phrases to reinforce the strength of love. Then, the second meditation is an opportunity to focus on one strength – to simply follow your breathing and image one strength of your choice; you can then monitor your body and mind, moment-to-moment taking notice of what occurs in relation to this strength. [This latter exercise, while potentially more challenging because of its open-ended nature might require the practitioner to offer a reminder on the value of silence and listening to oneself; it also tends to work best if the participants have a particular concern or feeling about a specific strength that they are focusing on (see the earlier questions) and they can then bring mindfulness to watch their experience closely as they "sit with" the strength.]

   Preliminary inquiries. Before we begin, I want to make sure you have selected focal points for both meditations. Do you have a loving person in mind whom you feel has strongly expressed love and warmth toward you? And, do you have one character strength in mind that you can focus on after we complete the loving-kindness meditation?

3. *Loving-kindness meditation* (abbreviated, pause after each sentence). [Listen to Track 6 of the attached CD for an example of this meditation]. Think of a time when you felt deeply and genuinely loved by someone. Call forth a particular moment in time. Feel the warmth in this moment. Image the person offering you the love in detail. Picture the situation you are in. Allow yourself to be open to the experience of love. Take notice of the sen-

sations in your body, your heart. Stay with this for a moment. Now, image and say these loving-kindness meditation phrases to yourself (see Handout 1.4). [Practitioner reads through these four lines at least twice with long pauses in between each line.]

4. *Transition.* Offer a pause and invitation for the participants to return to their breath anchor, let go of the last experience, and become fully in the present moment.

5. *Strength-exploration meditation* (abbreviated). [Listen to Track 7 of the attached CD for an example of this meditation]. Now, let's use our mindfulness to focus in on one character strength – the strength you selected prior to the meditation. As you follow your breathing, bring your full attention to that one strength. You can do this in any way you like. People do this in a variety of ways – the important aspect of the experience is to keep your focus on the strength. You might image it, picture it in motion, consider what it symbolizes, reflect on a past situation in which you used it, or simply just breathe with the word. (Pause). When your mind wanders, simply bring it back to the strength. What does this strength mean to you? Be open to what your body and mind intuitively decide to do. Be curious about your body and mind and the moment-to-moment experience. Be open to small changes in your thinking, feeling, memories, ideas, and body. Rather than judging what happens, do the best you can to practice being curious and open to your experience. If your mind seems to trail too far off, simply bring it back to focusing on the character strength.

6. *Debriefing.*
   - What struck you about this experience?
   - What did you become aware of in either meditation?
   - Did you feel love in your body, and if so, where?
   - What happened as you focused on one character strength and became open to the moment-to-moment experience with it?
   - Which exercise resonated more with you? Why do you suppose that was?
   - Which one brings forth additional curiosity and interest, pushing you to investigate further?

V Virtue Circle

VI Suggested Homework Exercises

- Loving-kindness meditation, 1 ×/day (Handout 5.4)
  - Or, practice the strength-exploration meditation with one strength
- Character strengths breathing space exercise
- Tracking mindfulness/strengths experiences (Handout 5.1)
- Character strengths 360 exercise (strengths interviews II): Ask several people in your life to: (a) Name the strengths they see in you and (b) Share an example of when they have seen you use that strength (Handout 5.2)
- Complete the character strengths brainstorm worksheet for one of your strengths (Handout 5.5)

Homework Exercises Review

- Participants are encouraged to practice either the GMM of loving-kindness meditation or the strength-exploration meditation exploring one specific character strength. Some participants might alternate from day to day while others will focus solely on one for the week.
- The character strengths brainstorm worksheet[1] is offered as a way for individuals to dig into the nuances of one particular strength. It's a nice lead-in for next week's session which begins to look at overuse and underuse of strengths. Participants who complete this worksheet will be better equipped for the following session.
  - I also bring participants' attention to the final question on the worksheet which is to describe the strength in 6 words. Note that next week, participants will be invited to share the 6 words with the group and the group will attempt to guess what strength the person is describing.

---

[1] I'd like to give credit to strengths educator and author Jenny Fox-Eades, who inspired earlier versions of this worksheet that were then used with success in workshops around the world by the VIA Institute on Character.

- Character strengths 360 exercise: In companies around the world, "360 evaluations" have become the standard for offering employees feedback on their work; the 360 evaluations are assembled from the employee's supervisor, team members, colleagues, and the employee themselves. Feedback on character strengths can work in a similar way. For this exercise, participants are invited to hand out as many of the character strengths 360 forms as they are comfortable giving to people. Participants are encouraged to pass them along to individuals in different life domains, e.g., family, social, work, school, spiritual, etc. Each participant can use the character strengths 360 exercise tracking form (Handout 5.3) as a way to monitor the feedback they receive and begin to make sense of it. There is a spot for participants to write the first name or initials of the person offering the feedback, the primary domain in which this person knows the participant, and then boxes for the participant to check-off the strengths this person spotted. Participants can also check-off the strengths noted by the VIA Survey. Notice there are three main categories participants might attempt to glean insights from as they consider their VIA Survey results alongside the character strengths 360 results:
  1. *Strong signature strengths:* those strengths noted high by both oneself and others.
  2. *Possible blind spots:* those strengths noted high by others only, thus represent areas that the individual might be "blind" to or less aware of.
  3. *Potential opportunities:* those strengths noted high by oneself only, thus represent avenues of future expression with others.

  In order for some participants to receive feedback from distant family and friends, permission can be given to participants to scan the character strengths 360 and send it in electronic form to people in their life (note that this permission is granted only for use with this exercise). This gives flexibility to individuals to offer it face-to-face or by e-mail. It is up to each recipient to determine how many strengths they will check off; if a participant is concerned about this or if one of their recipients expresses difficulty with the open-endedness of the exercise, then the participant might advise each person to limit the selections to five to seven strengths.

This is one of the most popular activities of MBSP, so encourage participants to enjoy the experience. Indeed, it's very interesting to see what emerges. Some participants compile additional files that further examine people's responses and their own results on the VIA Survey.

Some participants express concern that it will be difficult to ask various people to offer feedback to them about their positive qualities. Facilitators can normalize this experience in that it can feel awkward at first and encourage participants to offer a good rationale for why they are asking the person for the feedback. For example:

> I'm participating in an 8-week course focused on learning about mindfulness and about strengths. As part of the course, we are passing out this list of character strengths and inviting important people in our lives to fill out the form on our behalf. I value your feedback and would appreciate your thoughts. The idea is to check off the strengths that you see as strongest in me. [Many people limit themselves to around 5 or so.] Then, write a sentence or two of rationale for how you have seen that strength in me. These are all positive qualities so there is nothing negative that you can say about me by completing this form.

VII Closing Meditation: Strength Gatha

- Consider another volunteer to offer a strengths gatha to the group. Ask them to read it slowly two times. If no one volunteers, close with the strengths gatha on the handout. Listen to Track 5 of the attached CD.

Handouts

- Handout 5.1: Tracking & Suggested Exercises (1 page)

- Handout 5.2: Character Strengths 360 (1 page; give 5–10 copies per participant)
- Handout 5.3: Character Strengths 360 Tracking Grid (1 page)
- Handout 5.4: Loving-Kindness Meditation (1 page)
- Handout 5.5: Character Strengths Brainstorm (1 page)

Additional Considerations

Comments

The first meditation on loving-kindness is traditionally explained as a practice that begins to shift over time. The natural progression – after becoming strong at being able to generate, feel, and send love to oneself – is to generate love and direct it toward other people. This "second" phase usually involves sending love towards one person – a loved one, a neutral person, and eventually a person to whom one has had conflict with. The "third" phase then involves directing the generated love toward all living beings. One client expressed amazement at how relatively easy it was to generate and deliberately pass loving-kindness to her mother-in-law. This led her to see her mother-in-law in a new way and to spot her character strengths when they were together. She found a feeling of appreciation for her mother-in-law's strengths of zest, creativity, and judgment and began to focus on the good things her mother-in-law does with these strengths.

The second (strength-exploration) meditation will involve mindful reflection for some participants. Amaro (2010) describes two ways of doing this sort of investigation: (1) toward a specific theme (e.g., creativity, teamwork, gratitude) and (2) toward whatever emerges on its own (e.g., a new idea about strengths use). The former type of investigation is what is practiced in Session 5 in that individuals choose a strength they are interested in studying, confused by, or wanting to work on; and simply observes what emerges. When the mind races off to unrelated topics, individuals bring the focus back to the strength. Note that sometimes the moment is too charged and further concentration practice (e.g., re-establishing the breath anchor) is necessary before returning to the strength.

Some research has found that those who are high in brooding (negatively ruminating about unpleasant or painful experiences) tend to respond better to breathing meditation and not loving-kindness meditation, whereas those who are low in brooding tend to respond better to loving-kindness practice (Barnhofer, Chittka, Nightingale, Visser, & Crane, 2010). This is one of the advantages of doing these two meditations back-to-back as their variety increases the likelihood that one will appeal to most individuals. MBSP practitioners might note this suggesting that those prone to rehearsing negative thoughts in their minds might benefit from extended focus on the breath followed by the focus on a strength of their choosing, as opposed to the guided loving-kindness practice. All participants are encouraged to practice both through the facilitation of the practitioner.

Questions to Consider

- What is the best question you asked someone in the strengths interview?
- Do you appreciate your character strengths? How might you express greater value for your own strengths?
- Do you verbally appreciate the character strengths of others? How might you express greater appreciation for others' strengths?
- Are you friendly toward yourself? Would you consider yourself a friend to yourself? What does it mean to be one's own best friend?
  - This became a prominent theme in one particular MBSP group, directly tapping into one's relationship with oneself. Exploring participant reactions and insights on this topic is fascinating.
- How is the group beginning to support one another? How might the group leader highlight or facilitate this further?
  - One MBSP participant explained that she was typically insecure about expressing herself through writing and thus had some hesitancy with writing and sharing the strengths gatha exercise. She explained that she had reviewed her gatha several

times and had some worry about how others may perceive it. She criticized herself for taking this approach. I reframed this as her using her strengths of prudence and social intelligence. This lifted her confidence to read her gatha aloud. After she shared the gatha, the group spotted several strengths in the content (the gatha) and the process (her sharing it).

Strength-Exploration Meditation (Case Example)

One MBSP practitioner concluded the loving-kindness meditation and then re-prompted the participants to consider one of their strengths to focus in on and observe in a careful, open-ended way. One man chose love of learning because it's a strength that is high for him at #3 but when he thinks about the strength he feels a sense of anxiety. This confuses him because, after all, it appears to be a signature strength. Thus, he decided to face this dynamic directly by making love of learning his focal point for the strength-exploration meditation.

As he focused on his love of learning, his anxiety returned. He could feel it in his gut and his racing heart. But he felt he could face this anxiety by using his breath anchor. As he did, a myriad of thoughts, memories, and ideas came forth. He allowed himself to observe the thoughts and memories, emerging and fading, popping up in his mind and transitioning out. He then investigated his thoughts looking for how these mental formations related to his signature strength. A pattern emerged. Every thought and memory seemed to have themes relating to pressure and intensity. He had received pressure from his parents to achieve and from his uncle to rise in success up the corporate ladder, regardless of the impact on others. What played in his mind were the stories that related to achievement successes and failures, losing confidence in his studies, and a strong inner critic that told him that whatever he learned and did was "not quite good enough."

His love of learning had been expressed many times throughout his life according to what others wanted for him rather than what he wanted for himself. At the conclusion of the meditation, he realized he needed to continue this strength-exploration practice on his love of learning strength so he could explore different pathways where he might best express this strength in an authentic way.

Practice Trap

Some practitioners tend to gravitate toward their own areas of interest and run the risk of not attending to what the individuals in the group need most. In this session, practitioners often really like the structure, intentionality, and approach of the loving-kindness meditation. It is great for practitioners to show this interest and passion for particular meditations; however, too much focus on this meditation can lead to an oversight or under-focus on the strength-exploration meditation portion. This is important because some participants prefer the "silence with a focus" approach of the strength-exploration meditation as opposed to the structured, loving-kindness meditation.

Lesson learned: Stay mindful to one's own needs, interests, hopes, and plans as well as the group members' potential needs, interests, hopes, and plans.

MBSP Handout 5.1

Session 5: Valuing Your Relationships

Tracking and Suggested Exercises

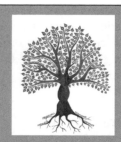

Suggested Exercises/Homework This Week:

- Loving-kindness meditation, 1×/day (see Handout 5.4) or the strength-exploration meditation, 1×/day. Also consider alternating between the two each day.
- Character strengths breathing space exercise
- Track your experiences below
- Character strengths 360 exercise (Strengths interviews II): Give Handout 5.2 to several people in your life to comment on your strengths. Track your findings in Handout 5.3. What stands out?
- Complete the character strengths brainstorm worksheet on one of your strengths (Handout 5.5)

Day/Date	Type of Practice & Time Length	Obstacles to My Practice	Strengths Used	Observations/Comments
Tuesday Date:				
Wednesday Date:				
Thursday Date:				
Friday Date:				
Saturday Date:				
Sunday Date:				
Monday Date:				
Tuesday Date:				

MBSP Handout 5.2

Session 5:

Character Strengths 360

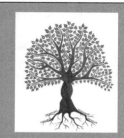

Step 1

Below are 24 character strengths. Which of these **most strongly** describes who this person is and how they operate in their life? Check off those strengths that you **most clearly** see in them.

____ **Creativity:** ingenuity; sees & does things in new/unique ways; original & adaptive ideas

____ **Curiosity:** novelty-seeker; takes an interest; open to different experiences; asks questions

____ **Judgment:** critical thinker; analytical; logical; thinks things through

____ **Love of Learning:** masters new skills & topics; passionate about knowledge & learning

____ **Perspective:** wise; provides wise counsel; sees the big picture; integrates others' views

____ **Bravery:** valorous; does not shrink from fear; speaks up for what's right

____ **Perseverance:** persistent; industrious; overcomes obstacles; finishes what is started

____ **Honesty:** integrity; truthful; authentic

____ **Zest:** enthusiastic; energetic; vital; feels alive and activated

____ **Love:** gives and accepts love; genuine; values close relations with others

____ **Kindness:** generous; nurturing; caring; compassionate; altruistic; nice

____ **Social Intelligence:** aware of the motives and feelings of oneself & others, knows what makes other people tick

____ **Teamwork:** a team player; community-focused, socially responsible; loyal

____ **Fairness:** just; does not allow feelings to bias decisions about others

____ **Leadership:** organizes group activities; encourages and leads groups to get things done

____ **Forgiveness:** merciful; accepts others' shortcomings; gives people a second chance

____ **Humility:** modest; lets accomplishments speak for themselves; focuses on others

---

___ **Prudence:** careful; wisely cautious; thinks before speaking; does not take undue risks

___ **Self-Regulation:** self-controlled; disciplined; manages impulses & emotions

___ **Appreciation of Beauty & Excellence:** awe; wonder; marvels at beauty & greatness

___ **Gratitude:** thankful for the good; expresses thanks; feels blessed

___ **Hope:** optimistic; future-minded; has a positive outlook

___ **Humor:** playful; enjoys joking and bringing smiles to others; lighthearted

___ **Spirituality:** religious and/or spiritual; practices a faith; purpose- & meaning-driven

Step 2
On the back of this page, give a brief rationale or example of how you have seen this person display each strength you checked off.

MBSP Handout 5.3
Session 5:
Character Strengths 360 Tracking Grid

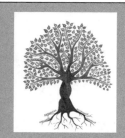

Name of Person:											
Domain (Work, Home, School, Social):											*Your VIA Survey Results*
VIA Character Strengths (spotted)										*Total:*	
1 Creativity											
2 Curiosity											
3 Judgment											
4 Love of Learning											
5 Perspective											
6 Bravery											
7 Perseverance											
8 Honesty											
9 Zest											
10 Love											
11 Kindness											
12 Social Intelligence											
13 Teamwork											
14 Fairness											
15 Leadership											
16 Forgiveness											
17 Humility											
18 Prudence											
19 Self-Regulation											
20 Appreciation of Beauty & Excellence											
21 Gratitude											
22 Hope											
23 Humor											
24 Spirituality											

Strong Signature Strengths (noted by self and others)				**Possible Blind Spots** (noted by others only)				**Potential Opportunities** (noted by self only)			
1		3		1		3		1		3	
2		4		2		4		2		4	

MBSP Handout 5.4

Session 5:

Loving-Kindness Meditation

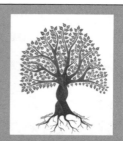

General

Loving-kindness practice, often called "metta," is a type of meditation that involves generating and directing one's capacity for love/kindness toward oneself, toward other people, and toward all living beings. The origins of this practice date back over 2,500 years to Buddhism.

Research

The science of loving-kindness and related practices of self-compassion have exploded. Research has found links with the building of resilience and personal resources over the long-run. Benefits that are emerging from this practice include: feelings of happiness, optimism and curiosity; decreased anxiety, depression, and rumination; fewer feelings of failure and inferiority; less self-criticism, perfectionism, anger and closed-mindedness; stronger buffers against negative social comparison and public self-consciousness; greater social connectedness, emotional intelligence and wisdom; improved initiative and mastery of goals.

Practice

Loving-kindness involves directing mindfulness toward specific character strengths within you. Some ideas for practicing loving-kindness meditation follow. Create an intention to be loving and kind to yourself – to treat yourself with compassion. You might begin this exercise by thinking back to a moment in time when you felt deeply and genuinely loved by someone; as you recall this specific experience of love, reflect on how you felt this love. Where do you feel it in your body? Is there an image that is associated with this? State the meditation/gatha below to yourself; allow yourself to "feel" and experience each line in a deep way. It might be helpful to form a pleasant image for each phrase as you say it.

Loving-Kindness Meditation (gatha on the strengths of love and kindness)

May I be filled with loving-kindness,

May I be safe from inner and outer dangers,

May I be well in body and mind,

May I be at ease and happy.

Additional Resources

Loving kindness: The Revolutionary Art of Happiness (Sharon Salzberg, 1995)
The Mindful Path to Self-Compassion (Christopher Germer, 2009)
Self-Compassion: Stop Beating Yourself Up and Leave Insecurity Behind (Kristin Neff, 2011)

MBSP Handout 5.5

Session 5:

Character Strengths Brainstorm Worksheet

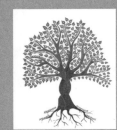

Choose one character strength. What does it look like?

What does it mean to have or express this strength?

What happens if you have too little (underuse of this strength)?

What happens if you have too much (overuse of this strength)?

When and where can you use this strength in your daily life?

What benefits does the strength bring to you and others?

Write about the strength in *6 words* without including the word itself. Two examples for curiosity include: "I open doors to unknown things" and "The art of making good questions."

Chapter 12

Mindfulness-Based Strengths Practice

Session 6: Mindfulness of the Golden Mean (Mindful Strengths Use)

To practice meditation, "what we need is a cup of understanding, a barrel of love, and an ocean of patience."

St. Francis de Sales

 Opening Story

A young couple became new parents to an energetic and delightful little boy. They worked hard to not take their parenting for granted, learning from their mistakes and trying to strike a balance between offering guidance/direction and allowing their son to explore and express himself. One day, when their son was just over two-years-old, he got a hold of some permanent markers that were sitting at the edge of a table. With lightning quickness, the boy scurried over to a freshly painted wall and began to use the wall as his canvas. He scribbled and scribbled with purpose and intensity. When he was done he threw the markers down and walked away.

When the parents came upon the wall, they were stunned. Giving pause, they looked at each other for a moment. They knew just what to do. They went to the store and purchased an appropriately sized frame. They pounded the frame into the wall, three-feet from the floor, "framing in" the entire set of scribbles created by their son.

Instead of putting soap to the wall to take away the action, they transformed it into a work of art.

 Structure for Session 6

I   Opening Meditation: Character Strengths Breathing Space or Strengths Gatha [3 min]
II   Practice Review [30 min]
III   Mindfulness of the Golden Mean [30 min]
IV   Fresh Look Meditation (Strengths Reframing of a Problem) [30 min]
V   Virtue Circle [20 min]
VI   Suggested Homework Exercises [6 min]
VII   Closing Meditation: Strengths Gatha [1 min]

Note. Times are approximates. This is for a 2-hour session; for a 1.5-hour session, it's advisable to eliminate the virtue circle and shorten each section accordingly

I Opening Meditation: Character Strengths Breathing Space or Strengths Gatha

II Practice Review

- While there is plenty to review, here is a way to structure some of the main ideas:
  - Setting aside the character strengths 360 exercise for a moment, what went well this week with your practice? Participants might discuss their practice with mindfulness or character strengths, strengths-spotting, the loving-kindness practice, or a focus on one particular character strength through meditation. Following this, it is generally an uplifting exercise to review what struck the participants in the character strengths brainstorm worksheet and have participants share the "6-word description" of the strength so that the other participants can guess it.
  - Character strengths 360 exercise review, in dyads or large group review. It's helpful to first gather comments about what struck participants most about the experience, and what they became more mindful of. The debriefing can be formalized with use of a white-board to write out at least three general areas for further discussion.
    - ○ *Strong signature strengths* (strengths that others see in you that you scored high on with the VIA Survey).
      - · Question: Do you realize how powerful/extraordinary these strong signature strengths are for you?
    - ○ *Possible blind spots* (strengths that others saw in you that you did not score as high on with the VIA Survey).
      - · Questions: What did you become mindful of that you were previously blind to? Does this give you ideas for strengths action you might take?
    - ○ *Potential opportunities* (strengths that others did not nominate as your highest strengths that you scored high on with the VIA Survey).

- Question: Is it possible that you're not bringing this strength forth enough in your life or in a particular life domain?
  - ○ There is, of course, a 4th category of *lost strengths*, which are those that neither you nor others saw as signature strengths. These are not weaknesses but are other capacities that are present in individuals. There's nothing wrong with discussing this category; however, it can become a distraction that misses the point about learning to wield one's best strengths to serve oneself and others. Can mindfulness be applied to boost lost strengths? Of course!
- Many times the character strengths 360 exercise leads individuals to "own" their highest strengths, especially those individuals who react with skepticism or disbelief to their initial VIA Survey results.
- Sometimes individuals receive feedback in which there are a large number of strengths checked off and the results seem moot. One MBSP participant noted a colleague checked off 20 strengths for her. At first, the woman felt the feedback was pointless as it didn't help her differentiate what her core qualities were. After further reflection, she reframed this as a positive in that this person must think highly of her and really like her.
- The feedback can offer an unexpected boost to relationships. A woman who already had a good relationship with her son received his 360 feedback and was struck by it. It was not that she couldn't believe he would spot certain strengths in her, but it was simply a different type of conversation to be having with him. It gave them a new appreciation for one another and a greater depth to their relationship.
- One gentleman was shocked that someone saw bravery in him. He'd always seen himself as less forthcoming, reserved, and not someone who exerts bravery (which comes up as a lesser strength for him), yet when this strength was spotted by two people, this gave him pause. Their feedback revolved around the man's courage that he brings to projects at work – that he faces challenges directly and does not

back down from negative feedback. This rationale of how they saw bravery in him was particularly important because it gave further credence to their observations.

- One woman was surprised (and disappointed) that people did not spot creativity as one of her highest strengths despite it being in her top 5 on the VIA Survey. This means that expression of creativity in relationships is a "potential opportunity" for her. She admitted she probably had suppressed her creativity, particularly at work, in order to conform to expectations and certain projects that were streamlined. However, she became determined to find ways to allow creativity greater expression at work. She noted she would begin expressing creativity more strongly during her next work project starting in a few days.
- In summary, this exercise brings a new dimension to how people see themselves. Some people feel a bit neutral to their strengths and are slower to warm up to the idea that they have various positive qualities existing in them. This tool, and the feedback it generates, offers individuals support and confirmation of what is best in them.

III   Mindfulness of the Golden Mean

Overview

- As we've discussed, there are two meta-approaches to the integration of mindfulness and character strengths – "strong mindfulness" (which involves bringing character strengths to help us maintain a mindfulness practice or to practice mindful living) and "mindful strengths use" (which involves bringing mindfulness to the practice of our strengths). We practiced the latter last week when we used mindfulness to be open to one particular strength. We will more explicitly tackle mindful strength use this week as we explore the dynamics and some of the positives and negatives involved in strengths use.

Strengths-Zone Continuum

- Each of the character strengths can be plotted on a continuum in which one side represents overuse because the strength is being expressed too strongly for the particular situation and the other side represents underuse because the strength is not being expressed strongly enough. See Handout 6.2 for sample language for overuse and underuse of each of the 24 strengths. Strengths overuse and underuse can cause significant problems in our lives. The optimal expression of a strength in a particular situation can be referred to as the *strengths zone*. Therefore, it is useful to consider strengths use according to the "golden mean of character strengths."

Golden Mean of Character Strengths

- The golden mean refers to expressing the right *combination* of character strengths to the right *degree* in the right *situation*. This concept originates from the philosophical work of Aristotle, who emphasized the virtue of balance among life activities. He emphasized a balance between excess and deficiency, which can then lead to the ultimate goal in life – personal happiness. Thus, the opposite of a strength can be viewed as both overuse and underuse (e.g., the opposite of curiosity is both nosiness and apathy). It's also important to note that there is no "absolute" mean, as strength expression is relative to the situation/context. The word "right" is relative to the individual and the context (it does not refer to the existence of one correct way or wrong way of using a strength).
  - Combination: We rarely use one strength in isolation at one time.
  - Degree: Character strength use is best viewed as a matter of degrees – more/less, higher/lower intensity.
  - Situation: Character strengths are always expressed in context, which varies according to factors in the individual and the environment.
- *Example:* A person high in the character strength of love will express their love differently if they are with an unemotional friend,

a jovial friend, or a mean friend; they may still express love but to a different degree. This expression will vary further if they are in an amusement park, a quiet restaurant, a funeral home, walking down a city street, or in the comfort of their own home.

- *Purpose:* What is the purpose to which we use our strengths? Is there an optimal purpose? If there is, one might say that the character strength expression is *for the benefit of self AND others*.

Reframing

- Reframing refers to offering a new perspective or angle to look at a situation. This different perspective can become a platform for a solution or better problem management. Sometimes reframing simply involves replacing one word in the individual's language or thought processes, e.g., "stubborn" becomes "perseverant" or "distractible" becomes "curious." Reframing may also take the form of pointing out the positive when the client only sees a negative, such as pointing out to a person who stays in an unhealthy relationship that they have levels of hope, perseverance, and bravery in their expectations that things will eventually get better. Reframing often gives the person an "ah-ha" moment, an insight into themselves, and an approach they can take to handle their issue.
- There are two simple steps for reframing with character strengths. Consider:
  - What strengths are being overused and underused?
  - What character strengths require greater mindfulness to bring balance to the situation? The strengths might help temper an overused strength, boost another strength, or combine in a synergistic way.
- *Example:* Consider John, a student who has a major paper due tomorrow but has spent all of his time doing Internet searches and reading books on the paper's topic and related topics. He has no outline and has not started the writing process. Ask the group to consider the strengths John might be overusing and underusing. Note that there is no wrong answer,

just different interpretations. Second, ask the group what strengths John might need to use to bring balance to this situation or to temper an overused strength.

- A few *possible* examples include: overusing love of learning (researching various subjects); overusing curiosity (tracking each new idea or related topic); overusing hope (thinking he can easily write the paper with little time left); underusing prudence (not putting together an outline, not managing his time wisely); underusing self-regulation (not managing his impulse of information-seeking); underusing kindness (putting extra pressure on himself might cause his body more duress).
- A few strengths that might be brought forth: zest and perseverance (finding ways to keep his energy up while starting and continuing the writing); hope (focusing on the goal, the positive things he has already done, and how he can use those positives to reach his goal); judgment (to temper his curiosity/love of learning and focus on the most salient tasks with his time remaining); perspective (to see the bigger picture of the whole paper amidst what he has already done and what remains); teamwork (enlist the help of a fellow student; set up an arrangement where the fellow student periodically checks in on him to ensure he is staying focused).

IV Fresh Look Meditation (Strengths Reframing of a Problem)

[Listen to Track 8 of the attached CD to hear the fresh look meditation]. Now, let's apply these concepts into a meditation experience. This approach will involve you selecting one minor problem or issue that you can bring to the "workbench" of your mind, where you can direct mindful energy of direct attention, openness, acceptance and curiosity toward the issue. I'll invite you to imagine the issue in detail, to welcome and be open to the thoughts and emotions that are present as you imagine it. You'll then have an opportunity to reflect on strengths you might be underusing or overusing with this problem and a way to take a different perspective. It's useful to consider what small problem you will focus on prior to beginning the meditation. Do you have a minor problem in mind that you'd like to work on?

One option here is to use Rumi's poem, "The Guest House," (see Box 12.1) at the beginning of this meditation to create an optimal space for the participants to "welcome" their problem.

Let's begin: Start by bringing our attention to our breathing for a few moments. (Pause). Anchor yourself closely to your breath; with each in-breath and out-breath you can feel your breath anchor becoming stronger, connecting you in the present moment. (Pause). Now, please call to mind the problem that you wish to focus on. Picture the details. Allow the problem to play forth in your mind like a story, like a movie – see the people involved, the environment. (Pause). Notice your body's reaction. Become aware of your body's sensations and your emotions right in this moment. What do you feel in your body? Breathe with the sensations and feelings. Perhaps you can allow yourself to accept these feelings as part of your present moment experience. (Pause). As you follow your breathing, mindfully reflect on what strengths you might be overusing or underusing with this problem. What is being overused? What is being underused? What strengths need to be brought forth? Continue to breathe, observing your moment-to-moment experience. (Long pause).

In a moment, I'll invite you to start the image or movie over and this time to replay the exact same image/movie but with one important difference. This time you will be using one of your strengths to help you better manage or solve this problem. Go ahead and restart your image/movie. Picture your successful use of strengths with this difficulty. Take note of how the difficulty is now managed or improved. (Pause). Return to your breath anchor.

Debriefing

Practitioners can note that a wide range of responses are often evident in a given group. The debriefing should not focus on inquiries to see

if individuals found a "solution" or "answer" to the problem since what matters most are the processes of reframing, mindfulness of overuse/underuse, and the use of mindfulness as a way to face challenges. Nevertheless, some individuals emerge with a new solution to their problem (often the source of their problem was avoidance), others garner insights around overuse, and others note the main thing they gained was a deeper perspective or a wider view of their problem.

Start with open-ended questions to allow participants to share at a level that is comfortable for them.

- What was that meditation like for you? What struck you?
- Were you able to picture a reframe of your problem?
- Did instances of overuse or underuse of strengths stand out to you? Was this a new insight for you? How so?
- Looking back at your experience, did you increase your level of acceptance to any degree? How might acceptance play a role in the future with this situation?

V   Virtue Circle

VI   Suggested Homework Exercises

- Fresh look meditation, 1 ×/day
- Character strengths breathing space exercise
- Track all mindfulness practices, including mindful walking, eating, driving, etc. (Handout 6.1)
- From mindless to mindful: Choose an area of your life where mindlessness has a negative impact. Practice bringing mindfulness and strengths to this area each day this week.

Homework Exercises Review

- Be sure to encourage the group to continue with a regular practice of mindfulness, taking note of what seems to bring them the greatest benefit, whether it is a structured meditation, strength-exploration meditation, movement-oriented meditation, or general sitting meditation.

- Practitioners may wish to bring in and read a copy of Rumi's poem "The Guest House" (see Box 12.1) during one of the meditations in today's session as it offers a wonderful metaphoric summary of this session's themes. The poem has been used in other mindfulness programs (e.g., Segal et al., 2002). It is interesting to include this in both the opening and closing meditations of this session. Generous pauses and silence for participants to sit with the poem are recommended.
  - The last exercise, from mindless to mindful, is interesting because it requires the individual to consider some activity that is daily (or almost daily) that they struggle with or are bothered by and that might benefit from greater mindfulness and strengths use. This is quite different from the "mindfulness of a routine activity" exercise practiced at Sessions 1 and 2 because people aren't typically bothered by "mindless teeth-brushing" or "autopilot-driven showering." However, something like "talking with my spouse," "participating at a work meeting," or "being around a difficult person at work," are likely to have a significant impact on the person's life. Often such struggles involve quite a bit of mindless reactivity and bad habits the individual has cultivated. This is an opportunity to cultivate a virtue, to make strength use more routine, and to use mindfulness to do so.
    - Example: A person who chooses "talking with my spouse" might make mindful listening and curiosity a priority in each interaction for a week.

Handouts

- Handout 6.1: Tracking & Suggested Exercises (1 page)
- Handout 6.2: Character Strengths Overuse/Underuse: Finding the Strengths Zone (1 page)

VII Closing Meditation

- If you haven't already used it, conclude with Rumi's "The Guest House" (see Box 12.1) woven into a brief mindful breathing meditation, or the character strengths breathing space, or a strengths gatha.

Box 12.1. The Guest House by Rumi

This being human is a guest house.
Every morning a new arrival.

A joy, a depression, a meanness,
some momentary awareness comes
as an unexpected visitor.

Welcome and entertain them all!
Even if they're a crowd of sorrows,
who violently sweep your house
empty of its furniture,

still, treat each guest honorably.
He may be clearing you out
for some new delight.

The dark thought, the shame, the malice.
meet them at the door laughing,
and invite them in.

Be grateful for whoever comes,
because each has been sent
as a guide from beyond.

Note. From Barks & Moyne (1997). Translation by Coleman Barks. Reprinted with the permission of Coleman Barks.

Additional Considerations

Problems vs. Aspirations

Problems are narrow and engage people only until the problem is solved or until it feels intractable. And problems carry an emotional, negative energy. Aspirations are expansive, inclusive, and inspiring. Therefore they are more engaging to more people for a longer period of time. Character strengths are fascinating in that they can be applied both to solving problems and to helping individuals seek and achieve aspirational goals. Character strengths can be directed to the past or future – or as with mindfulness, right into the present moment. This session helps participants deploy strengths with a problem while the next session begins to apply strengths to an aspiration or goal.

Step 1 and Step 2

One conceptualization in managing problems is that mindfulness is the first step and character strengths are the second step. Mindfulness opens the door so that character strengths can be brought in. For example, a person who becomes aware that they are running late all the time has just opened that first door of mindfulness that presents an opportunity for a change. But it doesn't make the change. The initiation of step two is the action or deliberate inaction that can be deployed. After building greater mindfulness, the individual might apply their prudence to become more conscientious or they might attempt to bring more mindfulness to their prudence in everyday life.

Cultivation Without Clinging

A construct often discussed in Buddhist psychology and the mindfulness literature is the phenomenon of attachment. As humans we frequently attach ourselves and cling to "things," to people, to positive feelings, and to certain experiences. When we do this, a part of us is not accepting the present moment, is trying to make something different, or is trying to control something to stay as it is. Mindfulness fosters an approach of nonclinging and nonattachment, the practice of "being," and acceptance of the moment as it is. Consider these ideas alongside the practice of strengths cultivation. Some individuals might attach themselves to one particular strength, desperate to create a certain emotion or experience. Mindful strengths use is thus a practice that involves cultivation without clinging. Individuals practice cultivating a "grateful mind" or a "prudent mind" but they do not cling to expectations of what this should look like and they do not reject present moment experiences that are less pleasant.

MBSP Handout 6.1

Session 6: Mindfulness of the Golden Mean

Tracking and Suggested Exercises

Suggested Exercises/Homework This Week:

- Fresh look meditation, 1×/day. As practiced in group: (1) Anchor mindfulness to breath; (2) image a life issue/challenge; (3) tune into thoughts/emotions/sensations in the present; notice in the image where strengths are overused/underused; (4) reframing: image your successful use of strengths to manage, balance, or resolve the issue/challenge; (5) breath anchor.
- Character strengths breathing space exercise, 1×/day, and as needed.
- Track all mindfulness practices, including mindful walking, eating, driving, etc. below.
- From mindless to mindful: Choose an area of your life where mindlessness has a negative impact on your life. Practice bringing mindfulness and strengths to it each day.

MBSP Handout 6.2

Session 6:

Character Strengths Overuse and Underuse

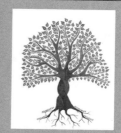

Strength	Overuse	Underuse	Core
Creativity	Eccentricity	Conformity	Originality that is adaptive
Curiosity	Nosiness	Disinterest	Exploration/seeking novelty
Judgment	Narrow-mindedness, cynicism	Unreflectiveness	Critical thinking & rationality
Love of Learning	Know-it-all	Complacency	Systematic deepening (of knowledge)
Perspective	Overbearing	Shallowness	The wider view
Bravery	Foolhardiness	Cowardice	Facing fears, confronting adversity
Perseverance	Obsessiveness	Fragility	Keep going, overcome all obstacles
Honesty	Righteousness	Phoniness	Being authentic
Zest	Hyperactive	Sedentary	Enthusiasm for life
Love	Emotional promiscuity	Emotional isolation	Genuine, reciprocal warmth
Kindness	Intrusiveness	Indifference	Doing for others
Social Intelligence	Over-analyzing	Obtuse or clueless	Tuned in, then savvy
Teamwork	Dependant	Selfishness	Collaborative, participating in a group effort
Fairness	Detachment	Partisonship	Equal opportunity for all
Leadership	Despotism	Compliant	Positively influencing others
Forgiveness	Permissive	Merciless	Letting go of hurt when wronged
Humility	Self-deprecation	Baseless self-esteem	Achievement does not elevate worth
Prudence	Stuffiness	Sensation seeking	Wise caution
Self-Regulation	Inhibition	Self-indulgence	Self-management of vices
Appreciation of Beauty & Excellence	Snobbery or Perfectionism	Oblivion	Seeing the life behind things
Gratitude	Ingratiation	Rugged individualism	Thankfulness
Hope	Pollyanna-ism	Negative	Positive expectations
Humor	Giddiness	Overly serious	Offering pleasure/laughter to others
Spirituality	Fanaticism	Anomie	Connecting with the sacred

Chapter 13

Mindfulness-Based Strengths Practice
Session 7: Authenticity and Goodness

*The most authentic thing about us is our capacity to create, to overcome, to endure,
to transform, to love and to be greater than our suffering.*

Ben Okri, Nigerian poet & novelist

Opening Story[1]

Two men approached a wise sage with a heated debate. They were arguing about the true path to God. They turned to the sage for his counsel. "Please share your thoughts with me," offered the sage.

One man shared a strong case emphasizing that the true path to God was one of effort and energy. It is built on being good to others and following the way of the Law. The sage listened carefully. "Is this the true path?" asked the man.

"You're right," replied the sage.

The second man, surprised at the sage's response, took his turn and offered an equally strong case. He explained the true path to God is one of total and complete surrender – a letting go in the purist of forms – to let go of all worldly things and live the sacred teachings fully in one's life. Again, the sage listened carefully. "Is this the true path?" the second man asked.

"You're right," replied the sage.

A third man who was listening, chimed in with great surprise, "Wait a minute, they can't both be right?!"

The sage paused, then turned to him: "You're right, too."

Structure for Session 7

I   Opening Meditation: Signature Strengths Breathing Space [5–10 min]
II   Practice Review [10 min]
III Strengths Branding [20 min]
IV A Strengths Model Toward Authenticity and Goodness [25 min]
V   Meditations: Best Possible Self and/or Defining Moments Exercise [30 min]
VI Virtue Circle [20 min]

---

1 This classic story has been shared in many forums and has seen various adaptations. One version of this story can also be found in Kornfield and Feldman (1996).

Note. Times are approximates. This is for a 2-hour session; for a 1.5-hour session, it's advisable to eliminate the virtue circle and shorten each section accordingly

I　Opening Meditation: Signature Strengths Breathing Space

This new meditation (see Handout 7.3 and listen to Track 9 of the attached CD) is introduced in the opening meditation as a way of bridging the previous session's focus on using strengths with a problem and also as a way to provide another tool for managing challenges. It brings together a variety of ideas from previous weeks and the current session – the application of signature strengths, the use of gathas, using the breathing space, and the aware-explore-apply model. This exercise also highlights one of the most important takeaways of MBSP which is to bring greater awareness to the nuances and uses of our signature strengths, including how they might be used at challenging times. To increase the strength of this meditation, it is suggested that it is repeated as the closing meditation for this session as well.

II　Practice Review

- Review: What worked well for you this week? How have you been employing an approach of mindful strengths use?
- Check in on specific examples of the mindless to mindful exercise, reframing a problem, and the fresh look meditation. Some individuals, who did not have time to collect responses and review their character strengths 360 exercise last week, may wish to spend time on it this week.

III　Strengths Branding

- *Instructions:* Here is a fairly brief challenge that will help you delve into and explore mindful strengths use. The exercise involves exploring the idea of "branding" yourself with a two-word phrase. Choose one of your signature strengths, perhaps the one that resonates with you most strongly. Make sure it's a strength you are high in and that you care deeply about. Merge it with mindfulness and describe your life with this strength. One way to start this exploration is to write, at the top of a piece of paper, the word "mindful" or "mindfully" in front of one of your signature strengths. For example, "mindful hope" or "mindfully hopeful;" "mindful curiosity" or "mindfully curious;" "mindfully fair" or "mindful fairness." Then brainstorm what this phrase means to you. How does it play out in your daily life? How does it describe who you are? For example, you might discuss how you express this signature strength in the world, how you combine the strength with different strengths in each setting, how you watch closely for times of overuse and underuse, and the way that mindfulness supports your use of the strength.
  - The group facilitator should offer a personal example. See an example and discussion of this exercise in Chapter 5.
  - Please take a moment now to reflect and jot down some ideas, and then we'll explore this further in dyads.
- It can be noted that participants might choose to apply this approach to many of their strengths. At the same time, the "branding" should not pigeonhole them into a strength, instead this is just one way to practice mindful strengths use. The intention is that fleshing out the details of this specific branding will open them up to a greater mindfulness of their strengths across contexts and situations.

IV　A Strengths Model Toward Authenticity and Goodness

- These last two sessions are about taking stock in what has struck participants most in this course so far, what has had the biggest impact, and how the insights and practices might be applied to their life goals and mindful living.

- Primer on a strengths process model: aware-explore-apply (A-E-A): This is an easy, user-friendly model for working with your character strengths. It serves as an overview for the strengths process that individuals use to develop character strengths. Mindfulness is involved at each phase. See Handout 7.2.
  - **1. Aware:** The first step of any change process – whether self-directed change or practitioner-supported change – is awareness. This crucial step involves understanding the language of strengths and seeing some of the strength labels as being attributed to oneself. This step answers the question, "What are my strengths?" and begins to answer the question, "What strength was I just using?" Such strength awareness leads to greater strength access.
  - **2. Explore:** This is the phase in which the individual connects the strength labels in a deeper way to their past and current experiences. It begins to shed some light on who the person really is and what really makes them tick. This step involves solitary reflection, pondering, and journaling, as well as interpersonal discussion and co-exploration.
  - **3. Apply:** This step involves the individual beginning to use their strengths in their daily life. This is the action phase – shifting from reflecting and thinking to doing. This phase manifests throughout MBSP but most strongly in these last two sessions. It begins to answer the question: How will mindfulness and character strengths make your life and those you interact with better?
    - *Authenticity* (a better "you"): Will MBSP help you become a better you: stronger at being yourself, more authentic, more consistent across life domains? Will you find ways to be more true to who you are (your core identity) – that is, to your signature strengths?
    - *Goodness* (a better "person"): Will MBSP help you become a better person: doing good for others, looking for the betterment of society, and being a

better citizen of the world? Will you find ways to use *all* of your strengths more fully to benefit others?
    - These two concepts of authenticity and goodness are offered as elements that individuals might be striving toward. The alignment of mindfulness and character strengths is important for both. Authenticity and goodness are related and in MBSP are viewed equally in terms of importance (thus the word "and" in the session's title becomes the crucial word). Focusing on one is likely to boost the other (e.g., if I'm being authentically true to myself and expressing my signature strengths fully, it's likely I'm bringing benefit and goodness to others). Some people resonate more with either the concept of goodness or the concept of authenticity and therefore choose to focus their attention more closely on that construct.
  - **Maintain:** If there is time, in the spirit of these last two sessions, one might add a final step of "Maintain" to refer to maintaining strengths use. Thus, the model becomes A-E-A-M. A couple questions that address this phase of the strengths process include:
    - How will you continue to use mindfulness and character strengths each month?
    - One year from now, what practices do you want to still be practicing?
- Note to facilitators: Just as the opening story in this chapter illustrates, the purpose is *not* to draw a philosophical or moralistic discussion about authenticity and goodness. Rather the purpose is for individuals to explore their personal intentions, take stock in their life, and consider how they want to "be" moving forward.
  - MBSP practitioners do *not* pretend to be an authority on goodness nor do they attempt to impose their own morals/values on others as that is very personal for each individual. If a practitioner were to take such an approach, they would be practicing "anti-MBSP," if there were such a thing. In this context, goodness refers to a

theme noted throughout MBSP, that of mindfully expressing one's strengths for the betterment of both oneself *and* others. Each individual will need to make decisions as to what that betterment or goodness means to them personally.

V Meditation(s)

Setting Up the Exercises

Usually time can be made to explain both of the following positive psychology exercises to people, allowing them to choose one to practice in the group. Following an explanation of each, meditation space can be offered for people to practice while the facilitator might offer brief reminders and tips about each during the silence. If there is less time, get a majority vote on practicing one or the other in the group. A final option is to simply lead the best possible self exercise, which is more widely known and has a good research base.

- Each of these can be viewed as guided mindfulness meditations, thus during the experience, awareness of the moment-to-moment experience (body sensations, emotions, thoughts) and breath awareness should be applied liberally.
- Each exercise helps individuals deepen their thinking about what matters most and therefore can support their reflections on self-growth actions they might take.
- Both of these exercises are described in full with examples at separate blog entries found at: http://blogs.psychcentral.com/character-strengths

Best Possible Self Exercise

- Listen to Track 10 of the attached CD as an example. This exercise involves two basic steps: visualizing yourself at a future moment in time having accomplished your goals, and considering the character strengths you'll need to deploy to make that vision a reality.
- Steps:
  1. Take a few minutes to select a future time period (e.g., 6 months, 1 year, or 5 years from now) and imagine that at that time

you are expressing your best possible self strongly. Visualize your best possible self in a way that is very pleasing to you and that you are interested in.
     o Imagine it in close details where you have worked hard and succeeded at accomplishing your life goals. You might think of this as reaching your full potential, hitting an important milestone, or realizing one of your life dreams. The point is not to think of unrealistic fantasies, rather, something that is positive and attainable.
  2. After you have a fairly clear image, think about the character strengths that will be involved in making your best possible self a reality. What character strengths will be the key pathways for you?

Defining Moments Exercise

- This exercise involves looking to your past for one moment in time that was a pivotal or defining moment for you, reflecting on the moment, and considering the character strengths you used in that moment. While this is not yet a research-supported exercise, it is hypothesized that this exercise offers a boost to well-being and self-confidence, strengthens a connection between identity and character strengths, and encourages individuals to savor their past experiences.
- This exercise has four basic steps:
  - *Defining moment:* Name one moment in time that has had a positive effect on you. Preferably, choose a moment in which you took action in some way. You have had many moments that have contributed to your identity. This moment does not have to be dramatic, simply any moment that has had a meaningful impact on you.
  - *Character strengths:* Name the character strengths you used in that situation. Which character strengths did you bring forth? Be able to provide evidence for how they were expressed.
  - *Identity:* Explore how this moment has shaped who you are. How has this moment contributed to your identity? No matter

how small, how has it affected your view of yourself?

— *Courage:* Reflect on your use of courage to mobilize your strengths in that moment. Many individuals rally their bravery strength in order to take action in their defining moment – this action might be to deploy one's signature strengths or to use a strength that is less familiar. In these instances, the strength of bravery often becomes a meta-strength (a higher-order strength that helps to mobilize other strengths). In addition, other strengths might have served as a "meta-strength" in the defining moment, such as perspective, leadership, spirituality, love, or self-regulation.

Debriefing

- Encourage people to share what struck them with either exercise. Invite them to jot down anything they'd like to remind themselves in relation to this exercise or sketch out any clear image that became apparent to them.

VI   Virtue Circle

VII   Suggested Homework Exercises

- Meditation, 1 ×/day: Your choice!
- Signature strengths breathing space: 1 ×/day
- Track (and/or journal) your experiences (Handout 7.1)
- Maintaining your practice:
  - Complete the goal-setting worksheet (Handout 7.5)
  - Consider your mindfulness/strengths supports
  - Consider your "bells" of mindfulness and "cues" to strengths use

Homework Exercises Review

- The participants are encouraged to reflect on those practices that have engaged them most over the weeks and to practice working with

them this week. This may set the stage for their future goals and practices.

- The importance of maintenance with one's mindfulness/strengths practice following this program should not be a new topic for the participants, rather it should be a topic that they are beginning to shift in – from a reflecting stage to a planning stage. Two ways to help facilitate this shift are the goal-setting worksheet and the building in of formal cues and supports.
  - *Worksheet* (Handout 7.5): This is self-explanatory in which an individual makes clear one or two life goals or mindfulness/strengths goals, and they list what they will need to do to reach the goal. The meditations/exercises from today's session should help facilitate this. Character strengths are explained as either the *pathways* to help reach the goal or as the *goal itself* (i.e., either the means or the ends). Mindfulness can be viewed in the same way.
  - *Supports:* How will participants be supported with their mindfulness/strengths practice following this MBSP course? Will they be part of a meditation community (sangha), become more connected with the VIA Institute and its strengths programming, receive support/encouragement from family/friends, etc.?
  - *Bells/cues:* These are external, environmental reminders to return to the present moment and to consider character strengths use.
    - As discussed in the course, there are many "bells" that naturally emerge in our environment that can wake us from autopilot and bring us back to the present moment. Participants may wish to consciously select a bell – literally (e.g., a church bell) or symbolically (e.g., a baby's cry, a cell phone ring, a person smiling). Something random and intermittent is generally most effective. Whenever they hear that "bell," this can be a call to mindfulness with whatever they are doing and a call to consider using their strengths with the task at hand.

○ More formal reminders can be set up, such as the use of sticky notes or little sticker dots. These are then placed in various domains (work office, car, various rooms at home, etc.) and also act as a call to the present moment. An individual may choose to set up a specific goal when they view the cue in their environment, such as to use their curiosity in the moment, become more mindful of a "heart" strength, etc.

Handouts

- Handout 7.1: Tracking & Suggested Exercises (1 page)
- Handout 7.2: The Strengths Model: Aware-Explore-Apply (1 page)
- Handout 7.3: The Signature Strengths Breathing Space (1 page)
- Handout 7.4: Review and Reflections (2 pages)
- Handout 7.5: Goal Setting/Action Planning (2 pages)

VIII Closing Meditation

- Signature strengths breathing space

Additional Considerations

Best Possible Self (Examples)

Here are a few snapshots of responses to this exercise (these are provided in a brief, goal-oriented framework below):

- I can envision starting a family in a few years and we are spending quality time together vacationing and going to activities together in the city.
  - I will need to use my *prudence* strength to map out my long-term finances, my *perseverance* strength as my spouse and I "keep trying" to have children, and my *forgiveness* strength which will help me "let go" of any blame I might impose on

myself or my spouse as we encounter obstacles along the way.

- I see myself doing coaching work that is meaningful and fills me with a sense of purpose as I help people reach their dreams on a daily basis.
  - I will use my *love of learning* and *curiosity* strengths as I return to school to study new topic areas. I will also routinely use *social intelligence* by networking with people in the helping profession and staying open to emerging possibilities that might broaden my experiences.
- I have created a small business on the Internet, and with a few employees helping me, I've found a way to shift from unemployed to happily engaged in successful work.
  - I will need to use my strengths of *creativity* to bring forth my new product, my *judgment/critical thinking* to devise many different marketing pathways, and *teamwork* on a daily basis to help me remember that this enterprise is a team effort and not just me alone.

Best Possible Self (Research)

The best possible self exercise is one of the stronger happiness exercises because it is positive, future-oriented, and has research support. The exercise has been shown to boost people's positive emotions, happiness levels, optimism, and hope, improve coping skills, and elevate positive expectations about the future (Austenfeld & Stanton, 2008; Austenfeld, Paolo, & Stanton, 2006; King, 2001; Meevissen et al., 2011; Peters, et al., 2010; Shapira & Mongrain, 2010; Sheldon & Lyubomirsky, 2006). This exercise has also been found to significantly lower negative affect and for individuals low in mindfulness, it had a substantial effect on positive emotions (Seear & Vella-Brodrick, 2012).

Best Possible Self (Adjustment)

Some individuals might struggle with this exercise and feel it is too "extreme" to think of their *best* self. MBSP practitioners can be prepared to offer a more "reachable" version of this exercise, if a particular individual is struggling with it. Practitioners can invite the participant who is struggling to consider envisioning one thing that would be of value to them to reach or access in the future. Examples might include being more fair in how they treat their spouse, acting with greater bravery by speaking out at work, or treating in-laws with higher doses of kindness. Participants can then consider how they will use their strengths to bring about that "one thing" in the upcoming month or two.

Defining Moments Exercise (Example)

One MBSP practitioner was working individually with an adolescent girl who shared her defining moment as a time when she and her work-aholic father connected with one another. The context was the father had taken a day off for the first time in years just to spend it with her and they spent the day going to parks, restaurants, and talking. There was one particular moment when they were talking while sitting on some swings and she suddenly felt very connected and happy. When asked, she identified the character strength of love in the story and realized that despite his typically absent behavior, he did have a deep love and care for her. As the girl shared the story, she felt as if she was replaying the moment and was able to tap into the feeling of love again. Another strength emerged for her – that of forgiveness. She felt as if she could let go of tension and resentment she has felt toward him and view him in a new light (i.e., with greater perspective).

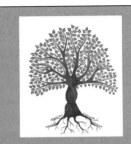

MBSP Handout 7.1

Session 7: Authenticity and Goodness

Tracking and Suggested Exercises

Suggested Exercises/Homework This Week:

- Suggested exercises/homework this week:
- Meditation, 1x/day: Your choice!
- Signature strengths breathing space (Handout 7.3)
- Track (and/or journal) your experiences below
- Maintaining your practice:
  - Complete the goal-setting worksheet (Handout 7.5)
  - Consider your mindfulness/strengths supports
  - Consider your "bells" of mindfulness and "cues" to strengths use

Day/Date	Type of Practice & Time Length	Obstacles to My Practice	Strengths Used	Observations/Comments
Tuesday Date:				
Wednesday Date:				
Thursday Date:				
Friday Date:				
Saturday Date:				
Sunday Date:				
Monday Date:				
Tuesday Date:				

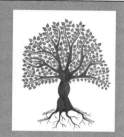

MBSP Handout 7.2

Session 7:

Aware-Explore-Apply

Attempting to improve or build upon a character strength is a process that involves three general steps: aware-explore-apply.

1. Aware

The first step of any change process – self-directed change or practitioner-guided change – is awareness. For strengths work, this crucial step involves understanding the language of strengths, the concepts, definitions, and seeing how they are attributed to oneself. This step answers the question, "What are my strengths?" and begins to answer, "What strength was I just using?"
• Mindfulness in this phase helps the individual shift from autopilot and strengths blindness to a place of greater awareness.

2. Explore

This phase is often skipped by individuals eager to begin making a quick change. It is important to first develop a deeper understanding of one's character strengths. Here, individuals begin to understand what their signature strengths are and how they have previously used them at times of suffering and success. This begins to shed some light on who they are and what really makes them tick. This phase typically involves solitary reflection, pondering, and journaling, as well as interpersonal discussion and co-exploration.
• Mindfulness in this phase helps the individual cultivate deeper insight into who they are and draw new connections with their past and current behaviors.

3. Apply

This is the action phase. After a sufficient amount of exploring, the individual is ready to set a goal and take action with character strengths. Typically, this involves setting a plan for the cultivation of a particular strength (e.g., boosting kindness) or of a strength approach (e.g., increase strengths-spotting in others). This usually is supported by the creation of a routine and/or a reminder or cueing system to stay on track with the new practice.
• Mindfulness in this phase helps the individual to stay connected to the question "What matters most?" and involves wise action as change is implemented.

Maintain: Repetition and Moving Forward

When working with strengths, remembering these three words (aware-explore-apply) is easy and straightforward and will provide a path for times when one feels "stuck" or confused.

As mindfulness and strengths work is an ongoing process, these phases should be repeated over time. Repetition underscores "practice and more practice" which is the key to developing character strengths and maintaining strong use. Without mindful awareness, the strengths use is likely to become stale and stagnant, ultimately leading to strengths erosion. Mindful awareness at each phase ignites the strengths work and creates a positive synergy of benefit.

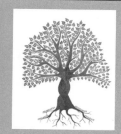

MBSP Handout 7.3

Session 7:

Signature Strengths Breathing Space

The signature strengths breathing space is a 3-step application exercise used to help individuals face the realities of the present moment with their highest strengths. This mindfulness meditation focuses on those strengths that are strongest in the individual. The individual then practices bringing them forth at positive and challenging times. This practice directly employs the aware-explore-apply model, a way of working with strengths. This model states that the first step in working with strengths is enhancing awareness and is followed by exploring that awareness to deepen understanding, and concludes with taking action.

Aware

As I establish a connection with my breathing, I tune in directly to one of my signature strengths, those strengths that are most core to who I am in this world. I allow myself to see the strength fully and clearly as I breathe.

Explore

As I continue to attend to my breathing which anchors me in this present moment, I explore my signature strength. I reflect on how I've used it in the past with success. I take notice of how it has contributed to the good in my life. I understand how it has helped others. I return my attention to the present moment.

Apply

As I breathe, I consider how I might use my signature strength in my present situation. I'm confident there is some way I can apply this strength in the present moment in my thinking, my feelings, or my actions. I use my breath to keep me focused on my strength and I stay open to new possibilities and growth. As I move forward, I breathe with my signature strength.

Optional: Strengths gatha to help support the signature strengths breathing space:

Breathing in, I am aware of my signature strength,

Breathing out, I explore my signature strength,

Inhaling, I breathe along with my current situation,

Exhaling, I apply my signature strength.

Note. This exercise is different from another MBSP exercise, the character strengths breathing space, which focuses on boosting three specific character strengths that are tied closely to different qualities of mindfulness.

MBSP Handout 7.4

Session 7:

Review and Reflections

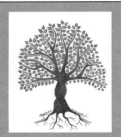

Take a moment to review the distance you have come since starting this Mindfulness-Based Strengths Practice program. Consider the core themes and main ideas we've been working with so far:

- Mindfulness and autopilot
- Your signature strengths
- Obstacles are opportunities
- Strong mindfulness AND mindful strengths use
- Valuing your relationships with others and yourself
- The golden mean AND facing difficulties with strength

In the first two sessions we focused on what is best in you and what might be a pathway for getting there and expressing those good qualities. We then focused on how when we bring forth our best qualities, not only will natural obstacles and challenges arise but we more closely notice the details in life. We then focused on widening and deepening our mindfulness and strengths practice, in part by considering how we might make our mindfulness practice stronger and find ways to bring mindfulness to our strengths practice. After the midway point, we considered a relationship we often don't pay attention to – the one with ourselves, and we practiced valuing ourselves (and others) and using a loving-kindness approach. In the most recent session, we brought the focus to difficulties or stressors in our lives and considered taking a strength-based approach to face these.

How are you doing with this process so far? What has stood out most to you? What has been most useful? Most surprising?

Session 7: Authenticity and goodness

- In terms of self-improvement and growth, will you be devoting your energy toward becoming better and stronger as a human being (e.g., trying to pay attention and build all 24 strengths)? The best possible self exercise may give you some good momentum toward this focus on becoming a "better person."
- Will you be devoting more focus toward becoming a better you – in other words, diving deeper into those strengths that are most core to who you are and finding ways to express them authentically in your life, work, and relationships? The defining moments exercise may give you some good momentum toward this focus on becoming a "better you."
- It is likely that a strong and dedicated approach toward one of these will lead to the other, but to focus explicitly on one for now might help you articulate your life vision and goals.

Tracking Sheets

The tracking sheets are a way to continue your self-monitoring – keeping track of your meditation behaviors, challenges, insights, and your progress. Self-monitoring is a technique that is one of the most scientifically proven ways to make changes in our lives. If your self-monitoring has drifted off, start where you are … in the here and now! What patterns have you noticed in your tracking sheets? What is the status of your mindfulness practice at present?

Journaling

Keeping your ongoing journal is a way to continue the exploration of your experiences, feelings, and ideas in a deep way. There are no limits to where the journaling can take you. Research has found journaling to be an effective exercise for self-growth and for dealing with problems. While it is not necessary to re-read what you have written, it is sometimes interesting to do so. In general, what have you been saying to yourself in your journal? Have you been giving yourself any important advice? What is the most important thing you have learned about yourself through journaling?

Mindfulness Practice

How has your mindfulness practice been going? Bring yourself back to Session 1 and your mindfulness practice at that point – what has emerged or changed since then? Consider your formal practice with the body scan, sitting meditation, character strengths breathing space, standing/walking meditation, loving-kindness meditation, and facing problems with mindfulness and strengths. What practice do you like the most? Which is most beneficial to you? Which would you like to maintain as a regular practice in your life?

How about your mindful living? Have you been bringing more awareness to routines in your life? Have you brought mindfulness to places where mindlessness was causing you trouble? Consider all the many ways mindfulness can be applied in your life – mindful eating, listening, speaking, shopping, working, driving, bathing, dressing, computing, and consuming. Do you bring some level of awareness to these areas?

Character Strengths

There have been a number of strengths-based exercises you have participated in – both in the group and outside of the group. You have practiced a lot of strengths-spotting, both of strengths in yourself and in others. We've emphasized the importance of appreciating and valuing all of our strengths, particularly our signature strengths. You practiced using your signature strengths in new ways. You practiced finding ways to use your strengths to deal with obstacles to your mindfulness practice. Connecting with others outside of the group has been another important component – you conducted a strengths interview of someone about their own top strengths, as well as you asked various people to offer you perspective on your own strengths. Then, there have been other strengths-related activities such as creating a strengths/mindfulness gatha, considering the strengths of movie/television/book characters, the strengths of your role models (people who have most influenced you), and fleshing out your strengths on a brainstorm worksheet. So, where do you go from here with this strengths work? What will you continue?

As you reflect on the points above, just take notice of what strikes you most. You don't have to have an answer to every question. What stands out as an idea, intention, hope, or desired goal?

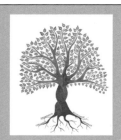

MBSP Handout 7.5

Session 7:

Goal Setting/Action Planning

Do you want to continue on this mindfulness/character strengths journey?

How will you maintain your practice?

These two questions can guide your thinking as you complete this worksheet and review Handout 7.4 (Review and Reflections). As you reflect on your journey so far, what stands out to you most? Is there any question, insight, or goal that seems to be "calling" you? What might be beneficial for you to work on in order to improve yourself? Does it relate to coming to know and express your true self better or does it relate to expressing more goodness in the world?

When you are ready to create an action plan, consider three components: An overall goal, activities you will do to reach the goal, and the character strength(s) you will use to get there. You might consider setting both a "life goal" and a mindfulness/strengths goal. A life goal might relate to your work, family, relationships, happiness, achievement, life engagement, meaning, or health. An example of each follows below:

Life Goal Example:

- Goal (what do you want?):
  - I want to become happier at work.
- Activities (how will you get there?):
  - I will share one thing about myself with a co-worker each day.
- Character strength(s) use (how will your strengths help you?):
  - I will use one of my signature strengths at work in a new way each day.
  - I will use my bravery strength to share my experiences with others.
  - I will use my perseverance to keep up with this task every day for 3 weeks.

Mindfulness Goal Example:

- Goal:
  - I want to become more mindful in my relationships at work.
- Activities:
  - I will practice the body mindfulness meditation for 30 minutes each day to help me maintain a good level of mindfulness of my internal experience.
  - Before difficult meetings at work, I will sit in my office and practice the character strengths breathing space to decompress and check-in with myself.
  - When I feel triggered or upset by others, I'll remind myself that they too have strengths I can notice. If appropriate, I'll practice strengths-spotting and strengths valuing in my interactions with them.
- Character strength(s) use:
  - I will use my kindness and curiosity strengths to keep motivated with the meditations and when I'm conversing with my work colleagues.

My Life Goal:

- Goal:

  _____

- Activities:

  _____

  _____

  _____

- Character strength(s) use:

  _____

  _____

  _____

My Mindfulness Goal:

- Goal:

  _____

- Activities:

  _____

  _____

  _____

- Character strength(s) use:

  _____

  _____

  _____

Chapter 14

Mindfulness-Based Strengths Practice
Session 8: Your Engagement With Life

I am unable to make the days longer, so I strive to make them better.

Henry David Thoreau

 Opening Story

During one series of MBSP groups, I became curious about how one participant was "receiving" the material. This was a tall, thin, middle-aged woman. She was a shy group member, not sharing very much. In dyad and small group exercises, she shared "lightly" and attempted to place the emphasis on others by asking them questions or distracting the conversation to topics relating to city news. When she did speak, it tended to be self-deprecatory and pessimistic. During many of the input/lecture portions of the sessions, she frequently displayed a puzzled look on her face. At the same time, she never missed a session and seemed to be putting forth effort to learn. I wondered if she was struggling with the material. I decided to politely pull the woman aside to check-in with her to see how she was doing.

"How are you doing with this mindfulness and character strengths work?" I asked with curiosity.

She immediately explained that following a divorce several years ago, she had lost touch with what was meaningful in her life and had lost touch with herself. She explained how she has been riding on autopilot for years, not doing anything new, just going through the motions. She then went on to explain how she was coming to realize how important her spirituality, gratitude, and kindness strengths were to her and that she had let them fade in her life. She was now beginning to bring these back to the center of her life. "I am *re-claiming* what is most important to me and about me," she shared.

My curiosity was quenched.

 Structure for Session 8

I   Opening Meditation: Signature Strengths Breathing Space Exercise [3–5 min]
II   Practice Review [30 min]
III   Your Engagement with Life [20 min]
IV   Sacred Object Meditation [20 min]
V   Golden Nuggets [15 min]
VI   Virtue Circle [20 min]

Note. Times are approximates. This is for a 2-hour session; for a 1.5-hour session, it's advisable to eliminate the virtue circle and shorten each section accordingly

I   Opening Meditation

- Signature strengths breathing space exercise, or an abridged version of the group's favorite meditation from the course.

II   Practice Review

- Before reviewing the goal-setting sheets and homework, "take stock" by reviewing the key themes, practices, and insights from the MBSP course.
    - Write a couple of columns on the board – "Key themes" and "MBSP practices" – and ask the group what has stood out most to them over the eight weeks.
    - Jot down the responses; the facilitator can ensure that every major mindfulness practice (e.g., listening, speaking, eating, etc.) is accounted for and every major strengths exercise has been considered (e.g., strengths-spotting, strengths interview, you at your best, etc.). In terms of themes, you might add any of the session titles from Sessions 1 through 8 that the group does not explicitly mention or allude to.
- In dyads or as a full group, invite participants to share their goal-setting worksheet. Those that did not complete it might refer to the board and speak to the practice that they feel most enthused or encouraged by and/or is a practice they would most like to bring regularly into their daily life.
- Solicit feedback from other group members about the participants' goals/plans and share your own feedback, placing emphasis on mindfulness and character strengths as pathways for reaching the goal.
    - If appropriate, ask participants about what kind of support they will need in order to stay on the path. Who will support them in their life?
    - At this point in MBSP, it is likely the practitioner and the participants have considered or discussed the potential of follow-up after Session 8. Will there be any follow-up needed for this group? Booster session? MBSP retreat? (Chapter 15 discusses these latter two approaches).

III   Your Engagement with Life

- Group strengths (this practice was initiated in Session 4): Ask the group about what they think the strengths of their group-as-a-whole are. What character strength would best describe their group? There might be one or more strengths that stand out, e.g., there was always high energy and enthusiasm so it's "the zest group." This could be based on those strengths that the most participants endorsed as signature strengths. In other instances, this could be the strengths that were spotted the most by group members. Finally, group strengths can emerge as the result of the constellation of strengths expressed by the participants, for example, a group that shows a high degree of forgiveness, humility, love, and hope might wish to sum themselves up as "the spirituality group."
- The session title – Your Engagement with Life – characterizes what ultimately happens when we live our life from our signature strengths and with greater mindfulness. We become more engaged and connected with who we are, with who we are with, and with our present moment activities. Typically, an "engage-

ment" is a commitment to another person. This theme applies to each participant's commitment to themselves and the life they would like to live. Participants can use mindfulness to "touch" life deeply, to "touch" their character strengths, and to engage fully in all areas of life (Nhat Hanh, 1992).

- Review the key reminders sheet (Handout 8.1). This can also be viewed as an MBSP tipsheet.

Suggestions for Moving Forward

- Return your attention back to the present moment with curiosity/openness/acceptance a billion more times in your life.
- Implement goals in which you can use your strengths to help you get the most out of life. Maintain a mindfulness practice that you resonate most with. Maintain a practice of strengths awareness, exploration, and use for yourself and with others.

IV   Sacred Object Meditation

- The purpose of this meditation is to offer an experience that brings the core themes of MBSP together and offers a "transitional object" for the participants to take with them as a special reminder of mindfulness, character strengths, and their fellow group members.
- I start by choosing one person randomly and presenting a bag to them in which they reach in and choose one object. I then go around the room to the other participants. The bag contains various stones, each with one character strength word engraved on it (each participant gets to keep the stone they select). I then lead participants in a beginner's mind meditation (e.g., similar to the raisin but placing emphasis on the visual/touch senses). In the meditation, I spend time focusing on the breath anchor, and the value of mindfulness in daily life. I reference the journey the group has been on together and that they can continue to tap into their strengths resources to meet their goals. I go through the themes of past sessions

and relate them as ongoing work on the journey of life (e.g., mindfulness of autopilot, facing obstacles with strengths, etc.). I reference the object they are holding as a cue for the strengths and mindfulness practice, as a symbol of this journey, and as a symbol of the vulnerability and imperfections that we can embrace and accept.

- Other options:
  - Purchase some kind of item that has strength words written on it.
  - Have participants create something with a strength word on it.
  - Sanctify an object (Goldstein, 2007): Invite participants to select one object on their person that they cherish most (e.g., wedding ring, necklace, watch, bracelet, coin, photo in wallet, etc.). Or, participants can be invited in Session 7 to bring in any small object that is precious to them. Invite the participants to hold the object in their hand as the meditation begins. Lead a focus on breath and body awareness emphasizing the breath anchor and use of character strengths with mindfulness. Emphasize that they can imbue the object with a sense of sacredness by focusing on the object in the present moment and naming it as precious, dear, blessed, special, holy, and/or cherished. Invite them to connect the object with their heart. Embed in additional themes mentioned earlier. Then, explain that this sacred object can serve as a mindfulness and strengths cue; when they see this object, they will be called back to what matters most, that it is a cue back to the present moment, a cue for them to consider their strengths in the moment.

V   Golden Nuggets

- Ask the group: "What is the most crucial 'nugget' that you learned in this course that you intend to hold close to you from this point forward? Said another way, what's your best learning from the course? Share it with mindful speech – you might share it as a phrase, a sentence, or a few sentences.

- For this exercise, it is very important to involve every group member. Start with a volunteer, then go around in a circle where each person shares briefly (e.g., it might only be a 30-second share each).
- Facilitators are encouraged to write down each nugget that is shared as this can inform them as they reflect on the MBSP group experience as a whole, help them understand what matters most to participants, and may serve to guide them in future MBSP group experiences.

VI Virtue Circle

VII Suggested Homework Exercises

- Since this is the final MBSP session, there is no formal homework exercise to review. However, the point should be emphasized that the participants' "homework" is to apply mindfulness and character strengths for the rest of their lives. Rather than being at the end, they are really at the beginning, and have the opportunity to keep on looking upon themselves, others, and their life with fresh eyes.
- For those groups that will be doing a MBSP retreat or booster session (discussed in Chapter 15), the practitioner might offer ideas and exercises to consider in the interim.

Handouts

- Handout 8.1: Key Mindfulness and Character Strengths Reminders (1 page)
- Handout 8.2: MBSP Qualitative Feedback Form (3 pages)

VIII Closing Meditation

- Abridged version of the group's favorite mindfulness meditation, along with comments about using strengths and mindfulness along their life journey.

IX Qualitative Feedback Form (Handout 8.2)

- Allow extra time (usually about 10 minutes) in the session for participants to fill out this review of the MBSP course, the impact that it had on them, and their practices.
- This should be given *after* the closing meditation, therefore the group has technically concluded by the time they fill out the form.
- The information participants provide is very valuable and helps to inform future MBSP groups that the practitioner might facilitate. MBSP group facilitators are encouraged to share this feedback with Ryan Niemiec (rmjn@sbcglobal.net).

Additional Considerations

Regarding "Obstacles"

As the group sessions progress, the participants might come to a particular insight – that there really are no obstacles. What has come to be viewed as a barrier or a practice hurdle is merely part of life experience. We face the vicissitudes of life and mindfulness allows participants to see experiences as they are – as fodder for the practice. Such a realization generates a profound acceptance for oneself, others, and what it means to be "living" this life.

Sacred Object Meditation (Research)

Many studies reflect positive correlations between spirituality and well-being; however, little research has been done on interventions that actually increase an aspect of the spirituality strength known as sacred moments. Many scholarly works have discussed the importance and relevance of connecting with the sacred, e.g., Anthony de Mello (1978) and Roger Walsh (1999). In one study, Goldstein (2007) defined sacred moments as having two components: (1) a spiritual quality involving a feeling of connection with and support from the transcendent (e.g., God, higher power, all of life), a connection with others, purpose, gratefulness, awe, compassion, mercy, and/or a deep sense of inner peace; and (2) involvement of descriptive qualities such as precious, dear, blessed, cherished, and/or holy. Examples of this vary per each individual, ranging from the individual perceiving a sacred moment with a higher power describing it as blessed, to the person hiking and feeling a sense of awe in the natural world describing it as a cherished moment.

This study was a randomized controlled trial with an intervention and control group. For the first three days of the three-week experiment, the intervention group practiced a mindfulness strategy, and starting on Day 4, participants sanctified a sacred, tangible or nontangible object of their choosing (sanctification was defined as reimbuing the object with a sense of what was considered by the individual to be precious, dear, blessed, special, holy, and/or cherished qualities). Participants then spent 5 minutes per day starting with a mindfulness practice followed by turning attention to that which is sacred in the object for a time period determined by each individual. The control group spent 5 minutes per day reflecting on and writing about daily activities (an already proven intervention). Both groups were to do the activity 5 days per week.

Both interventions were effective in boosting psychological well-being. Significant increases were found in satisfaction with life, positive affect, positive relations with others, and purpose in life as well as a decrease in perceived stress. The increase in life satisfaction was sustained at six-week follow-up. For 89% of the intervention group, the exercise was effective in creating a sacred moment, while 11% found it obstructive; 100% found they could cultivate sacred moments in their life.

Golden Nugget Examples

Participants report a wide range of insights/benefits. Here are a *few* examples:

- My strengths are becoming more automatic. It's as if I'm reformulating parts of my auto-pilot mind.
- I learned I don't need to shy away from obstacles. Mindfulness and strengths are all I need to face challenges that come up.
- For me, personal growth means to repeatedly choose to integrate strengths and conscious living.
- When I become self-judging, I bring my mindfulness to this. I call upon my signature strengths.
- It's ironic that mindfulness is actually a fast track. I solve problems and get things done more quickly now, even though mindfulness is about slowing down. My rationale is that mindfulness helps us see what's most important and so we go right toward it. We take a straight line rather than the crooked, meandering path of avoidance.
- I use my strengths gatha daily and have merged it with the breathing space exercise.
- When I go into a negative spiral, I catch myself and say "Stop! Aware! Go to your signature strengths!"
- It's another way of being. I now am proactive with obstacles.
- My best possible self is within me, and it is within reach.

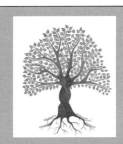

MBSP Handout 8.1

Session 8:

Your Engagement With Life

Mindfulness and Character Strength – Key Reminders

- Notice your mind's autopilot tendencies. Embrace this capacity of your mind. Catch your AP-ASAP.

- Return your attention back to the present moment with openness and curiosity a billion[1] more times in your life.

- Bring awareness to your character strengths often; accept and value your strengths; find ways to express them regularly in your life.

- Practice spotting and overtly valuing the strengths of others, at good times and difficult/stressful times.

- Face your mindfulness practice (and the obstacles that come up) as an opportunity to deepen your connection with yourself/others/the world.

- Face your problems by using your strengths. Consider how you may have overused or underused several strengths and understand how you can deploy your strengths to temper overuse and/or better manage the problem.

- Implement goals in which you can use your strengths to help you get the most out of life.

- Bring mindfulness and strengths into your daily routines. Never give up on finding new ways to express your signature strengths in your life.

- Maintain a mindfulness practice that you resonate most with. Use your strengths to stick with it.

- Return to "beginner's mind" (seeing things as if for the first time) at least once every day.

---

[1] One should not take this statement light. To highlight how big of a number a billion is consider the difference between a million and a billion: A million seconds is 12 days; a billion seconds is 31 years!

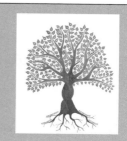

MBSP Handout 8.2

Session 8: MBSP Qualitative Feedback Form

1. As you consider this group, please circle whether each of the following were "too much," "not enough," or "just right."

	Too much	Not enough	Just right
The amount of time per session (2 hours):	❏	❏	❏
Amount of time for whole-group discussions:	❏	❏	❏
Amount of time for one-on-one discussions (dyads):	❏	❏	❏
Amount of time practicing meditation:	❏	❏	❏
Amount of time receiving information on a topic:	❏	❏	❏
Amount of time for the virtue circle:	❏	❏	❏
Amount of homework exercises given:	❏	❏	❏
The number of sessions in the program (8):	❏	❏	❏
Time spent on integrating mindfulness & strengths:	❏	❏	❏

2. On a 1–10 scale where 1 is "not important" and 10 is "extremely important," how important would it be for your learning to attend *all 8* of these 8 classes? _____

3. In this course, I cared most about (circle one):
   ❏ Learning about character strengths
   ❏ Learning about mindfulness
   ❏ Learning about the integration

4. My favorite mindfulness meditation practice: _____

5. My favorite strengths activity/practice: _____

6. On average, how much of the homework did you do each week (be sure to consider meditations, strengths activities, interviews, tracking/journaling, etc.):

   ❏ 0%   ❏ 10%   ❏ 25%   ❏ 40%   ❏ 50%   ❏ 60%   ❏ 75%   ❏ 90%   ❏ 100%

7. Which of the following did you practice regularly? (check all that apply)

❏ Journaling   ❏ Tracking/monitoring your behaviors/practices

❏ Mindfulness meditation   ❏ Working with strengths

❏ Reflecting on past experiences with strengths   ❏ Observing your and others' strengths

❏ Asking others for feedback   ❏ Discussing strengths with others

❏ Planning out your practices   ❏ Appreciating others' strengths

8. Which of the following do you believe is true for you? (check all that apply)

❏ Knowledge of character strengths will make my mindfulness practice stronger.

❏ Knowledge of mindfulness will help my character strength use and expression.

❏ The integration of mindfulness and character strengths is essential for practicing either one.

❏ None of the above

9. As a result of this group, I (check off all that apply or leave blank):

❏ Started a new mindfulness practice   ❏ Have deepened my mindfulness practice

❏ Overcame more obstacles in my mindfulness practice   ❏ Am aware of my signature strengths

❏ Use my strengths to deal with my problems/difficulties   ❏ Use my strengths more often

❏ Spot strengths in others frequently   ❏ Verbally appreciate strengths more in others

❏ Use mindfulness to face my problems/difficulties   ❏ I made no changes because of this group

10. What are the major obstacles to your mindfulness practice? (Check all that apply):

❏ Not enough time/too busy   ❏ Often forgot to practice/schedule

❏ Did not see the purpose in practicing   ❏ Mind wandered too much

❏ Wanted to avoid painful sensations   ❏ Wanted to avoid difficult emotions

❏ Wanted to avoid troubling thoughts/memories   ❏ Kept falling asleep

❏ It was not very helpful/I don't see the point   ❏ Too bothered by the external (e.g., noises)

❏ Other: _____

11. As you think about the "virtue circle," were there any benefits of this experience? Please explain:

_____

_____

_____

12. Please *rank-order* what was *most* beneficial to your overall learning and growth in terms of mindfulness and character strengths (give a 1 to the most beneficial, 2 to the second most beneficial, and so on):

    ___ Homework exercises/practice (outside group)   ___ Discussions with whole group

    ___ One-on-one activities (in group)   ___ Meditations (in group)

    ___ Lecture/input periods (in group)   ___ Virtue circle (in group)

13. Has this course had a positive effect on one of your relationships? If so, please share:

_____

_____

_____

14. What effect (if any) did this program have on any of the following?

	A lot higher/better			No change		A lot worse/lower	
Your overall well-being	7	6	5	4	3	2	1
Your sense of who you are	7	6	5	4	3	2	1
Your engagement with life tasks	7	6	5	4	3	2	1
Your sense of accomplishment	7	6	5	4	3	2	1
Your meaning in life	7	6	5	4	3	2	1
Your sense of purpose	7	6	5	4	3	2	1
The quality of your relationships	7	6	5	4	3	2	1
Your management of stress	7	6	5	4	3	2	1
Your management of problems	7	6	5	4	3	2	1

15. What has struck you most about this course? Please share below:

_____

_____

_____

Thank you for your time!

Chapter 15

Additional MBSP Features and Adaptations for Different Settings/ Populations

Cultivate Virtue in yourself,
And Virtue will be real.
Cultivate it in the family,
And Virtue will abound.
Cultivate it in the village,
And Virtue will grow.
Cultivate it in the nation,
And Virtue will be abundant.
Cultivate it in the universe,
And Virtue will be everywhere.

Lao Tsu

 Chapter Snapshot

MBSP is potentially for everyone. It should not be limited to any one population, setting, culture, or delivery method. Future research will reveal if certain populations or particular modalities benefit more significantly than others. This chapter begins with some optional features that practitioners might include along with the 8-week MBSP group in order to enhance the program. These additional features include:

- The MBSP retreat
- Optional tools between MBSP sessions
- Booster sessions

The chapter also offers tentative suggestions to consider in making optimal adjustments to the MBSP program. Further research in each area is needed to determine efficacy. Suggestions are offered for the following:

- Cultural considerations
- Modalities
  - Individual (one-on-one) MBSP
  - Couples MBSP
  - Online MBSP
- Settings
  - Schools/Education
  - Organizations/Business

Opening Story[1]

This following poetic story was written by an MBSP participant who is a writer and educator. During the group, she explained that she was experiencing a "writer's block." Throughout the MBSP group experience, she practiced creative writing and exploration but she hadn't yet put what she really wanted to on paper. Then, in the space of the MBSP retreat (discussed later in this chapter), the words poured out. With mindfulness and heartfulness, a story unfolded. She then read the story to the group during the Virtue Circle. The group was stunned, not only by the beauty and meaning but by the fact that she wrote the story in less than 45 minutes. Since then, the words have been flowing as she continues to work on her stories for children.

"Tree Opus"

Tree stood
sturdy
tall
unbending

one day Bird
came to live in Tree
and made a hole
to its heart

Bird's songs echoed
thru its branches
so sweet the music
Tree wept tears of rain

for many years Tree
echoed Bird's songs
but no one heard

one Spring Tree asked Bird
I sing your song
yet no one hears

Bird said,
find your own song
and flew away

Tree stood in silence
and asked its heart
will you help me
find my song?

Heart said
just be silent
and you will hear
your voice

Tree was silent

many Falls
and cold icy Winters
Tree remained silent

one day
Tree was tired of waiting
and yelled throughout the forest
Who am I?

everything changed

thousands of buds
appeared on Tree's branches

leaves
Unfurling
bountiful shades of green

melodies rang out throughout the forest
joyful songs singing

Maple, Maple
you are a Maple Tree
full of color and life

come practice with us
so we may sing together
In harmony

Tree did

now when Bird comes
Tree plays leaf music
rustling with wind and rain

in harmony with Bird

and if you are quiet
you, too
will hear Tree sing

Author:
Marti Kwiatkowski

---

[1] This opening story, "Tree Opus," is used here with the written permission of Marti Kwiatkowski. Marti is the sole author of the story.

Optional Features of MBSP

The MBSP Retreat

This is an optional but recommended part of MBSP. There are logistic issues that preclude many practitioners from being able to lead a retreat. Also, many practitioners may not feel comfortable leading this kind of experience.

A sample MBSP retreat schedule can be seen in Handout 15.1. After participants arrive, a brief introduction is offered to set up the event. Some key themes to include in the introduction and observations of previous MBSP retreats follow.

Retreat Introduction Themes
- Discuss schedule, silence, free time.
- Explain that the intention of the retreat is not to introduce new material, instead it is to engage fully in practices. That said, a retreat experience is often "new" to many participants.
- The retreat offers an opportunity for solitude, silence, extended practice, and an exploration of strengths and mindfulness practices.
- It's helpful to gently set some guidelines to help participants separate temporarily from the outside world and engage fully. One suggestion is to preclude the use cell phones and electronic devices. This is aligned with the reality that participants have carved out space for themselves to reconnect with who they are and to replenish themselves and not to be tempted by work or outside influences.
- The value of space (see Chapter 5); emphasis on creating space for oneself; each moment matters (e.g., turning a doorknob, preparing food) and can be viewed as sacred. There is potential in each moment to practice mindfulness and engage one's character strengths.
- Exploring and expanding: Many people come back from a retreat and say, "I deepened my practice." This is because individuals take time to explore their mind and their present moment and expand each meditation practice.
- Explain the purpose of retreats: Opportunity to slow down and replenish oneself; to remind oneself of one's strengths/goodness; to apply and practice mindful living; to practice bringing strengths such as one's curiousness, pru-

dence, creativity, kindness, love, and fairness to one's mindfulness practice.
- Create a strength intention: Consider your hopes and intentions for the day; ask yourself why are you here today? Write down one word you'd like to embody to get there. For example, someone who said they wanted to have more peace wrote down "self-regulation"; another who wanted to explore their reactivity wrote down "curiosity"; someone who wanted to deepen their courage to face the stress of their life wrote down "bravery"; another person wanted to figure out how to better deal with their mother-in-law and wrote down "kindness."

Retreat Observations
- Following the introduction, there is a shift to mindfulness exercises. It is usually helpful to offer two or three practices in a row to help participants engage and deepen.
- The experience of retreats is often a brand new or relatively new experience for people. Therefore, the use of new material has the tendency to distract from the present moment as it elicits questions in which participants look to the leader for answers. The retreat facilitator should emphasize that the priority is self-discovery.
- Silence is very important: during exercises, free time, in between activities, and during meals. As always, it is embedded in the virtue circle.
- Participants benefit from the use of the bell periodically for random cueing to the present moment.
- Offering ideas for spending free time (e.g., during the period of "mindful strengths use") is very helpful for many participants.
- Leaf meditation: This meditation addressing "little things matter" is useful for those groups that did not have time for it during the MBSP sessions. It involves the facilitator bringing in several leaves or participants going outside to select one leaf object. The facilitator then leads a meditation of beginner's mind focusing on taking notice of the visual details and use of senses with the leaf. A connection is drawn between the leaf and the tree it came from, and the transitory nature of life is highlighted.

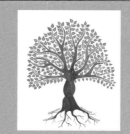

MBSP Handout 15.1
MBPS Retreat Schedule

Every morning, when we wake up, we have 24 brand-new hours to live. We have the capacity to live in a way that these 24 hours will bring peace, joy, and happiness to ourselves and others.

Thich Nhat Hanh

Schedule:

8:00–8:30:	Arrival and settling in
8:30:	The character strengths breathing space Welcome, retreat orientation Strength intentions
9:00:	Strong mindfulness: Breath & body meditation
9:30:	Strong mindfulness: Walking meditation
10:15:	*Mindful strengths use
11:30:	Mindful food preparation (or free time)
12:00:	Mindful eating: in silence and strength
1:00:	Virtue circle: Mindful listening, mindful speech, strengths-spotting
1:45:	The signature strengths breathing space
2:00:	Mindful departure

Noble Silence:

- Please respect the quietness that others are pursuing by limiting talking.

*Possible Mindful Strengths Use Ideas (free time to practice with your strengths)

- Choose one of your signature strengths and use it in a new way
- Write out your best possible self and the strengths that will be pathways to getting there. Or, draw or create something that represents your best possible self.
- Write out a moment in time that shaped who you are (defining moments exercise).
- Write a letter to someone in which you use one of the 24 strengths (e.g., gratitude letter, forgiveness letter, spirituality letter).
- Draw or create something that depicts one of your strengths in a symbolic way.

Themes of the leaf meditation: the preciousness of life; noticing the little details along with the bigger view of life; interconnection with the leaf (see Session 3 and Box 9.2 for further details).

Optional Tools Between MBSP Sessions

Between MBSP sessions, participants return to the business of daily life and naturally shift into autopilot. Participants may report high energy the day or two after an MBSP session, but often there is a mid-week drift or loss of energy. The homework exercises and practices are designed to help participants stay focused in developing mindfulness and strengths knowledge/use. The following are some adjunctive approaches that can assist participants in between sessions.

E-Mail Tips
Some participants find it useful for practitioners to offer them a reminder of the MBSP they are engaging in. This might come in the form of an e-mail message to the group that offers one reminder from the last group session, an inspiring quote, or a tip about staying focused with one of the homework assignments. Some MBSP participants may even quote a study in a user-friendly way, for example, sharing more details about the research on how using signature strengths in new ways leads to significant, lasting increases in happiness (Gander et al., 2012a), or how the focus on specific life satisfaction strengths is also of benefit to happiness (Proyer, Ruch, & Buschor, 2012).

Cues
Participants might be encouraged to spontaneously create a concrete cue for mindfulness or character strengths. Participants sometimes decide to print up quotes, key exploratory questions, or a strength-based picture and post it near their computer or somewhere they often pass by. There are a number of suggestions practitioners might make in relation to participants keeping their signature strengths at the forefront of their mind, such as writing them out on several sticky notes and posting them in different rooms of their home.

Strengths Cards
Some MBSP practitioners might have access to strengths cards or other products that have the strength words on them. Practitioners can have each participant in the group randomly choose one card *after* a particular session and place the card somewhere in their home. Whenever the participant sees the card, they shift their mindfulness to the given strength, remind themselves this is a capacity within them, and query themselves as to whether it would be useful to bring forth this strength more strongly in the current situation they are in or later that day. Note that in most settings it is generally not recommended that strengths cards be formally integrated into MBSP sessions as this can distract from the topic at hand or mislead participants into thinking that focusing on a randomly chosen strength card is more important than deploying one's signature strengths.

Mindful Bell
In our technology-driven world, we are surrounded by electronic devices. So, why not use them to our mindful advantage? One of the best ways to do this is to download a mindfulness bell to one's computer or other device. This can be set to chime randomly or at a particular interval (e.g., hourly). Each time the individual hears the sound of the bell, this is a call to return to the present moment. One bell can be found at this site: www.mindfulnessdc.org/mindfulclock.html

Organizing Binder
Many MBSP group leaders decide to create a binder or notebook to hand participants at Session 1 in an attempt to help participants organize the materials. This then becomes not only a cue that can be placed in a prominent place in their home, but is a useful resource to review between sessions.

Recording Devices
Some participants may have difficulty remembering a particular meditation practice (especially those that are homework assignments) and decide not to purchase mindfulness CDs. Therefore, practitioners are encouraged to invite any participant to bring in a recording device to do a live recording of the body scan, breathing space, or other meditation experience during the group so

that it can be replayed for home practice. This approach also helps to reinforce the importance of "practice." Note that this is encouraged only for the meditation portion of MBSP and not discussion periods. Participants, therefore, are not placed in an uncomfortable position where their voice might be recorded and confidentiality is broken.

Optional Purchases

These are described in Chapter 6 and include books, interpretive reports, and CDs. Some practitioners may decide to require one or more of these purchases prior to Session 1 of MBSP.

Booster Sessions

Many MBSP participants will want to continue the group sessions following the 8-week program. Sometimes this highlights the enjoyment participants experienced or reflects the sadness of letting go. Nevertheless, it is often useful to offer what is referred to as booster sessions. A booster session is a specially designed session that occurs a certain period of time after Session 8 (e.g., one or two months later) and serves as both a check-in and a refresher. It is also an opportunity to continue the practice.

- **Check-in:** Participants report to the group on progress they have made, the new (and old) obstacles they have encountered, the supports they are using, and their goal progress. The maintenance of gains and structure of practice are discussed.
- **Refresher:** The practitioner reviews key focus areas of MBSP as well as the main insights that emerged, specific to this particular group. Mindfulness practices and strengths-spotting exercises are conducted and serve as a reminder and a boost for the participants as well.

While booster sessions are traditionally not used to offer extensive new material, participants tend to appreciate new "flavors" of practices while keeping to the routine structure and practice of the MBSP groups. One exercise that usually aligns well with booster sessions is called "imagined travel" (Glück & Baltes, 2006). Box 15.1 offers a basic script that has been adapted to fit MBSP. This meditation exercise has been found to boost

wisdom-related knowledge, as it involves building upon the accumulating wisdom that participants have already been cultivating. It underlies the teaching point and popular adage that the participants already have within them the necessary knowledge to make wise choices.

Box 15.1. Imagined Travel

Take a moment to re-connect with your breath anchor. Bring to mind a current difficulty, meditation obstacle, or a small challenge in your life. As you follow your breathing, imagine that you are traveling around the world and stopping in various places to learn from the different cultures and people. At each stop, allow yourself to gain new perspectives and ideas, learning fresh ways of seeing the obstacle or challenge. See your obstacle through the eyes of others. Gain from their perspective. Take note of the variety of character strengths the people display. With each breath in, take in the wisdom. (Pause). As you travel from place to place, notice the differences in the values and context of each place. Allow bits and pieces to provide you a new perspective on life. How does it assist you with your current life challenge? (Pause). Bring this wisdom with you as you return your focus to the present moment.

Cultural Adaptations

Even though MBSP focuses on the universal, human phenomena of mindfulness and character strengths, practitioners will need to consider if adjustments need to be made to create an optimal fit for their particular culture. In general, practitioners from other cultures have *not* needed to make significant adjustments to "fit" MBSP to their cultural norms or to become more aligned with the values/customs of their country.

In many instances, the adjustments that are made are subtle – such as changing the title of "virtue circle" to "strengths circle" in many countries, as well as eliminating the bowing ritual. For certain exercises, greater explanation needs to be offered for increased clarity and comfort of the participants. For example, some individuals from certain cultures may react with discomfort at the idea of telling a story of "You at your best," as this may feel awkward or immodest. Therefore, additional explanation may be warranted around how this is an opportunity to explore strengths, to spot strengths, to open oneself up to someone, and to practice mindful speech/listening, in addition to reviewing the benefits of the exercise to both oneself and the other. In these situations, practitioners might explain that participants can share a time when "things went well," a situation of happiness, or a time when they were successful. Participants are also reminded that MBSP is an opportunity for them to move outside of their comfort zone, to "stretch" themselves, and to experiment with new ways of perceiving themselves.

Practitioners should be mindful of the impact of sociological processes and history in their culture and the potential impact this has on the psyche of participants. One example is the Law of Jante, found in Scandinavian countries (e.g., Denmark, Sweden), and refers to a pattern of discouraging others from standing out as an achiever among a group. This mindset, which is more prevalent among certain subgroups, includes particular rules that underlie this mindset, including: "You shall not think that you are wiser than us," "You shall not think that you are good at anything," and "You shall not think that anyone cares about you." A similar phenomenon found in Australia, UK, New Zealand, and Canadian cultures, referred to as "tall poppy syndrome," occurs when individuals of genuine merit are criticized and resented because of their talents or achievements that elevate them above others. Of course, these social phenomena do not characterize every individual in these cultures, however, they are important processes that affect group dynamics and underpin the attitudes and approaches of many individuals.

Practitioners should also be mindful of the dynamics present in cultures that tend toward individualism and those that tend toward collectivism. At the same time, practitioners should be careful to not attempt to "over-correct" or adjust MBSP too much because of this. For example, it is probably *not* a good idea to eliminate the virtue circle simply because one is conducting MBSP in an individualist culture. In fact, based on the

feedback thus far from both MBSP practitioners and participants in individualist and collectivist cultures, it is important to allow time for individuals to explore and express their personal character strengths *and* time to explore and discuss strengths as a group and experience group exercises.

Modalities

There are a variety of modalities that practitioners employ to help people – meeting with people individually, meeting with couples, and meeting with participants online. Each of these MBSP modalities have shown initial promise, however, systematic research is needed to test the adaptation of MBSP with each.

Individual Work (One-on-One)

Some practitioners will be more comfortable experimenting with MBSP with individuals before attempting it in a group format. This allows practitioners to become more familiar with the material, the flow of the content, the meditations and experiential exercises, and the handling of common questions that come up. On the other hand, some practitioners who do not work with groups may wish to apply MBSP in their individual counseling, coaching, supervision, or psychotherapy work.

There are adjustments to consider when shifting MBSP to individual work. Box 15.1 offers a general adapted structure for individual sessions. Times may need to be altered based on the agreed-upon framework between the practitioner and client. Here are some suggestions and observations for working with individuals:

- In general, shift from 2-hour sessions to 1-hour sessions.
- One-on-one situations are set up for increased dialog. Take advantage of this and tailor the material, questions, and experiential exercises to the individual's goals, interests, and problems, including debriefing on each experience. This approach allows for more immediate feedback.
- In some ways, there is more pressure on the individual to complete homework exercises and build in practices (i.e., it's easier to "hide"

from the facilitator in a group format). This can intensify the work for individuals. As the pressure increases, more time can be taken for mindfulness and strengths practices to face and manage the tension in the moment.

- It is easier to write out individualized reminders (e.g., strengths prescriptions) and individually tailor recordings of meditations conducted.
- There are more opportunities to discuss and work directly with the individual's character strengths, as well as adapt to their level of mindfulness experience.
- Since there is no virtue circle, the practitioner becomes the only source of feedback for strengths-spotting, strengths valuing, and modeling of mindful living and mindfulness practice. The practitioner might keep each of these in mind during each session. In addition, the character strengths 360 homework exercise for Session 6 becomes pivotal.

Box 15.2. General Structure for Individual MBSP Sessions

- Opening meditation [5 min]
  - Character strengths breathing space exercise, breathing meditation, signature strengths breathing space, walking meditation, or strengths gatha
- Discussion [15 min]
  - Review of homework practices and applications with mindfulness and strengths
- Input and life application [15 min]
  - New material and discussion of relevance/use to daily life, problems, and goals
- Experiential [15 min]
  - The centerpiece MBSP experience for the session (see Chapter 6 for details)
  - Debriefing
- Homework practices for next week [5 min]
- Closing meditation [5 min]
  - Character strengths breathing space exercise, breathing meditation, signature strengths breathing space exercise, walking meditation, or strengths gatha

---

Couples Work

Here are some adaptations to consider for those practitioners working with couples:

- A two-hour meeting might be too long for some couples and one-hour meetings may not allow for enough time, especially considering the work involves three parties to which the concepts can be applied – two individuals and the couple itself. It seems that 1.5-hour meetings is sufficient for a solid 8-week MBSP program for couples. The structure in Box 15.2 might be used and the times adjusted accordingly.
- The homework review of practices is usually a discussion of individual practices but also the couple-as-a-team. When there are time limitations to only hear from one in the dyad, the other can be encouraged to practice strengths-spotting while listening.
- Include the mindful speech/mindful listening intervention for couples described in detail in Chapter 4, Box 4.1.
- Include mindful touch. This can be as simple as having the couple hold hands during the character strengths breathing space exercise or other activities. During the loving-kindness meditation, each individual practices sending and receiving love to their partner and makes note of the felt experience of this.
- Include mindful communication within the MBSP exercises. For example, when doing the statue meditation have the couple face one another.
- During particular strengths exercises or other activities, the couple is encouraged to close their eyes to enhance the depth that mindful listening (and speech) can have.
- Spending time in Session 2 and later sessions reviewing parallel strengths and unique strengths is recommended. Which strengths are shared by the couple in their top 7? Which are the unique strengths in which only one of the individuals is high on? Encourage couples to remember these parallel and unique strengths of one another. Explore the dynamics of how these similarities and differences contribute to the couple's well-being and distress.
- Include discussion of character strengths at high points and low points in the relationship. For example, one couple working with MBSP

got married midway through the MBSP program. This offered a myriad of high points (e.g., moments during the ceremony and reception) and low points (e.g., stressful moments of last-minute planning and unexpected hiccups) and the mindful use of character strengths in each of these instances.

- Additional creative adaptations can be made such as for the character strengths 360 exercise in which the couple can invite individuals to nominate the character strengths viewed in the couple as a unit and how they relate to one another, rather than having individuals offer nominations of the couple as individuals.
- There are trade books that address healthy, loving, or mindful communication that can be recommended as supplemental materials. Some examples include: Nhat Hanh (2006), Gottman (1994), Grayson (2003), and Kahn (1995).
- See Appendix C for a diagram of certain groupings of character strengths among a couple –the strongest shared strengths of the couple, the supportive strengths, and the unique strengths of each individual in the couple.

Online

MBSP has had some initial success in an online format using Skype technology. Exercises, meditations, and lecture material are able to be conducted in an online format for participants to understand. This includes exercises such as the raisin exercise, mindful breathing, body scanning, standing meditation, and various strengths exercises. An adjustment might be made for walking meditation (Session 4) in which participants listen to instructions while practicing mindful standing and then walk for a designated time period (e.g., 10 minutes) to which the sound of the bell can invite participants back to their computers. The statue meditation (Session 3) is ideally done with visual capability (e.g., through Skype) so that all participants can observe the other participants and group leader during the experience.

A minimum requirement is a quality audio connection. Glitches in the audio or visual technology can become a major barrier. Another barrier for facilitators to be attuned to is that if participants are facing a sensitive topic or experiencing difficulty in sharing, they can easily "escape" from the group claiming they're experiencing "technology problems." On the positive side, some reports express that online programs can provide an opportunity to deepen mindful listening as the use of certain senses decreases. Some group members find that this leads to enhanced motivation in order to compensate for any barrier created by technology in that a virtuous circle of positivity emerges from the home practices and live work in group.

In some instances, the participants' responses can be just as strong online and it's possible the program might be able to have a similar impact online compared with live. Online platforms such as e-Mindful have successfully demonstrated the application of mindfulness online (Wolever et al., 2012), where online delivery was equivocal to in-person delivery and both were superior to controls in improving perceived stress, sleep quality, and measures of heart rate variability. In addition, the online delivery had a much higher program completion percentage than did the live program.

Other research on web-based training of mind-body programs have found these technologies to be well-received by participants and reveal positive results. Web-based programs have shown the impact of mindfulness in reducing stress (Krusche, Cyhlarova, King, & Williams, 2012), improving mental health and decreasing pain catastrophizing (Gardner-Nix, Backman, Barbati, & Grummitt, 2008), establishing a long-term impact of mindfulness after three months (Gluck & Maercker, 2011), and decreasing stress, depression, and anxiety among a relaxation response group (Hoch et al., 2012).

Settings

Regardless of the setting that a practitioner is applying MBSP, maintaining a sensitivity to the population is essential. For example, if an individual is working on a medical unit in a hospital, then stories, examples, and meditations from MBSP should be tailored to medical situations, conditions, and physical symptoms, when possible.

There are an increasing number of positive psychology programs in business, education, and other settings; however, too often the approach is one that attempts to "throw everything but the kitchen sink" at the students or employees. Such approaches are vulnerable to more shallow coverage of the topic areas. An alternative approach is to focus in strongly on one or two evidenced-based areas and embed this work into the program and setting. MBSP is set up to take such an approach.

Schools/Education

Mindfulness has been integrated into school curricula along with the training of students and teachers in many schools around the world; this has elicited a number of psychological, cognitive, and social benefits. In a review of 14 studies that integrated mindfulness training with students in elementary school or high school, the following improvements were noted: working memory, attention, academic skills, social skills, emotional regulation, self-esteem, mood, anxiety, stress, and fatigue (Meiklejohn et al., 2012). For a review of mindfulness and acceptance based interventions for children and adolescents, see Twohig, Field, Armstrong, and Dahl (2010).

The application of character strengths in schools has also had a recent surge. Carmel Proctor and Jenny Fox Eades (2011) created Strengths Gym, which is a program revolving around the use of the 24 character strengths with students in primary and secondary schools, including different exercises and programs for each grade level. Strengths Gym has been evaluated with favorable results: A study of 319 adolescent students between the ages of 12–14 were divided into two groups in which ⅔ received character strengths-builder activities and strengths challenges within the school curriculum (i.e., Strengths Gym), and ⅓ did not. Those who participated in strengths activities experienced increased life satisfaction compared to the control group (Proctor et al., 2011).

The first evidenced-based study of a classroom-based, positive psychology intervention, the Strath Haven project, included half of its lessons on VIA character strengths. Significant gains were found for student engagement in learning, school enjoyment, achievement, and social skills and most of these significant findings held steady for two years post-intervention (Seligman, Ernst, Gillham, Reivich, & Linkins, 2009). Character strengths have been used as the core of school-wide festivals and celebrations and at the heart of stories that teachers tell their students (Fox Eades, 2008). In addition, there are strengths-based guidebooks that consultants who work with teachers, parents, and schools can use (e.g., Yeager et al., 2011).

Here are some examples of other recent studies involving the use of character strengths in schools and with children and adolescents:

- In a longitudinal study of adolescents' transition to middle school, intellectual and temperance strengths predicted school performance and achievement, interpersonal strengths related to school social functioning, and temperance and transcendence strengths predicted well-being (Shoshani & Slone, 2012).

- In a study of children's adjustment to first grade, parents' intellectual, interpersonal, and temperance strengths related to their child's school adjustment, while the children's intellectual, interpersonal, temperance, and transcendence strengths related to first-grade adjustment (Shoshani & Ilanit Aviv, 2012).

- In a study of adolescents' character strengths and career/vocational interests, intellectual strengths were related to investigative and artistic career interests; transcendence and other-oriented strengths were related to social career interests; and leadership strengths were associated with enterprising career interests (Proyer, Sidler, Weber, & Ruch, 2012).

- In a study of adolescent romantic relationships, honesty, humor, and love were the most preferred character strengths in an ideal partner (Weber & Ruch, 2012a).

- Character strengths of the mind (e.g., self-regulation, perseverance, love of learning) were predictive of school success (Weber & Ruch, 2012b).

- In a study of the VIA Youth Survey, five strengths factors emerged and were independently associated with well-being and happiness (Toner, Haslam, Robinson, & Williams, 2012).

- Among high school students, other-oriented strengths (e.g., kindness, teamwork) predicted fewer depression symptoms while transcendence strengths (e.g., spirituality) predicted greater life satisfaction (Gillham et al., 2011).

- The most prevalent character strengths in very young children are love, kindness, creativity, curiosity, and humor (Park & Peterson, 2006a).
- When compared with US adults, youth from the US are higher on the character strengths of hope, teamwork, and zest, and adults are higher on appreciation of beauty and excellence, honesty, leadership, judgment (Park & Peterson, 2006b).
- Convergence of strengths between parents and child are modest except for spirituality where it is substantial (Peterson & Seligman, 2004)
- Character strengths with a developmental trajectory (least common in youth and increase over time through cognitive maturation) are appreciation of beauty and excellence, forgiveness, humility, and judgment (Park & Peterson, 2006a; 2006b).
- Focus groups with 459 high school students from 20 high schools found that students largely believe the 24 VIA strengths are acquired and that the strengths develop through ongoing experience; they particularly valued the strengths of love of learning, perspective, love, social intelligence, leadership, and spirituality (Steen et al., 2003).

The training of both character strengths and mindfulness in schools is well-represented in "The Happy Classrooms" program, created by the SATI team, coordinated by Ricardo Arguis Rey. This is an educational program in Spain that teaches students in preschool, primary, and secondary school. The program embeds teachings on mindfulness and character strengths into the classroom curriculum with the objectives of enhancing the personal and social development of students as well as the happiness of students, teachers, and families. The program is available in Spanish and is being translated into English and Chinese. More information can be found at http://catedu.es/psicologiapositiva/

The integration of MBSP into schools is an under-explored area. However, practitioners can learn from other mindfulness pioneers who have adapted established mindfulness programs in working with children and adolescents. One great example can be found in Semple, Lee, and Miller (2006) who made adjustments to MBCT in order to create MBCT-C (Mindfulness-Based Cognitive Therapy for Children), which has been used with children with a variety of psychological problems. In considering important developmental differences between children and adults, Semple, Lee, and Miller (2006) suggest three key tenets in adapting mindfulness to children (each of which should be at the forefront of the MBSP practitioner's mind): repetition enhances learning, variety increases children's interest, and most exercises should require active participation.

Those planning to integrate MBSP into schools will need to keep a few ideas in mind, such as:

- Keep the meditation exercises short (e.g., 30 seconds to 10 minutes, in many cases)
- Bring fun and laughter into the exercise
- Incorporate movement when possible
- Discuss and debrief each exercise
- Emphasize experiential learning
- Involve the family, when possible (e.g., consider adding in one session or conducting a booster session that includes the parents/caretakers).
  - This point also applies to the teachers, however, in some instances, it might be the teachers who are leading the MBSP program.
- Make adjustments to the virtue circle structure, e.g., instead of bowing, a "talking stick" can be used to indicate the speaker; any child that is not holding the "talking stick" practices "mindful listening."
- Specific guidance for homework exercises will need to be adjusted. For example, for younger children, the strengths interview questions will need to be adjusted and the interviewee might be a parent or caretaker.
- Consider conducting 1-hour sessions (this would double the quantity of sessions to 16 and allow for 2 weeks to cover each area).
- Prioritize the exploration of each student's unique signature strengths (empowering), rather than telling students what strengths they should have (authoritarian). The latter approach is taken in most programs because practitioners are eager to focus on certain strengths linked with achievement-oriented outcomes (e.g., perseverance). While well-intended, this can come at the expense of helping the student discover and apply their signature strengths.

To expand on these ideas, there are some general approaches MBSP practitioners will want to keep in mind and prioritize in each session. These revolve around the four core strands that comprise an essential character strengths-based intervention (Linkins, 2012):

1. Developing a character strengths language/lens
2. Recognizing and appreciating character strengths in others
3. Recognizing and appreciating one's own character strengths
4. Applying/developing one's own character strengths

Organizations/Business

In the organizational setting, executives, managers, and supervisors might be resistant to MBSP due to misconceptions about both mindfulness and character strengths. A review of earlier chapters that provide education, research, and practices on these topics is an important first step.

Practitioners should also become familiar with the various recent research findings that examine character strengths in organizations. For example:

- Workers experience more positive experiences at work and work-as-a-calling when they apply 4 or more signature strengths at work (Harzer & Ruch, 2012a).
- Alignment of character strengths at work: Regardless of which character strengths are used, the congruent use of strengths in the situational circumstances at work is important for fostering job satisfaction, pleasure, engagement, and meaning (Harzer & Ruch, 2012b).
- Employee engagement has 3 primary drivers: focusing strengths, managing emotions, and aligning purpose (from a 3-year, thematic analysis study by Crabb, 2011).
- The strengths of zest, perseverance, hope, and curiosity play a key role in healthy and ambitious work behavior (Gander, Proyer, Ruch, & Wyss, 2012b).
- In a unique study of top-level executive leaders of for-profit companies (studying only the strengths of honesty/integrity, bravery, perspective, social intelligence), each of these strengths were important for performance but honesty/integrity had the most contribution in explaining variance in executive performance (Sosik, Gentry, & Chun, 2012).
- Across occupations, curiosity, zest, hope, gratitude, and spirituality are the "Big 5" strengths associated with work satisfaction (Peterson, Stephens, Park, Lee, & Seligman, 2010).
- Workers who deploy their character strengths at work have higher job satisfaction and personal well-being (Littman-Ovadia & Davidovitch, 2010).
- Among volunteer and paid workers, endorsing strengths is related to meaning, but both endorsing AND deploying strengths is connected to well-being (Littman-Ovadia & Steger, 2010).
- A study of just the five wisdom strengths found them to be related to higher performance on a creative task and negatively related to stress (Avey, Luthans, Hannah, Sweetman, & Peterson, 2012).
- In a study of middle and senior managers, life satisfaction strengths, spiritual strengths, and community-building strengths do not appear to be overtly encouraged in the workplace; instead it is the temperance and hardworking strengths that are emphasized (Money, Hillenbrand, & Camara, 2008).
  - Top 10 (rank order) strengths expressed at work: honesty, judgment, perspective, fairness, perseverance, love of learning, leadership, zest, curiosity, social intelligence.
  - Bottom 5 (starting with lowest) strengths expressed at work: spirituality, appreciation of beauty and excellence, love, bravery, humility.
  - Strengths determined to be a "high match" with work demands: honesty, judgment, perspective, fairness, and zest.
  - Appreciation of beauty and excellence was the only strength determined to be a "low match" with work demands; the rest of the strengths were a "medium match."
  - Work demands required the individual to use *more* of the following strengths than what is natural for them: perseverance, love of learning, leadership, curiosity, self-regulation, and prudence.
  - Work demands required *less* of these strengths than what is natural for the indi-

vidual: social intelligence, gratitude, team-work, hope, humor, creativity, kindness, forgiveness, humility, bravery, love, appreciation of beauty and excellence, spirituality.

There is an emerging literature on the benefits of mindfulness programs in the workplace. Mindfulness-related programs have been effectively applied on worksites as a way to manage employees' stress (Limm et al., 2011; McCraty, Atkinson, & Tomasino, 2003; Mino, Babazono, Tsuda, & Yasuda, 2006; Wolever et al., 2012). Some argue that workplace mindfulness enhances social relationships in the workplace, and increases resilience and boosts task performance (Glomb, Duffy, Bono, & Yang, 2011). One program called Occupational Mindfulness was employed with managers and disability workers and yielded some good results (increases in positive affect and the "observing" component of mindfulness) and some unfavorable results (increases in stress, negative affect, anxiety, and decreases in job satisfaction) (Brooker et al., 2012).

The integration of mindfulness combined with character strengths, such as MBSP, into organizations, teams, and leadership development is an under-explored area. Those planning to adapt MBSP into organizations may need to make adjustments to fit the organizational culture. The following are examples of adaptations as well as potential topic areas for discussion and practice:

- Make adjustments to the virtue circle: Many organizations will prefer the title "strengths circle." The use of bowing can be substituted or extracted.
- Encourage mindful use of signature strengths each day. For example, research shows that four or more signature strengths used at work leads to more positive work experiences. This requires employees build self-awareness about how they bring forth who they are each day. This research finding can be adapted into an exercise in Session 2, which focuses on signature strengths. Practitioners might elicit discussion or add a homework assignment such as the following:
1. Examine those strengths that appear in your Top 7.

2. Examine your work-week with the following question: How many of these strengths am I regularly using during my work-day?
3. If you are using 4 or more, then commend yourself! You might consider how you can keep a daily awareness of this strengths use. If you are using 0–3 top strengths, start by adding in one more strength. Find a way to use one of your top strengths in a new way. Brainstorm with your supervisor. Journal about ways you've used your strengths at work in the past. Ask others to give you examples of when they've seen you express each of your top strengths.

- During group discussions, allow plenty of time for strengths-spotting and inquiry statements, especially if applying MBSP for a group of individuals from the same company or work team. Research among 60 strategic business management teams found that high performing teams include much higher levels of positive emotion and inquiry statements (seeking information) compared with negative emotion and self-advocacy statements (rebutting others and advocating for one's own view) (Losada & Heaphy, 2004).
- Address mindful teamwork: Those who work on a business team might be encouraged to be attuned to team-oriented self-talk: Consistent with the old saying, "there's no I in team," research has found that focusing on positive self-talk focused on the group's ability (e.g., "we are focused and ready") rather than the individual's ability (e.g., "I am focused and ready") led to greater success and individual/team confidence than focusing on one's personal ability (Son et al., 2011).
- Address mindful leadership: For certain business groups and leadership development programs, the topic of mindful leadership may become a crucial discussion point. The strengths branding exercise in Session 7 might be shifted to a discussion about how each participant can exert mindful leadership in their work.
  - Those who are in a position of leadership might speak to generating a greater mindfulness of their own strengths and those of their employees.
  - Those not in a position of leadership might explore how they can uniquely contribute

to the organization by bringing forth signature strengths they are uniquely high in or focus on those strengths that aren't expressed strongly in the company; these, too, are examples of mindful leadership.

- Build in specific workplace strategies into discussions and exercises:
  - Discuss ways to weave in work-breaks that use the 3-minute, character strengths breathing space exercise.
  - Practice strengths-spotting and expressing appreciation to colleagues about their strengths.
  - Start and end meetings by reviewing strengths and positive work experiences.
  - Target specific character strengths relating to well-being (healthy, ambitious work behavior is predicted by the character strengths of zest, perseverance, hope, and curiosity) (Gander, Proyer, Ruch, & Wyss, 2012b).
  - Place heavy emphasis on signature strengths: One of the primary drivers of employee engagement in organizations is the deployment of character strengths (Crabb, 2011). After taking the VIA Survey, employers and employees might co-explore one guiding question: What opportunities are there within the employee's job and the organization for the employee to play his or her signature strengths further?

- Create alignment of signature strengths: Strengths alignment with tasks can occur on at least two levels:
  1. The perspective of the employee: It's important to not only endorse but also deploy character strengths at work (Littman-Ovadia & Steger, 2010). Employees can find ways to express their signature strengths in any work task. Those who do are more likely to experience greater job satisfaction, pleasure, engagement, and meaning (Harzer & Ruch, 2012b).
  2. The perspective of the employer: Employers can take the perspective of examining current tasks that need to get done and aligning employees high in certain strengths that would best match the task. For example:
     - For a relationship-oriented task, someone high in love, kindness, or social intelligence might take the lead.
     - For tasks involving researching a new approach or conducting an Internet search, those high in creativity, love of learning, or curiosity might be a particularly good fit.
     - For tasks involving the team meeting a strict deadline, someone high in prudence or perseverance might be the best match.

Section IV: Resources

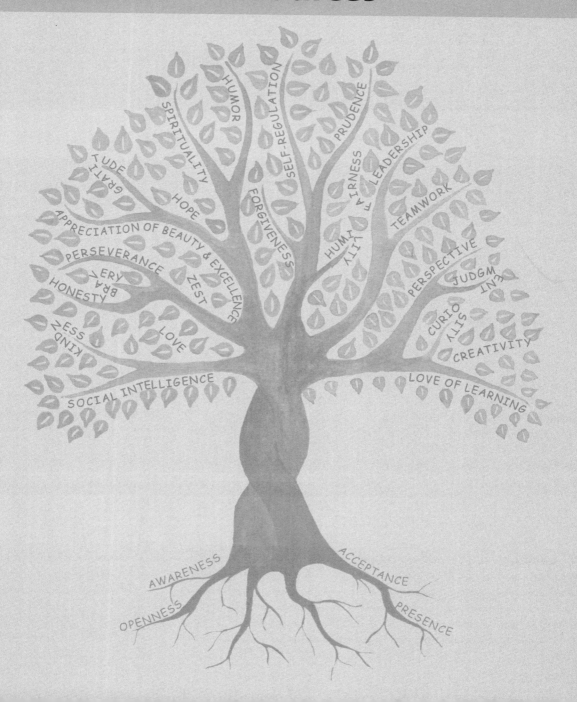

Appendix A
MBSP Audio CD Content

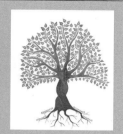

To complement the material presented in the book, many of the major exercises used in MBSP are available in audio format. An audio CD is enclosed in the printed book. The audio material is also available for customers of ebooks in the form of mp3 data at:

http://www.hogrefe.com/downloads/mindfulness-and-character-strengths/.

In order to access this material your login password is: T7253j989c

The audio content may be used by purchasers of this book for personal/professional use but not for any commerical use.

Disclaimer: All exercises and practices discussed in this book should be used with caution and be delivered under the guidance of a licensed professional.

Contents

1. Introduction
2. Body-Mindfulness Meditation
3. You at Your Best and Strengths-Spotting
4. Character Strengths Breathing Space
5. Strengths Gatha
6. Loving-Kindness Meditation
7. Strength-Exploration Meditation
8. Fresh-Look Meditation
9. Signature Strengths Breathing Space
10. Best Possible Self

Appendix B
General Tracking Sheet

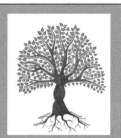

Day/Date	Type of Practice & Time Length	Obstacles to My Practice	Strengths Used	Observations/Comments
Monday Date:				
Tuesday Date:				
Wednesday Date:				
Thursday Date:				
Friday Date:				
Saturday Date:				
Sunday Date:				

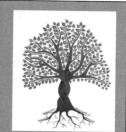

Appendix C

A Marriage of Character Strengths

For the newly married couple: X and Y:
- The 8 character strengths at the top are strengths that are core to who you are as individuals. They are likely to also be *core* to you as a couple.
- The 4 character strengths in the center are your highest *shared strengths* as a couple. Using these regularly may reveal your highest potential together.
- The 4 strengths outside of the circle are *supportive strengths*. These help you build on all the good you have as a couple.
- The strengths toward the bottom are your *unique strengths*, those that are uniquely high to each of you (humor for X, hope for Y). Use these to offer uniqueness and power to the marriage.

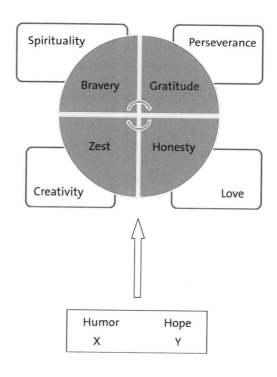

Appendix D

Mindfulness at the Movies[1]

Mindfulness is a construct that is so versatile it can be applied far and wide. It is particularly interesting to apply mindfulness to something that is universal. My longstanding interest in positive psychology movies and the movie-going experience is the perfect fit. The following discussion was adapted from a section of *Positive Psychology at the Movies 2* (Niemiec & Wedding, 2014).

There are at least seven levels of mindfulness that can be related to movies. Here is a discussion of each level and some accompanying film examples:

1. *Mindful approach by the viewer.* A viewer can approach a film with an attitude of mindfulness in which the viewer connects with their breath and is open to the experience of the film in the present moment. I've led over 70 special events with movies in which mindfulness meditation was deliberately threaded in as a core part of the structure of the movie-going experience. When used prior to watching a film, the intention of mindfulness is to help the viewer let go of the day's stressors and hassles (i.e., the past) and come fully into the present moment to appreciate the work of art they are about to witness. When used prior to movie discussions, a mindfulness exercise helps the participants to connect with one another, and become attentive to remnant images, sounds, characters, or bits of dialog that are floating around in their minds following the film.

2. *Mindfulness evoked in the viewer.* The characteristics of the film itself – images, sounds, music, actions – can elicit mindfulness in the viewer. In some cases this can lead the viewer to a deeper state of absorption and flow in which he or she is enveloped in the film, and in other cases this can lead to a state of self-consciousness in which the viewer is aware he or she is watching a film. The film *Holy Motors* (2012) is one good example. Many filmmakers are known for their ability to elicit this effect; some examples include the directors Federico Fellini, Luis Bunuel, and Jean Pierre-Jeunet.

3. *Mindfulness practice depicted.* The most common mindfulness meditation practice depicted in films is sitting meditation. The intriguing mystery/comedy *Zen Noir* (2006) depicts various types of meditation including mindful walking, mindful eating, mindful breathing, and the use of Zen koans – riddles used to awaken an individual from standard ways of thinking. Mindfulness of sound is well-portrayed by Björk's character in *Dancer in the Dark* (2000). The use of mindfulness to face pain and suffering directly is captured well in the documentary *Ram Dass, Fierce Grace* (2001) in which the well-known author of *Be Here Now* explains his stroke and how he used mindfulness to manage the symptoms.

Protagonists in *The Fountain* (2006), *Un Buda* (2005, Argentina), and *Tron: Legacy* (2010) are shown using formal meditation as a regular practice and as an approach to coping during times of great distress. At one point in the latter film, the protagonist, Kevin Flynn, turns to meditation immediately prior to a major event, referring to it as "knocking on the sky." *Kung Fu Panda* (2008) depicts the challenges of a meditation practice and the importance of humility to maintain it. *How to Cook Your Life* (2007, Australia), an independent film about a Buddhist chef, depicts mindful food preparation and discusses other aspects of mindfulness. Films explicitly depicting Buddhism typically show formal meditation, e.g., *Kundun* (1997), *Little Buddha* (1993), and *Spring, Summer, Autumn, Winter... And Spring* (2003). In one scene of *Why Has Bodhi-*

---

[1]   This appendix was adapted from a text that appears in *Positive Psychology at the Movies 2* (Niemiec & Wedding, 2014). Used with the permission of Hogrefe Publishing.

Dharma Left for the East? (1989), a student meditates on a rock in the middle of crashing cold rapids while steadying a rock on his head, giving the viewer a sense of meditation as interconnection with beauty and stillness. Implementation of full meditation programs in the prison system is well-depicted in *The Dhamma Brothers* (2008) and *Doing Time, Doing Vipassana* (1997).

The Karate Kid (1984; 2010) movies depict repetitious activities that are integral to training in karate. The protagonists do these practices (e.g., waxing cars using a circular hand motion or picking up a coat and placing it on a coat-rack in a certain way) mindlessly and reluctantly. They eventually learn the purpose of these actions and begin to perform them with greater mindfulness. This, in turn, helps their karate training.

4. *Mindfulness as character transformation.* While not as obvious as viewing a character practicing sitting meditation, character transformations are not difficult to notice in movies. Often this means the protagonist has developed mindful awareness that has led to insight and change. In many films, this is portrayed as a shift from autopilot to greater mindfulness. The protagonists in *Ikiru* (1952, Japan), *Stranger Than Fiction* (2006), *Pleasantville* (1998), *Waking Life* (2001), *Zorba the Greek* (1964), and *Peaceful Warrior* (2006) are strong examples of this deliberate shift in awareness that transforms who the individual is and their interactions with others. Rannulph Junnah in *Legend of Bagger Vance* (2000), the three team members championing a horse in *Seabiscuit* (2003), and the title character in *The Truman Show* (1998) are additional examples of characters that transform by making this shift in awareness.

Transformations can often be seen in films explicitly about the "life journey." For example, *About Schmidt* (2002), *The Straight Story* (1999), *Eyes Wide Shut* (1999), and *The Way* (2010) depict transformation from the journey. Whether a physical journey or not, this category of mindfulness in films depicts psychological change through the journey motif. The viewing of one's own suffering with mindfulness can lead to the awareness of others'

suffering, as noted in *Son of the Bride* (2001, Argentina) and *Biutiful* (2010). In the latter film, the character Uxbal realizes his time is limited after he is diagnosed with prostate cancer, and he struggles to do good, atone, and help others. Mindfulness in motion is exhibited by Colter, a soldier in *Source Code* (2010) who develops his attention as the film progresses; he is open to novelty, develops razor-sharp distinctions as his mission becomes more complex, is sensitive to contexts, and embodies an orientation to the present (Clyman, 2011).

The phenomenon of *beginner's mind* is a transformation in which an individual shifts their perception to viewing people, places, and things as if they were seeing them for the "first time." *Unknown White Male* (2005) is a fascinating depiction of the true story of Douglas Bruce, a man who turned himself into the police claiming total amnesia. Bruce experiences everything in life anew – his "first" fireworks, snowfall, and seeing the ocean in which he becomes so overwhelmed in awe that he weeps upon seeing it. He displays an eagerness to learn "everything" – to re-invent himself. Beginner's mind is also demonstrated clearly in the approach taken by several young boys when they come across a ping pong ball for the first time in *Mongolian Ping Pong* (2005), and in *The Gods Must Be Crazy* (1980) when the bushmen of the Kalahari desert come across a Coke bottle.

5. *Moments of mindfulness.* In movies, the character transformation often culminates into a particular, sometimes dramatic, moment. It might be a single line in a conversation or a small part of a scene. Ricky Fitts attempts to capture these moments as he films a dead bird, a frozen woman, and a floating piece of trash in *American Beauty* (1999). Another example of a crucial moment is displayed by Todd Anderson (Ethan Hawke) and his fellow students who stand on the desks proclaiming "O Captain, My Captain" to their fired but inspirational teacher in *Dead Poets Society* (1989). A crucial moment of acceptance occurs in a conversation between two characters struggling in their committed relationship at the end of *Eternal Sunshine of the Spotless Mind*

(2004). *Lost in Translation* (2003) displays a scene of intimacy and sharing between two new friends who could turn their shared loneliness into a sexual experience but decide not to, instead having an encounter that is far more significant than a simple sexual encounter.

Mel Gibson's character in *Signs* (2002) comes to a crucial awareness at a critical moment and instructs his brother to "swing away"; this simple instruction saves a family from an alien invasion. Such scenes are often turning points or climactic moments in the film as they indicate character insights or a crucial action taking place. External mindfulness is apparent in *Pulp Fiction* (1994) when Butch (Bruce Willis) returns to his home after betraying his boss, Marcellus Wallace. Butch knows there is now a "hit" on him so he uses exquisite mindful caution as he slowly and careful turns door knobs and walks through the house; close-up shots intensify the suspense and highlight his mindfulness. External mindfulness of beauty can be seen in moments experienced by protagonists in the opening scene of *My Life Without Me* (2003) and in several scenes with Gil (Owen Wilson) in Woody Allen's *Midnight in Paris* (2011).

6. *Symbolic images.* Some cinematic images are particularly symbolic. This representation might be used by the filmmaker as a "symbol of mindfulness" for the viewer and/or the characters in the film. Perhaps there is no better example of this than the classic paper trash scene in *American Beauty* (1999). Other examples include the floating feather in *Forrest Gump* (1994), the color blue in Kieslowski's *Blue* (1993), and the cherry blossoms in *The Last Samurai* (2003).

7. *Rhapsodies of mindfulness.* Jon Kabat-Zinn uses the phrase "rhapsody of mindfulness" to refer to Thoreau's classic novel *Walden* because the entire novel relates to or describes the mindfulness experience. There are also movies that are rhapsodies of mindfulness. These are films that simultaneously depict mindfulness themes throughout and make overt and covert attempts to deepen awareness in the viewer. In such films, everything is interconnected, much like an epic poem. The nonverbal films *Baraka* (1992) and *Samsara* (2012) illustrate rhapsodies of mindfulness, as does *Alone in the Wilderness* (2004) and *Into Great Silence* (2005, France), a film in which Carthusian monks practice contemplation in solitude and quietude, exhibiting mindfulness in all actions of their daily life. Less obvious rhapsodies would include *Amelie* (2001) (the tagline of which is "She'll change your life") and *American Beauty* (1999). In the latter, the film's tagline – and at one point in the production it was the title – is "Look Closer." This might be viewed as a call to those viewers who believe they have "figured" out the film (or their own lives) to look deeper. This film reminds the viewer that we need not look any further than ourselves to discover the present moment and the beauty of the moment. The protagonist, Lester, is "trapped" in life and is mindlessly sleepwalking through his days until he realizes that it's never too late to "wake up" and get his life back. This emergence of mindfulness is juxtaposed with the character of Ricky Fitts, someone who sees the "life behind things," meaning that he uses a high level of trait mindfulness to look deeply at life and tune into what most people overlook.

It's a great thing when you realize you still have the ability to surprise yourself. Makes you wonder what else you can do that you've forgotten about.

Lester in *American Beauty*

Appendix E

Character Strengths Q & A

In order to understand character strengths in a deeper way, MBSP practitioners might spend extra time reviewing Chapter 2. What follows are some common questions, mostly pertaining to specific character strengths, that are asked by both practitioners and participants in MBSP.

Which character strengths are most common around the world?

The most prevalent character strengths in human beings in descending order are honesty, fairness, kindness, judgment, curiosity, and gratitude (McGrath, in press; Park et al., 2006).

Which character strengths are least common around the world?

The least prevalent character strengths in human beings are zest, spirituality, prudence, humility, and, lastly, self-regulation (McGrath, in press; Park et al., 2006).

Are some strengths more naturally connected with happiness than others?

Some character strengths repeatedly show a strong connection with life satisfaction. These are (starting with the highest): zest, hope, gratitude, curiosity, and love (e.g., Park et al., 2004).

What if I'm not high in one of these strengths that connect strongly with happiness?

The above research points us in a direction but is not intended to offer a prescription. Note that whenever you are deciding to focus on a strength, you are probably using energy/enthusiasm (zest) and a positive outlook for something good to happen (hope), thus, the highest life satisfaction strengths are right there with you whether you are mindful of it or not. Also, remember that focusing on your signatures strengths (regardless of which strengths are signature strengths for you) is linked with a good happiness boost (Gander et al., 2012a; Seligman et al., 2005), so that is an important route to always consider. Finally,

some individuals might indeed decide to deliberately pursue one of the life satisfaction strengths as that also has been shown to help people boost their happiness (Proyer et al., 2012).

What is the difference between curiosity and love of learning?

These two character strengths commonly co-occur for individuals as a dyad that appears in their signature strengths; however, it is not always the case because there are important distinctions. Curiosity is a pursuit of novelty and newness while love of learning is the pursuit of deep learning and knowledge. While curiosity might initially draw people to a new pathway of knowledge, it is love of learning that sustains them and helps them dig into the material in a systematic way.

What is the difference between love and kindness?

There is a fair amount of overlap and a high correlation between these two strengths. One way to distinguish them is to view those high in love as valuing close relationships and expressing warmth and genuineness to others, while kindness refers to doing thoughtful things for others, being generous with one's time, and showing compassion to those in need.

Why is there a strength called "judgment"? Isn't that overtly negative?

The word judgment has been used by many philosophers in history to connote a virtue. In the VIA Classification, judgment does not mean judgmental or being harshly critical. Judgment is critical thinking and that is the main area being measured with this strength. This means the individual uses reason and logic to analyze the details of situations, problems, and ideas. They are able to view things from many different angles. In this vein, people high in the judgment/critical thinking strength are expressing a dimension of open-mindedness.

How should we frame strengths such as humility and prudence so that those who have them as signature strengths can see their potential?

First, explain that these are *strengths*. Explore this with the individual to help them see these strengths and to "own" them as such. Emphasize discussions that focus on the relevance of these strengths in their life rather than irrelevance (or exceptions where they do not fit). These are virtuous qualities in the individual that have helped them significantly throughout their lives in many positive ways. These strengths have contributed strongly to who the person is today.

Prudence refers to being wisely cautious. Prudence gets a bad rap because individuals tend to think of the overuse of prudence (i.e., stuffiness) as prudence. However, when prudence is expressed in a balanced way, it is far from stuffiness; instead, it is being conscientious, planful, goal-oriented, and respectful to others. Explore with them the many ways that thinking things through, being cautious at times, thinking before acting, and approaching life with care and carefulness has served them well.

Humility tends to get "lost" or discarded in individuals' profiles. This is too bad as humility is a strong strength that refers to the individual having a strong sense of who they are and good self-esteem, yet they care enough about others to place the attention on them. It is the overuse of humility – self-deprecation – that is often the misinterpretation in regard to this strength. Humility has been linked with generosity and kindness, as well as individuals having more friends. Explore with them how focusing on other people, accomplishing things with quietude, choosing restraint over conceit, and not being boastful has served them in important ways.

What is meant by leadership? I was surprised to come out low on leadership because I am the head of my company.

Leadership can be viewed in terms of "Big L" (movers and shakers, those who are mayors, governors, or CEOs) and "small l" (everyday leaders). VIA measures the latter type of leadership. This refers to individuals who are good at organizing people and projects, those who give all subordinates a fair chance, and those who get ev-eryone in a group rallied around a common goal. Some people in important leadership positions may not have this as a signature strength and that's fine, as those in leadership positions might have people that work for them to help do all the organizing and managing of activities. Good leaders are those who are highly self-aware of their signature strengths, use them effectively to motivate those who work for them, and inspire the character strengths of others to do their best and contribute to the organization.

Why are there so many questions about religion? Does the VIA Survey distinguish between religion and spirituality?

The VIA Survey has only one question that uses the word religion/religious/religiousness in it. The other questions for the spirituality strength deal with various related constructs such as purpose, faith, calling, meditation or prayer practice, and viewing oneself as a spiritual person. In this way, the VIA Survey more closely addresses spirituality (defined by scholars in the field as a search or connection with "the sacred") than about whether one ascribes to a particular religion, engages in religious rituals, or goes to church/mosque/temple every week.

The VIA Survey finds that I'm high in creativity, but I don't feel creative. I don't make creative things like others do. Please explain.

There are many forms of creativity and many ways to express it. The popular conception of creativity is that this strength is for the artists, musicians, and writers. Those individuals are often creative, they tend to create creative "products," and they might have creativity as a signature strength, but creativity is more varietal than making creative things. The VIA Survey focuses on the trait of creativity and closely looks at creative thinking. Specifically, this refers to what's called divergent thinking – being able to think of many ways to solve a problem or to do a certain task. In this vein, creativity helps the individual to build new knowledge and to integrate new ideas with old ideas because they are always doing internal brainstorms and thinking "outside the box." Many very creative people might not ever create a tangible product.

Appendix F: Website Resources

Mindfulness-Based Strengths Practice (MBSP)

www.viacharacter.org/mindfulness
Articles, research, trainings, free audios, MBSP practitioners, and the latest MBSP info

www.ryanniemiec.com
About, services, workshops, books, articles

Character Strengths

www.viacharacter.org
VIA Institute on Character

www.viame.org
VIA Survey of Character Strengths

www.viapros.org
Extensive resources on character strengths

www.youtube.com/VIAStrengths
YouTube channel on character strengths

www.positivepsychologynews.com
Positive Psychology News Daily articles

blogs.psychcentral.com/character-strengths
Ryan Niemiec, PsychCentral

www.psychologytoday.com/blog/what-matters-most
Ryan Niemiec, Psychology Today

www.psychologytoday.com/blog/quite-character
Neal Mayerson, Psychology Today

www.viapros.org/www/en-us/training/viapioneersspeakerseries.aspx
Free talks: VIA Pioneers Speaker Series

Mindfulness

www.iamhome.org
Thich Nhat Hanh & The Mindfulness Bell

www.umassmed.edu/cfm/stress/index.aspx
Mindfulness-Based Stress Reduction

www.jonkabat-zinn.com
Mindfulness CDs by Jon Kabat-Zinn

www.mbct.com or **www.mbct.co.uk**
Mindfulness-Based Cognitive Therapy

www.mindfulexperience.org
Monthly mindfulness research summaries

www.self-compassion.org
Resource on self-compassion

www.mindandlife.org
The Mind & Life Institute

http://link.springer.com/journal/12671
Scientific journal: *Mindfulness*

www.mindful.org
Magazine: "Mindful"

References

Albers, S. (2003). *Eating mindfully*. Oakland, CA: New Harbinger Publications.

Allen, M., Bromley, A., Kuyken, W., & Sonnenberg, S. J. (2009). Participants' experiences of mindfulness-based cognitive therapy: It changed me in just about every way possible. *Behavioural and Cognitive Psychotherapy, 37,* 413–430.

Allport, G. W. (1921). Personality and character. *Psychological Bulletin, 18,* 441–455.

Amaro, A. (2010). Thinking II: Investigation, the use of reflective thought. *Mindfulness, 1*(4), 265–268.

American Psychiatric Association. (1994). *Diagnostic and statistical manual of mental disorders* (4th ed.). Washington, DC: Author.

American Psychological Association (Producer). (2004). *APA Psychotherapy Videotape Series VI: Mindfulness-based cognitive therapy for depression with Zindel V. Segal* [DVD]. Available from the American Psychological Association.

Aquinas, T. (1989). *Summa theologiae: A concise translation* (T. McDermott, Ed. & Trans.). Westminster, MD: Christian Classics. (Original work completed 1265–1273).

Aristotle (2000). *Nicomachean ethics* (R. Crisp, Trans.). Cambridge, UK: Cambridge University Press. (Original work composed 4th century BCE)

Astin, J. A. (1997). Stress reduction through mindfulness meditation: Effects on psychological symptomatology, sense of control, and spiritual experiences. *Psychotherapy and Psychosomatics, 66,* 97–106.

Austenfeld, J. L., Paolo, A. M., & Stanton, A. L. (2006). Effects of writing about emotions versus goals on psychological and physical health among third-year medical students. *Journal of Personality, 74* (1), 267–286.

Austenfeld, J. L., & Stanton, A. L. (2008). Writing about emotions versus goals: Effects on hostility and medical care utilization moderated by emotional approach coping processes. *British Journal of Health Psychology, 13,* 35–38.

Averill, J. R. (1992). The structural bases of emotional behavior: A metatheoretical analysis. *Review of Personality and Social Psychology, 13,* 1–24.

Avey, J. B., Luthans, F., Hannah, S. T., Sweetman, D., & Peterson, C. (2012). Impact of employees' character strengths of wisdom on stress and creative performance. *Human Resource Management Journal, 22*(2), 165–181.

Avey, J. B., Wernsing, T. S., & Luthans, F. (2008). Can positive employees help positive organizational change? *Journal of Applied Behavioral Science, 44,* 48–70.

Baer, R. A. (2003). Mindfulness training as a clinical intervention: A conceptual and empirical review. *Clinical Psychology: Science and Practice, 10,* 125–143.

Baer, R. A. (2010). *Assessing mindfulness and acceptance processes in clients: Illuminating the theory and practice of change*. Oakland, CA: New Harbinger.

Baer, R. A., Carmody, J., & Hunsinger, M. (2012). Weekly change in mindfulness and perceived stress in a mindfulness-based stress reduction program. *Journal of Clinical Psychology*. Advance online publication. doi: 10.1002/jclp.21865.

Baer, R. A., & Lykins, E. L. M. (2011). Mindfulness and positive psychological functioning. In K. M. Sheldon, T. B. Kashdan, & M. F. Steger (Eds.), *Designing positive psychology: Taking stock and moving forward* (pp. 335–348). New York, NY: Oxford University Press.

Baer, R. A., Lykins, E. L. B., & Peters, J. R. (2012). Mindfulness and self-compassion as predictors of psychological wellbeing in long-term meditators and matched nonmeditators. *Journal of Positive Psychology, 7*(3), 230–238.

Baer, R. A., Smith, G. T., Hopkins, J., Krietemeyer, J., & Toney, L. (2006). Using self-report assessment methods to explore facets of mindfulness. *Assessment, 13,* 27–45.

Baker, L., & McNulty, J. (2011). Self-compassion and relationship maintenance: The moderating roles of conscientiousness and gender. *Journal of Personality and Social Psychology, 100*(5), 853–873.

Baliki, M. N., Geha, P. Y., Apkarian, A. V., & Chialvo, D. R. (2008). Beyond feeling: Chronic pain hurts the brain, disrupting the default-mode network dynamics. *Journal of Neuroscience, 16,* 1398–1403.

Barber, L., Maltby, J., & Macaskill, A. (2005). Angry memories and thoughts of revenge: The relationship between forgiveness and anger rumination. *Personality and Individual Differences, 39,* 253–262.

Barnard, L. K., & Curry, J. F. (2011). Self-compassion: Conceptualizations, correlates, and interventions. *Review of General Psychology, 15,* 289–303.

Barnes, S., Brown, K. W., Krusemark, E., Campbell, W. K., & Rogge, R. D. (2007). The role of mindfulness in romantic relationship satisfaction and response to relationship stress. *Journal of Marital and Family Therapy, 33*, 482–500.

Barnhofer, T., Chittka, T., Nightingale, H., Visser, C., & Crane, C. (2010). State effects of two forms of meditation on prefrontal EEG asymmetry in previously depressed invidividuals. *Mindfulness, 1,* 21–27.

Batson, C. D., Chang, J., Orr, R., & Rowland, J. (2002). Empathy, attitudes, and action: Can feeling for a member of a stigmatized group motivate one to help the group? *Personality and Social Psychology Bulletin, 28*(2), 1656–1666.

Bauer, J. J., McAdams, D. P., & Pals, J. L. (2008). Narrative identity and eudaimonic well-being. *Journal of Happiness Studies, 9,* 81–104.

Baumeister, R. F., Bratslavsky, E., Finkenaeuer, C., & Vohs, K. D. (2001). Bad is stronger than good. *Review of General Psychology, 5*(4), 323–370.

Baumeister, R. F., Matthew, G., DeWall, C. N., & Oaten, M. (2006). Self-regulation and personality: How interventions increase regulatory success, and how depletion moderates the effects of traits on behavior. *Journal of Personality, 74*(6), 1773–1802.

Baumeister, R. F., & Tierney, J. (2011). *Willpower: Rediscovering the greatest human strength.* New York: Penguin.

Baumeister, R. F., & Vohs, K. D. (2004). *Handbook of self-regulation: Research, theory, and applications.* New York: Guilford.

Bayda, E. (2002). *Being zen: Bringing meditation to life.* Boston: Shambhala.

Beckman, H. B., Wendland, M., Mooney, C., Krasner, M. S., Quill, T. E., Suchman, A. L., & Epstein, R. M. (2012). The impact of a program in mindful communication on primary care physicians. *Academic Medicine, 87*(6), 815–819.

Beitel, M., Ferrer, E., & Cecero, J. J. (2005). Psychological mindedness and awareness of self and others. *Journal of Clinical Psychology, 61*(6), 739–750.

Bennett-Goleman, T. (2001). *Emotional alchemy: How the mind can heal the heart.* New York: Harmony Books.

Benson, H. (1975). *The relaxation response.* New York: Avon.

Berne, E. (1964). *Games people play.* New York: Ballantine Books.

Bieling, P. J., Hawley, L. L., Bloch, R. T., Corcoran, K. M., Levitan, R. D., Young, L. T., MacQueen, G. M., & Segal, Z. V. (2012). Treatment-specific changes in decentering following mindfulness-based cognitive therapy versus antidepressant medication or placebo for prevention of depressive relapse. *Journal of Consulting and Clinical Psychology, 80*(3), 365–372.

Bihari, J., & Mullan, E. (2012). Relating mindfully: A qualitative exploration of changes in relationships through mindfulness-based cognitive therapy. *Mindfulness.* Advance online publication. doi: 10.1007/s12671-012-0146-x

Birnie, K., Speca, M., & Carlson, L. E. (2010). Exploring self-compassion and empathy in the context of mindfulness-based stress reduction (MBSR). *Stress and Health: Journal of the International Society for the Investigation of Stress, 26,* 359–371.

Bishop, S. R., Lau, M., Shapiro, S. L., Carlson, L., Anderson, N. D., Carmody, J., ... Devins, G. (2004). Mindfulness: A proposed operational definition. *Clinical Psychology: Science and Practice, 11,* 230–241.

Biswas-Diener, R. (2006). From the equator to the North Pole: A study of character strengths. *Journal of Happiness Studies, 7,* 293–310.

Biswas-Diener, R. (2010). *Practicing positive psychology coaching: Assessment, diagnosis and intervention.* New York: John Wiley & Sons.

Biswas-Diener, R. (2012). *The courage quotient.* San Francisco, CA: Jossey-Bass.

Biswas-Diener, R., Kashdan, T. B., & Minhas, G. (2011). A dynamic approach to psychological strength development and intervention. *Journal of Positive Psychology, 6*(2), 106–118.

Black, D. S. (2010). Mindfulness research guide: A new paradigm for managing empirical health information. *Mindfulness, 1*(3), 174–76.

Block-Lerner, J., Adair, C., Plumb, J. C., Rhatigan, D. L., & Orsillo, S. M. (2007). The case for mindfulness-based approaches in the cultivation of empathy: Does nonjudgmental, present moment awareness increase capacity for perspective-taking and empathic concern? *Journal of Marital and Family Therapy, 33,* 501–516.

Bohlmeijer, E., Prenger, R., Taal, E., & Cuijpers, P. (2010). The effects of mindfulness-based stress reduction therapy on mental health of adults with a chronic medical disease: A meta-analysis. *Journal of Psychosomatic Research, 68*(6), 539–544.

Bohy, N. (2010). A qualitative study of mindfulness-based relationship enhancement and its contributions to relationship resilience. *Dissertation Abstracts International, 71.*

Borders, A., Earleywine, M., & Jajodia, A. (2010). Could mindfulness decrease anger, hostility, and aggression by decreasing rumination? *Aggressive Behavior, 36*(1), 28–44.

Borghans, L., Duckworth, A. L., Heckman, J. J., & ter Weel, B. (2008). The economics and psychology of personality traits. *Journal of Human Resources, 43*(4), 972–1059.

Bowen, S., Chawla, N., Collins, S., Witkiewitz, K., Hsu, S.,Grow, J., ... Marlatt, A. (2009). Mindfulness-based relapse prevention for substance use disorders: A pilot efficacy trial. *Substance Abuse, 30*, 205–305.

Bowen, S. & Marlatt, G. A. (2009). Surfing the urge: Brief mindfulness-based intervention for college student smokers. *Psychology of Addictive Behaviors*, 23(4), 666–671.

Bowen, S., Witkiewitz, K., Dillworth, T. M., Chawla, N., Simpson, T. L., Ostafin, B. D., ... Marlatt, G. A. (2006). Mindfulness meditation and substance use in an incarcerated population. *Psychology of Addictive Behaviors, 20*(3), 343–347.

Bowlin, S. L., & Baer, R. A. (2012). Relationships between mindfulness, self-control, and psychological functioning. *Personality and Individual Differences, 52*(3), 411–415.

Boyatzis, R., & McKee, A. (2005). *Resonant leadership: Renewing yourself and connecting with others through mindfulness, hope, and compassion.* Boston, MA: Harvard Business School Publishing.

Brach, T. (2003). *Radical acceptance: Embracing your life with the heart of a Buddha.* New York, NY: Bantam.

Brahm, A. (2006). *Mindfulness, bliss, and beyond: A meditator's handbook.* Boston: Wisdom Publications.

Breen, W. E., Kashdan, T. B., Lenser, M. L., & Fincham, F. D. (2010). Gratitude and forgiveness: Convergence and divergence on self-report and informant ratings. *Personality and Individual Differences, 49*, 932–937.

Brewer, J. A., Worhunsky, P. D., Gray, J. R., Tang, Y.-Y., Weber, J., & Kober, H. (2011). Meditation experience is associated with differences in default mode network activity and connectivity. *Proceedings of the National Academy of Sciences, 108*, 20254–20259.

Brickman, P., & Campbell, D. T. (1971). Hedonic relativism and planning the good society. In M. H. Appley (Ed.), *Adaptation level theory: A symposium* (pp. 287–302). New York: Academic Press.

Bridges, L. J., Denham, S. A., & Ganiban, J. M. (2004). Definitional issues in emotional regulation research. *Child Development, 75*(2), 340–345.

Brooker, J., Julian, J., Webber, L., Jeffrey Chan, J., Shawyer, F., & Meadows, G. (2012). Evaluation of an occupational mindfulness program for staff employed in the disability sector in Australia. *Mindfulness.* Advance online publication. doi: 10.1007/s12671-012-0112-7

Brotto, L. A., Erskine, Y., Carey, M., Ehlen, T., Finlayson, S., Heywood, M., ... Miller, D. (2012). A brief mindfulness-based cognitive behavioral intervention improves sexual functioning versus wait-list control in women treated for gynecologic cancer. *Gynecologic Oncology, 125*(2), 320–325.

Brown, K. W., & Kasser, T. (2005). Are psychological and ecological well-being compatible? The role of values, mindfulness, and lifestyle. *Social Indicators Research, 74*, 349–368.

Brown, K. W., & Ryan, R. M. (2003). The benefits of being present: Mindfulness and its role in psychological well-being. *Journal of Personality and Social Psychology, 84*(4), 822–848.

Brown, K. W., Ryan, R. M., & Creswell, J. D. (2007). Mindfulness: Theoretical foundations and evidence for its salutary effects. *Psychological Inquiry, 18,* 211–237.

Bryant, F. B., & Veroff, J. (2007). *Savoring: A new model of positive experience.* Mahwah, NJ: Lawrence Erlbaum Associates.

Buber, M. (1958). *I and thou.* New York: Scribners.

Buckingham, M., & Clifton, D. O. (2001). *Now, discover your strengths: How to develop your talents and those of the people you manage.* London, UK: Simon & Schuster.

Caldwell, K. L., Baime, M. J., & Wolever, R. Q. (2012). Mindfulness based approaches to obesity and weight loss maintenance. *Journal of Mental Health Counseling, 34*, 269–282.

Caldwell, K., Harrison, M., Adams, M., Quin, R. H., & Greeson, J. (2010). Developing mindfulness in college students through movement-based courses: Effects on self-regulatory self-efficacy, mood, stress, and sleep quality. *Journal of American College Health, 58*(5), 433–442.

Carlson, E. N. (2013). Overcoming the barriers to self-knowledge: Mindfulness as a path to seeing yourself as you really are. *Perspectives on Psychological Science, 8*(2), 173–186.

Carmody, J., & Baer, R. A. (2008). Relationships between mindfulness practice and levels of mindfulness, medical and psychological symptoms and well-being in a mindfulness-based stress reduction program. *Journal of Behavioral Medicine, 31*, 23–33.

Carmody, J., & Baer, R. A. (2009). How long does a mindfulness-based stress reduction program need to be? A review of class contact hours and effect sizes for psychological distress. *Journal of Clinical Psychology, 65*(6), 627–638.

Carmody, J., Baer, R. A., Lykins, E. L. B., & Olendzki, N. (2009). An empirical study of the mechanisms of mindfulness in a mindfulness-based stress reduction program. *Journal of Clinical Psychology, 65*(6), 613–626.

Carmody, J., Reed, G., Kristeller, J., & Merriam, P. (2008). Mindfulness, spirituality, and health-related symptoms. *Journal of Psychosomatic Research, 64*, 393–403.

Carrigan, H. L. (Ed.) (2001). *Eternal wisdom from the desert: Writings from the desert fathers*. Brewster, MA: Paraclete Press.

Carson, J. W., Carson, K. M., Gil, K. M., & Baucom, D. H. (2004). Mindfulness-based relationship enhancement. *Behavior Therapy, 35*(3), 471–494. doi: 10.1016/s0005-7894 (04)80028-5

Carson, J. W., Carson, K. M., Gil, K. M., & Baucom, D. H. (2006). Mindfulness-based relationship enhancement (MBRE) in couples. In R. A. Baer (Ed.), *Mindfulness-based treatment approaches: Clinician's guide to evidence base and applications.* (pp. 309–331): San Diego, CA: Elsevier Academic Press.

Carson, J. W., Carson, K. M., Gil, K. M., & Baucom, D. H. (2007). Self-expansion as a mediator of relationship improvements in a mindfulness intervention. *Journal of Marital and Family Therapy, 33*(4), 517–528.

Cattron, R. (2008). *Beauty and mindfulness*. Unpublished manuscript, Lewis-Clark State College.

Cawley, M. J., Martin, J. E., & Johnson, J. A. (2000). A virtues approach to personality. *Personality and Individual Differences, 28*, 997–1013.

Chambers, R., Gullone, E., & Allen, N. B. (2009). Mindful emotion regulation: An integrative review. *Clinical Psychology Review, 29*, 560–572

Chatzisarantis, N. L. D., & Hagger, M. S. (2007). Mindfulness and the intention: behavior relationship within the theory of planned behavior. *Personality and Social Psychology Bulletin, 33*(5), 663–676.

Chiesa, A., & Malinowski, P. (2011). Mindfulness-based approaches: Are they all the same? *Journal of Clinical Psychology, 67*(4), 404–424.

Chiesa, A., & Serretti, A. (2009). Mindfulness-based stress reduction for stress management in healthy people: A review and meta-analysis. *Journal of Alternative & Complementary Medicine, 15*(5), 593–600.

Chiesa, A., & Serretti, A. (2011). Mindfulness based cognitive therapy for psychiatric disorders: A systematic review and meta-analysis. *Psychiatry Research, 187*(3), 441.

Chodron, P. (1997). *When things fall apart: Heart advice for difficult times*. Boston: Shambhala.

Cloninger, C. R. (2007). Spirituality and the science of feeling good. *Southern Medical Journal, 100* (7), 740–743.

Clyman, J. (2011). Mindfulness in motion. [Review of the motion picture *Source code*]. *PsycCRITIQUES, 56*(44).

Coffey, K. A., Hartman, M., & Fredrickson, B. L. (2010). Deconstructing mindfulness and constructing mental health: Understanding mindfulness and its mechanisms of action. *Mindfulness, 1*(4), 235–253.

Cohn, M. A., & Fredrickson, B. L. (2010). In search of durable positive psychology interventions: Predictors and consequences of long-term positive behavior change. *Journal of Positive Psychology, 5*, 355–366.

Colzato, L. S., Ozturk, A., & Hommel, B. (2012). Meditate to create: the impact of focused-attention and open-monitoring training on convergent and divergent thinking. *Frontiers in Psychology. 3*, 116. doi: 10.3389/fpsyg.2012.00116

Costa, P. T., Jr., & McCrae, R. R. (1992). *Revised NEO Personality Inventory (NEO PI-R) and NEO Five-Factor Inventory (NEO-FFI): Professional manual*. Odessa, FL: Psychological Assessment Resources.

Cowger, E. L., & Torrance, E. P. (1982). Further examination of the quality changes in creative functioning resulting from meditation (zazen) training. *The Creative Child and Adult Quarterly, 7*(4), 211–217.

Covington, M. V. (1999). Caring about learning: The nature and nurturing of subject-matter appreciation. *Educational Psychologist, 34*(2), 127–136.

Crabb, S. (2011). The use of coaching principles to foster employee engagement. *The Coaching Psychologist, 7*(1), 27–34.

Craighead, L. W., & Allen, H. N. (1995). Appetite awareness training: A cognitive behavioral intervention for binge eating. *Cognitive and Behavioral Practice, 2*, 249–270.

Crane-Okada, R., Kiger, H., Anderson, N. L., Carroll-Johnson, R. M., Sugerman, F., Shapiro, S. L., & Wyman-McGinty, W. (2012). Mindful movement program for older breast cancer survivors: A pilot study. *Cancer Nursing, 35*(4), e1–e13.

Csikszentmihalyi, M. (1997). *Finding flow: The psychology of engagement with everyday life*. New York: Basic Books.

Dahlsgaard, K., Peterson, C., & Seligman, M. E. P. (2005). Shared virtue: The convergence of valued human strengths across culture and history. *Review of General Psychology, 9*(3), 203–213.

Dalai Lama, & Cutler, H. C. (1998). *The art of happiness.* New York: Riverhead.

Davidson, R. J., & Begley, S. (2012). *The emotional life of your brain.* New York: Hudson Street Press.

Davidson, R. J., Kabat-Zinn, J., Schumacher, J., Rosenkranz, M., Muller, D., Santorelli, S. F., ... Sheridan, J. F. (2003). Alterations in brain and immune function produced by mindfulness meditation. *Psychosomatic Medicine, 65*, 564–570.

Davis, D. E., Worthington, E. L., & Hook, J. N. (2010). Humility: Review of measurement strategies and conceptualization as personality judgment. *Journal of Positive Psychology, 5*(4), 243–252.

Dekeyser, M., Raes, F., Leijssen, M., Leysen, S., & Dewulf, D. (2008). Mindfulness skills and interpersonal behaviour. *Personality and Individual Differences, 44*(5), 1235–1245.

Delgado, L. C., Guerra, P., Perakakis, P., Viedma, M. I., Robles, H., & Vila, J. (2010). Human values education and mindfulness meditation as a tool for emotional regulation and stress prevention for teachers: An efficiency study. *Behavioral Psychology/Psicología Conductual: Revista Internacional Clínica y de la Salud, 18*(3), 511–532.

De Mello, A. (1978). *Sadhana: A way to God: Christian exercises in Eastern form.* St. Louis, MO: The Institute of Jesuit Sources.

DeValve, M. J., & Quinn, E. (2010). Practical poetry: Thich Nhat Hanh and the cultivation of a problem-oriented officer. *Contemporary Justice Review, 13*, 191–205.

Diener, E., Emmons, R. A., Larsen, R. J., & Griffin, S. (1985). The Satisfaction With Life Scale. *Journal of Personality Assessment, 49*, 71–75.

Diener, E., Lucas, R. E., & Scollon, C. N. (2006). Beyond the hedonic treadmill: Revising the adaptation theory of well-being. *American Psychologist, 61*(4), 305–314.

Diener, E., Wirtz, D., Tov, W., Kim-Prieto, C., Choi, D., Oishi, S., & Biswas-Diener, R. (2009). New measures of well-being: Flourishing and positive and negative feelings. *Social Indicators Research, 39,* 247–266.

Diessner, R., Rust, T., Solom, R., Frost, N., & Parsons, L. (2006). Beauty and hope: A moral beauty intervention. *Journal of Moral Education, 35*, 301–317.

Dimberg, U., Andréasson, P., & Thunberg, M. (2011). Emotional empathy and facial reactions to facial expressions. *Journal of Psychophysiology, 25*, 26–31.

Djikic, M., & Langer, E. J. (2007). Toward mindful social comparison: When subjective and objective selves are mutually exclusive. *New Ideas in Psychology, 25,* 221–232.

Dunn, B. R., Hartigan, J. A., & Mikulas, W. L. (1999). Concentration and mindfulness meditations: Unique forms of consciousness? *Applied Psychophysiology & Biofeedback, 24*, 147–165.

Dunn, R., Callahan, J. L., Swift, J. K., & Ivanovic, M. (2012). Effects of pre-session centering for therapists on session presence and effectiveness. *Psychotherapy Research, 23*(1), 78–85.

Dweck, C. (2006). *Mindset: The new psychology of success.* New York, NY: Ballantine Books.

Easterlin, B. L., & Cardena, E. (1999). Cognitive and emotional differences between short- and long-term Vipassana meditators. *Imagination, Cognition and Personality, 18*(1), 68–81.

Eberth, J., & Sedlmeier, P. (2012). The effects of mindfulness meditation: A meta-analysis. *Mindfulness, 3*(3), 174–189.

Eisenberg, N., & Spinrad, T. L. (2004). Emotion-related regulation: Sharpening the definition. *Child Development, 75*, 334–339.

Elgin, D. (1993). *Voluntary simplicity: Toward a way of life that is outwardly simple, inwardly rich.* New York: William Morrow.

Elston, F., & Boniwell, I. (2011). A grounded theory study of the value derived by women in financial services through a coaching intervention to help them identify their strengths and practice using them in the workplace. *International Coaching Psychology Review, 6*(1), 16–32.

Emanuel, A. S., Updegraff, J. A., Kalmbach, D. A., & Ciesla, J. A. (2010). The role of mindfulness facets in affective forecasting. *Personality and Individual Differences, 49*, 815–818.

Emmons, R. A. (2007). *Thanks!: How the new science of gratitude can make you happier.* New York: Houghton Mifflin Company.

Emmons, R. A., & McCullough, M. E. (2003). Counting blessings versus burdens: An experimental investigation of gratitude and subjective well-being in daily life. *Journal of Personality and Social Psychology, 84*, 377–389.

Evans, D. R., Baer, R. A., & Segerstrom, S. C. (2009). The effects of mindfulness and self-consciousness on persistence. *Personality and Individual Differences, 47*(4), 379–382.

Feldman, G., Greeson, J., Renna, M., & Robbins-Monteith, K. (2011). Mindfulness predicts less texting while driving among young adults: Examining attention- and emotion-regulation motives as potential mediators. *Personality and Individual Differences, 51*(7), 856–861.

Feldman, G., Greeson, J., & Senville, J. (2010). Differential effects of mindful breathing, progressive muscle relaxation, and loving-kindness meditation on decentering and negative reactions to repetitive thoughts. *Behaviour Research & Therapy, 48*(10), 1002–1011.

Fjorback, L. O., Arendt, M., Ornbøl, E., Fink, P., & Walach, H. (2011). Mindfulness-based stress reduction and mindfulness-based cognitive therapy: A systematic review of randomized controlled trials. *Acta Psychiatrica Scandinavica, 124*(2), 102–119.

Fluckiger, C., & Grosse Holtforth, M. (2008). Focusing the therapist's attention on the patient's strengths: A preliminary study to foster a mechanism of change in outpatient psychotherapy. *Journal of Clinical Psychology, 64*, 876–890.

Forest, J., Mageau, G. V. A., Crevier-Braud, L., Bergeron, L., Dubreuil, P., & Lavigne, G. V. L. (2012). Harmonious passion as an explanation of the relation between signature strengths' use and well-being at work: Test of an intervention program. *Human Relations, 65*(9), 1233–1252.

Fowers, B. J. (2008). From continence to virtue: Recovering goodness, character unity, and character types for positive psychology. *Theory & Psychology, 18*(5), 629–653.

Fox Eades, J. (2008). *Celebrating strengths: Building strengths-based schools.* Coventry, UK: Capp Press.

Franklin, B. (1962). *Autobiography of Benjamin Franklin.* New York: MacMillan.

Franklin, S. S. (2009). *The psychology of happiness.* New York: Cambridge University Press.

Fredrickson, B. (2001). The role of positive emotions in positive psychology: The broaden-and-build theory of positive emotions. *American Psychologist, 56*, 218–226.

Fredrickson, B. L., Cohn, M. A., Coffey, K. A., Pek, J., & Finkel, S. M. (2008). Open hearts build lives: Positive emotions, induced through loving-kindness meditation, build consequential personal resources. *Journal of Personality and Social Psychology, 95*(5), 1045–1062.

Fredrickson, B. L., & Losada, M. (2005). Positive affect and the complex dynamics of human flourishing. *American Psychologist, 60*(7), 678–686.

Friese, M., Messner, C., & Schaffner, Y. (2012). Mindfulness meditation counteracts self-control depletion. *Consciousness and Cognition, 21*(2), 1016–1022.

Fronsdal, G. (Trans.) (2005). *The dhammapada.* Boston, MA: Shambhala.

Gable, S., & Haidt, J. (2005). What (and why) is positive psychology? *Review of General Psychology, 9*(2), 103–110.

Gable, S. L., Reis, H. T., Impett, E. A., & Asher, E. R. (2004). What do you do when things go right? The intrapersonal and interpersonal benefits of sharing positive events. *Journal of Personality and Social Psychology, 87*(2), 228–245.

Galassi, J. P., & Akos, P. (2007). *Strengths-based school counseling: Promoting student development and achievement.* New York: Lawrence Erlbaum Associates.

Gander, F., Proyer, R. T., Ruch, W., & Wyss, T. (2012a). Strength-based positive interventions: Further evidence for their potential in enhancing well-being. *Journal of Happiness Studies.* Advance online publication. doi: 10.1007/s10902-012-9380-0

Gander, F., Proyer, R. T., Ruch, W., & Wyss, T. (2012b). The good character at work: An initial study on the contribution of character strengths in identifying healthy and unhealthy work-related behavior and experience patterns. *International Archives of Occupational and Environmental Health, 85*(8), 895–904.

Gardner-Nix, J., Backman, S., Barbati, J., & Grummitt, J. (2008). Evaluating distance education of a mindfulness-based meditation programme for chronic pain management. *Journal of Telemedicine and Telecare, 14*(2), 88–92.

Garland, E. L., Gaylord, S. A., & Fredrickson, B. L. (2011). Positive reappraisal mediates the stress-reductive effects of mindfulness: An upward spiral process. *Mindfulness, 2*(1), 59–67.

Garland, E., Gaylord, & Park, J. (2009). The role of mindfulness in positive reappraisal. *Explore: The Journal of Science and Healing, 5*(1), 37–44.

Garland, E. L., Schwarz, N. R., Kelly, A., Whitt, A., & Howard, M. O. (2012). Mindfulness-oriented recovery enhancement for alcohol dependence: Therapeutic mechanisms and intervention acceptability. *Journal of Social Work Practice in the Addictions, 12*(3), 242–263.

Geary, C., & Rosenthal, S. L. (2011). Sustained impact of MBSR on stress, well-being, and daily spiritual experiences for 1 year in academic health care employees. *Journal of Alternative and Complementary Medicine, 17*(10), 939–44.

Geller, S. M., & Greenberg, L. S., (2012). *Therapeutic presence: A mindful approach to effective therapy.* Washington, DC: American Psychological Association.

Germer, C. (2009). *The mindful path to self-compassion.* New York, NY: Guildford.

Gerzina, H.A., & Porfeli, E.J. (2012). Mindfulness as a predictor of positive reappraisal and burnout in standardized patients. *Teaching and Learning in Medicine, 24*(4), 309–314.

Geschwind, N., Peeters, F., Huibers, M., van Os, J., & Wichers, M. (2012). Efficacy of mindfulness-based cognitive therapy in relation to prior history of depression: Randomised controlled trial. *British Journal of Psychiatry, 201*(4), 320–325.

Gilbert, P. (2009). *The compassionate mind: A new approach to life's challenges*. London: Constable & Robinson.

Gilbert, P. (2010). *Compassion focused therapy: Distinctive features*. London: Routledge.

Gillham, J., Adams-Deutsch, Z., Werner, J., Reivich, K., Coulter-Heindl, V., Linkins, M., … Seligman, M.E.P. (2011). Character strengths predict subjective well-being during adolescence. *Journal of Positive Psychology, 6*(1), 31–44.

Giluk, T.L. (2009). Mindfulness, big five personality, and affect: A meta-analysis. *Personality & Individual Differences, 47*(8), 805–811.

Glomb, T.M., Duffy, M.K., Bono, J.E., & Yang, T. (2011). Mindfulness at work. In J. Martocchio, H. Liao, & A. Joshi (Eds.), *Research in personnel and human resources Management, 30*, 115–157.

Glueck, J., & Baltes, P.B. (2006). Using the concept of wisdom to enhance the expression of wisdom knowledge: Not the philosopher's dream but differential effects of developmental preparedness. *Psychology and Aging, 21*, 679–690.

Glueck, T., & Maercker, A. (2011). A randomised controlled pilot study of a brief, web-based mindfulness training. *BMC Psychiatry, 11*, 175.

Goldstein, E.D. (2007). Sacred moments: Implications on well-being and stress. *Journal of Clinical Psychology, 63*(10), 1001–1019.

Goldstein, J. (1976). *The experience of insight: A simple and direct guide to Buddhist meditation*. Boston, MA: Shambhala.

Goldstein, J. (2003). *Insight meditation*. Boston, MA: Shambhala.

Goleman, D. (1997). *Healing emotions: Conversations with the Dalai Lama on mindfulness, emotions, and health*. Boston: Shambhala.

Goleman, D. (2006). *Social intelligence: The new science of human relationships*. New York: Bantam Books.

Gottman, J. (1994). *Why marriages succeed or fail … and how you can make yours last*. New York: Simon & Schuster.

Govindji, R., & Linley, P.A. (2007). Strengths use, self-concordance and well-being: Implications for strengths, coaching and coaching psychologists. *International Coaching Psychology Review, 2*(2), 143–153.

Grant, A.M., & Schwartz, B. (2011). Too much of a good thing: The challenge and opportunity of the inverted u. *Perspectives on Psychological Science, 6*(1), 61–76.

Grayson, H. (2003). *Mindful loving: 10 practices for creating deeper connections*. New York: Gotham Books.

Grepmair, L., Mitterlehner, F., Loew, T., Bachler, E., Rother, W., & Nickel, M. (2007). Promoting mindfulness in psychotherapists in training influences the treatment results of their patients: A randomized, double-blind, controlled study. *Psychotherapy and Psychosomatics*, 76, 332–338.

Grossman, P., Niemann, L., Schmidt, S., & Walach, H. (2004). Mindfulness-based stress reduction and health benefits: A meta-analysis. *Journal of Psychosomatic Research, 57*(1), 35–43.

Gunaratana, H. (2002). *Mindfulness in plain English*. Boston, MA: Wisdom Publications.

Hamilton, N.A., Kitzman, H., & Guyotte, S. (2007). Enhancing health and emotion: Mindfulness as a missing link between cognitive therapy and positive psychology. *Journal of Cognitive Psychotherapy: An International Quarterly, 20*(2), 123–134.

Harnett, P.H., Whittingham, K., Puhakka, E., Hodges, J., Spry, C., & Dob, R. (2010). The short-term impact of a brief group-based mindfulness therapy program on depression and life satisfaction. *Mindfulness, 1*, 183–188.

Hart, W., Albarracin, D., Eagly, A.H., Brechan, I., Lindberg, M.J., & Merrill, L. (2009). Feeling validated versus being correct: A meta-analysis of selective exposure to information. *Psychological Bulletin, 135*(4), 555–588.

Harzer, C., & Ruch, W. (2012a). When the job is a calling: The role of applying one's signature strengths at work. *Journal of Positive Psychology, 7*(5), 362–371.

Harzer, C., & Ruch, W. (2012b). The application of signature character strengths and positive experiences at work. *Journal of Happiness Studies*. Advance online publication. doi: 10.1007/s10902-012-9364-0

Hayes, A.M., & Feldman, G. (2004). Clarifying the construct of mindfulness in the context of emotion regulation and the process of change in therapy. *Clinical Psychology: Science and Practice, 11*(3), 255–262.

Hayes, S.C., Luoma, J.B., Bond, F.W., Masuda, A., & Lillis, J. (2006). Acceptance and commitment therapy: Model, processes, and outcomes. *Behaviour Research and Therapy, 44*, 1–25.

Hayes, S. C., Strosahl, K. D., & Wilson, K. G. (1999). *Acceptance and commitment therapy.* New York: Guilford.

Hayes, S. C., Wilson, K. W., Gifford, E. V., Follette, V. M., & Strosahl, K. (1996). Experiential avoidance and behavioral disorders: A functional dimensional approach to diagnosis and treatment. *Journal of Consulting and Clinical Psychology, 64*, 1152–1168.

Headey, B., Schupp, J., Tucci, I., & Wagner, G. G. (2010). Authentic happiness theory supported by impact of religion on life satisfaction: A longitudinal analysis with data for Germany. *Journal of Positive Psychology, 5*(1), 73–82.

Heppner, W. L., & Kernis, M. H. (2007). Quiet ego functioning: The complementary roles of mindfulness, authenticity, and secure high self-esteem. *Psychological Inquiry, 18*, 248–251.

Hoch, D. B., Watson, A. J., Linton, D. A., Bello, H. E., Senelly, M., Milik, M. T., … Kvedar, J. C. (2012). The feasibility and impact of delivering a mind-body intervention in a virtual world. *PLoS ONE, 7*(3), e33843.

Hoeksma, J. B., Oosterlaan, J., & Schipper, E. M. (2004). Emotion regulation and the dynamics of feelings: A conceptual and methodological framework. *Child Development, 75*, 354–360.

Hofmann, S. G., Grossman, P., & Hinton, D. E. (2011). Loving-kindness and compassion meditation: Potential for psychological interventions. *Clinical Psychology Review, 31*, 1126–1132.

Hofmann, S. G., Sawyer, A. T., Witt, A. A., & Oh, D. (2010). The effect on mindfulness-based therapy on anxiety and depression: A meta-analytic review. *Journal of Consulting and Clinical Psychology, 78*, 169–183.

Hong, P., Lishner, D., & Han, K. (2012). Mindfulness and eating: An experiment examining the effect of mindful raisin eating on the enjoyment of sampled food. *Mindfulness.* Advance online publication. doi: 10.1007/s12671-012-0154-x

Honore, G. (2005). *In praise of slow.* London, UK: Orion Publishing.

Horowitz, M. J. (2002). Self- and relational observation. *Journal of Psychotherapy Integration, 12*(2), 115–127.

Howell, A. J., Dopko, R. L., Passmore, H. A., & Buro, K. (2011). Nature connectedness: Associations with well-being and mindfulness. *Personality and Individual Differences, 51*(2), 166–171.

Hurley, D. B., & Kwon, P. (2012). Savoring helps most when you have little: Interaction between savoring and uplifts on positive affect and satisfaction with life. *Journal of Happiness Studies.* Advance online publication. doi: 10.1007/s10902-012-9377-8

Huston, D. C., Garland, E. L., & Farb, N. A. S. (2011). Mechanisms of mindfulness in communication training. *Journal of Applied Communication Research, 39*(4), 406–421.

Hutcherson, C. A., Seppala, E. M., & Gross, J. J. (2008). Loving-kindness meditation increases social connectedness. *Emotion, 8*(5), 720–724.

Jamison, C. (2006). *Finding sanctuary: Monastic steps for everyday life.* Collegeville, MN: Liturgical Press.

Jarden, A., Jose, P., Kashdan, T., Simpson, O., McLachlan, K., & Mackenzie, A. (2012). [International Wellbeing Study]. Unpublished raw data.

Jazaieri, H., Jinpa, G. T., McGonigal, K., Rosenberg, E. L., Finkelstein, J., Simon-Thomas, E., … Goldin, P. R. (2012). Enhancing compassion: A randomized controlled trial of a compassion cultivation training program. *Journal of Happiness Studies.* Advance online publication. doi: 10.1007/s10902-012-9373-z

Johnson, D. P., Penn, D. L., Fredrickson, B. L., Kring, A. M., Meyer, P. S., Catalino, L. I., & Brantley, M. (2011). A pilot study of loving-kindness meditation for the negative symptoms of schizophrenia. *Schizophrenia Research, 129*(2/3), 137–140.

Jong, H. W. (2012). Mindfulness and spirituality as predictors of personal maturity beyond the influence of personality traits. *Mental Health, Religion, & Culture, 16*(1), 38–57.

Kabat-Zinn, J. (1982). An outpatient program in behavioral medicine for chronic pain patients, based on the practice of mindfulness meditation. *General Hospital Psychiatry, 7*(1), 71–72.

Kabat-Zinn, J. (1990). *Full catastrophe living.* New York, NY: Dell.

Kabat-Zinn, J. (1994). *Wherever you go, there you are.* New York, NY: Hyperion.

Kabat-Zinn, J. (2003). Mindfulness-based interventions in context: Past, present, and future. *Clinical Psychology: Science and Practice, 10*(2), 144–156.

Kabat-Zinn, J. (2005). *Coming to our senses.* New York, NY: Hyperion.

Kabat-Zinn, J., Lipworth, L., & Burney, R. (1985). The clinical use of mindfulness meditation for the self-regulation of chronic pain. *Journal of Behavioral Medicine, 8*(2), 163–190.

Kabat-Zinn, J., Massion, A. O., Kristeller, J., Peterson, L. G., Fletcher, K., Pbert, L., … Santorelli, S. F. (1992). Effectiveness of a meditation-based stress reduction program in the treatment of anxiety disorders. *American Journal of Psychiatry, 149*, 936–943.

Kabat-Zinn, M., & Kabat-Zinn, J. (1997). *Everyday blessings: The inner work of mindful parenting.* New York: Hyperion.

Kahn, M. (1995). *The tao of conversation.* Oakland, CA: New Harbinger.

Kaplan, K. H., Goldenberg, D. L., & Galvin-Nadeau, M. (1993). The impact of a meditation-based stress reduction program on fibromyalgia. *General Hospital Psychiatry, 15*(5), 284–289.

Kashdan, T. B. (2007). Social anxiety spectrum and diminished positive experiences: Theoretical synthesis and meta-analysis. *Clinical Psychology Review, 27*, 348–365.

Kashdan, T. (2009). *Curious? Discover the missing ingredient to a fulfilling life.* New York, NY: HarperCollins.

Kashdan, T. B., Afram, A., Brown, K. W., Birnbeck, M., & Drvoshanov, M. (2011). Curiosity enhances the role of mindfulness in reducing defensive responses to existential threat. *Personality and Individual Differences, 50*, 1227–1232.

Kashdan, T. B., McKnight, P. E., Fincham, F. D., & Rose, P. (2011). When curiosity breeds intimacy: Taking advantage of intimacy opportunities and transforming boring conversations. *Journal of Personality, 79,* 1369–1401.

Kashdan, T. B., & Rottenberg, J. (2010). Psychological flexibility as a fundamental aspect of health. *Clinical Psychology Review, 30*, 865–878.

Kass, S. J., VanWormer, L. A., Mikulas, W. L., Legan, S., & Bumgarner, D. (2011). Effects of mindfulness training on simulated driving: Preliminary results. *Mindfulness, 2*(4), 236–241.

Kasser, T. (2006). Materialism and its alternatives. In M. Csikszentmihály & I. S. Csikszentmihály (Eds.), *A life worth Living: Contributions to positive psychology* (pp. 200–214). Oxford, UK: Oxford University Press.

Kee, Y. H., & Wang, C. K. J. (2008). Relationships between mindfulness, flow dispositions and mental skills adoption: A cluster analytic approach. *Psychology of Sport and Exercise, 9*, 393–411.

Keng, S. L., Smoski, M. J., Robins, C. J., Ekblad, A. G., & Brantley, J. G. (2012). Mechanisms of change in mindfulness-based stress reduction: Self-compassion and mindfulness as mediators of intervention outcomes. *Journal of Cognitive Psychotherapy, 26*(3), 270–280.

Keyes, C. L. M. (2002). The mental health continuum: From languishing to flourishing in life. *Journal of Health and Social Behavior, 43,* 207–222.

Khong, B. S. L. (2011). Mindfulness: A way of cultivating deep respect for emotions. *Mindfulness, 2* (1), 27–32.

Kiken, L. G., & Shook, N. J. (2011). Looking up: Mindfulness increases positive judgments and reduces negativity bias. *Social Psychological and Personality Science, 2,* 425–431.

Killingsworth, M. A., & Gilbert, D. T. (2010). A wandering mind is an unhappy mind. *Science, 330,* 932.

King, A. (2001). The health benefits of writing about life goals. *Personality and Social Psychology Bulletin, 27*(7), 798–807.

Kingston, T., Dooley, B., Bates, A., Lawlor, E., & Malone, K. (2007). Mindfulness-based cognitive therapy for residual depressive symptoms. *Psychology and Psychotherapy: Theory, Research, and Practice, 80*, 193–203.

Kornfield, J. (1993). *A path with heart.* New York, NY: Bantam Books.

Kornfield, J. (2005). Foreword. In G. Fronsdal (Trans.), *The dhammapada* (pp. ix–x). Boston: Shambhala.

Kornfield, J. (2008). *The art of forgiveness, loving-kindness, and peace.* New York, NY: Bantam.

Kornfield, J., & Feldman, C. (1996). *Soul food: Stories to nourish the spirit and the heart.* New York, NY: HarperCollins.

Kristeller, J. L. (2003). Mindfulness, wisdom, and eating: Applying a multi-domain model of meditation effects. *Constructivism in the Human Sciences, 8* (2), 107–118.

Kristeller, J. L., & Hallett, C. B. (1999). An exploratory study of a meditation-based intervention for binge eating disorder. *Journal of Health Psychology, 4*, 357–363.

Kristeller, J. L., & Johnson, T. (2005). Cultivating loving kindness: A two-stage model for the effects of meditation on compassion, altruism, and spirituality. *Zygon: Journal of Religion and Science, 40* (2), 391–408.

Kristeller, J. L., & Wolever, R. Q. (2011). Mindfulness-based eating awareness training for treating binge eating disorder: The conceptual foundations. *Eating Disorders: The Journal of Treatment and Prevention, 19*, 49–61.

Kristeller, J. L., Wolever, R. Q., & Sheets, V. (2013). Mindfulness-based eating awareness training (MB-EAT) for binge eating: A randomized clinical trial. *Mindfulness.* doi: 10.1007/s12671-012-0179-1

Krusche, A., Cyhlarova, E., King, S., & Williams, M. G. (2012). Mindfulness online: A preliminary evaluation of the feasibility of a web-based mindfulness course and the impact on stress. *BMJ Open, 2*(3), e000803.

Kuan, T. (2008). *Mindfulness in early Buddhism: New approaches through psychology and textual analysis of Pali, Chinese and Sanskrit sources.* New York, NY: Routledge.

Kuzminski, A. (2007). Pyrrhonism and the Madhyamaka. *Philosophy East and West, 57*(4), 482–511.

Lakey, C. E., Kernis, M. H., Heppner, W. L., & Lance, C. E. (2008). Individual differences in authenticity and mindfulness as predictors of verbal defensiveness. *Journal of Research in Personality, 42* (1), 230–238.

Lambert, N. M., Gwinn, A. M., Fincham, F. D., & Stillman, T. F. (2011). Feeling tired? How sharing positive experiences can boost vitality. *International Journal of Wellbeing, 1*(3), 307–314.

Langer, E. (1989). *Mindfulness.* Reading, MA: Addison-Wesley.

Langer, E. (1997). *The power of mindful learning.* Reading, MA: Addison-Wesley.

Langer, E. (2006). *On becoming an artist.* New York: Ballantine Books.

Langer, E. (2009). Mindfulness versus positive evaluation. In S. J. Lopez & C. R. Snyder (Eds.), *Oxford handbook of positive psychology* (pp. 279–293). New York: Oxford University Press.

Langer, E. J., Delizonna, L., & Pirson, M. (2010). The mindlessness of social comparisons and its effect on creativity. *Psychology of Aesthetics, Creativity, and the Arts, 4*, 68–74.

Langer, E. J., & Imber, L. (1980). Role of mindlessness in the perception of deviance. *Journal of Personality and Social Psychology, 39*(3), 360–367.

Lau, M. A., Bishop, S. R., Segal, Z. V., Buis, T., Anderson, N. D., Carlson, L., ... Devins, G. (2006). The Toronto Mindfulness Scale: Development and validation. *Journal of Clinical Psychology, 62*(12), 1445–1467.

Lazar, S. W., Kerr, C. E., Wasserman, R. H., Gray, J. R., Greve, D. N., Treadway, M. T., ... Fischl, B. (2005). Meditation experience is associated with increased cortical thickness. *Neuroreport, 16,* 1893–1897.

Ledesma, D., & Kumano, H. (2009). Mindfulness-based stress reduction and cancer: A meta-analysis. *Psycho-oncology, 18*(6), 571–579.

Lee, T. M., Leung, M. K., Hou, W. K., Tang, J. C., Yin, J., So, K. F., Lee, C. F., & Chan, C. C. (2012). Distinct neural activity associated with focused-attention meditation and loving-kindness meditation. *PLoS One, 7*(8), e40054.

Levesque, C., & Brown, K. W. (2007). Mindfulness as a moderator of the effect of implicit motivational self-concept on day-to-day behavioral motivation. *Motivation and Emotion, 31*, 284–299.

Levine, M. (2009). *The positive psychology of Buddhism and yoga: Paths to a mature happiness.* New York, NY: Routledge.

Lillis, J., Hayes, S. C., Bunting, K., & Masuda, A. (2009). Teaching acceptance and mindfulness to improve the lives of the obese: A preliminary test of a theoretical model. *Annals of Behavioral Medicine, 37*, 58–69.

Limm, H., Gundel, H., Heinmuller, M., Marten-Mittag, B., Nater, U. M., Siegrist, J., & Angerer, P. (2011). Stress management interventions in the workplace improve stress reactivity: A randomized controlled trial. *Occupational and Environmental Medicine, 68*, 126–133.

Linehan, M. M. (1993). *Cognitive-behavioral treatment of borderline personality disorder.* New York, NY: Guilford.

Linkins, M. (2012). *Thriving classrooms teacher training module: Theory and practice.* Unpublished manual, Mayerson Academy, Cincinnati, OH.

Linkins, M., Niemiec, R. M., Mayerson, D., & Gillham, J. (in press). Through the strengths lens: A framework for educating the heart. *Journal of Positive Psychology.*

Linley, A. (2008). *Average to A+: Realising strengths in yourself and others.* Coventry, UK: CAPP Press.

Linley, P. A., & Harrington, S. (2006). Strengths coaching: A potential-guided approach to coaching psychology. *International Coaching Psychology Review, 1*(1), 37–46.

Linley, P. A., Nielsen, K. M., Gillett, R., & Biswas-Diener, R. (2010). Using signature strengths in pursuit of goals: Effects on goal progress, need satisfaction, and well-being, and implications for coaching psychologists. *International Coaching Psychology Review, 5*(1), 6–15.

Littman-Ovadia, H., & Davidovitch, N. (2010). Effects of congruence and character-strength deployment on work adjustment and well-being. *International Journal of Business and Social Science, 1* (3), 138–146.

Littman-Ovadia, H., & Steger, M. (2010). Character strengths and well-being among volunteers and employees: Toward an integrative model. *Journal of Positive Psychology, 5*(6), 419–430.

Liu, X., Wang, S., Chang, S., Chen, W., & Si, M. (2012). Effect of brief mindfulness intervention on tolerance and distress of pain induced by cold-pressor task. *Stress & Health.* Advance online publication. doi: 10.1002/smi.2446.

Ljótsson, B., Hedman, E., Lindfors, P., Hursti, T., Lindefors, N., Andersson, G., & Rück, C. (2011). Long-term follow-up of internet-delivered exposure and mindfulness based treatment for irritable bowel syndrome. *Behaviour Research and Therapy, 49*, 58–61.

Logghe, I. H. J., Verhagen, A. P., Rademaker, A. C. H. J., Bierma-Zeinstra, S. M. A., van Rossum, E., Faber, M. J., & Koes, B. W. (2010). The effects of Tai Chi on fall prevention, fear of falling and balance in older people: A meta-analysis. *Preventive Medicine: An International Journal Devoted to Practice and Theory, 51*(3–4), 222–227.

Louis, M. C. (2011). Strengths interventions in higher education: The effect of identification versus development approaches on implicit self-theory. *Journal of Positive Psychology, 6*(3), 204–215.

Losada, M. (1999). The complex dynamics of high performance teams. *Mathematical and Computer Modelling, 30*(9–10), 179–192.

Losada, M., & Heaphy, E. (2004). Positive organizational scholarship. *American Behavioral Scientist, 47*, 740–765.

Luks, A. (1991). *The healing power of doing good: The health and spiritual benefits of helping others.* New York: Fawcett Columbine.

Lutz, A., Brefczynski-Lewis, J. A., Johnstone, T., & Davidson, R. J. (2008). Voluntary regulation of the neural circuitry of emotion by compassion meditation: Effects of expertise. *PLoS One, 3*(3), e1897.

Lutz, A., Dunne, J. D., & Davidson, R. J. (2007). Meditation and the neuroscience of consciousness: An introduction. In P. D. Zelazo, M. Moscovitch, & E. Thompson (Eds.), *The Cambridge handbook of consciousness* (pp. 499–511). Cambridge, UK: Cambridge University Press.

Lyubomirsky, S. (2008). *The how of happiness: A scientific approach to getting the life you want.* New York, NY: Penguin Press.

Madden, W., Green, S., & Grant, A. M. (2011). A pilot study evaluating strengths-based coaching for primary school students: Enhancing engagement and hope. *International Coaching Psychology Review, 6*(1), 71–83.

Marchand, W. R. (2012). Mindfulness-based stress reduction, mindfulness-based cognitive therapy, and zen meditation for depression, anxiety, pain, and psychological distress. *Journal of Psychiatric Practice, 18*(4), 233.

Martin, R. (Ed.), & Morimoto, J. (Illus.). (1995). *One hand clapping: Zen stories for all ages.* New York: Rizzoli International Publishers.

Masicampo, E. J., & Baumeister, R. F. (2007). Relating mindfulness and self-regulatory processes. *Psychological Inquiry, 18*, 255–258.

Mayer, J. D., Chabot, H. F., & Carlsmith, K. (1997). Conation, affect, and cognition in personality. In G. Matthews (Ed.), *Cognitive science perspectives on personality and emotion* (pp. 31–63). Amsterdam: Elsevier.

Mazzucchelli, T. G., Kane, R. T., & Rees, C. S. (2010). Behavioral activation interventions for well-being: A meta-analysis. *Journal of Positive Psychology, 5*(2), 105–121.

McCullough, M. E., Root, L. M., & Cohen, A. D. (2006). Writing about the benefits of an interpersonal transgression facilitates forgiveness. *Journal of Consulting and Clinical Psychology, 74*(5), 887–897.

McCraty, R., Atkinson, M., & Tomasino, D. (2003). Impact of a workplace stress reduction program on blood pressure and emotional health in hypertensive employees. *Journal of Alternative and Complementary Medicine, 9*, 355–369.

McGrath, R. E. (in press). Character strengths in 75 nations: An update. *Journal of Positive Psychology.*

McKee, A., Boyatzis, R., & Johnston, F. (2008). *Becoming a resonant leader.* Boston, MA: Harvard Business Press.

Meevissen, Y. M. C., Peters, M. L., & Alberts, H. J. E. M. (2011). Become more optimistic by imagining a best possible self: Effects of a two week intervention. *Journal of Behavior Therapy and Experimental Psychiatry, 42*, 371–378.

Meiklejohn, J., Phillips, C., Freedman, M. L., Griffin, M. L., Biegel, G., Roach, A., ... Saltzman, A. (2012). Integrating mindfulness training into K-12 education: Fostering the resilience of teachers and students. *Mindfulness, 3*(4), 291–307.

Miller, J., Fletcher, K., & Kabat-Zinn, J. (1995). Three-year follow-up and clinical implications of a mindfulness meditation-based stress reduction intervention in the treatment of anxiety disorders. *General Hospital Psychiatry, 17*(3), 192–200.

Miller, W. R., & Rollnick, S. (1991). *Motivational interviewing: Preparing people to change addictive behavior.* New York, NY: Guilford Press.

Mino, Y., Babazono, A., Tsuda, T., & Yasuda, N. (2006). Can stress management at the workplace prevent depression? A randomized controlled trial. *Psychotherapy and Psychosomatics, 75*, 177–182.

Mirams, L., Poliakoff, E., Brown, R. J., & Lloyd, D. M. (2012). Brief body-scan meditation practice improves somatosensory perceptual decision making. *Consciousness and Cognition.*

Mitchell, J., Stanimirovic, R., Klein, B., & Vella-Brodrick, D. (2009). A randomised controlled trial of a self-guided internet intervention promoting well-being. *Computers in Human Behavior, 25*, 749–760.

Money, K., Hillenbrand, C., & Camara, N. D. (2008). Putting positive psychology to work in organizations. *Journal of General Management, 34*(2), 21–26.

Mongrain, M., & Anselmo-Matthews, T. (2012). Do positive psychology exercises work? A replication of Seligman et al. *Journal of Clinical Psychology, 68*(4), 382–389.

Moyers, B. (Producer) (1993). *Healing and the mind: Vol. 3. Healing from within* [Television broadcast]. New York, NY: David Grubin Productions and Public Affairs Television.

Mrazek, M. D., Smallwood, J., & Schooler, J. W. (2012). Mindfulness and mind-wandering: finding convergence through opposing constructs. *Emotion, 12*(3), 442–448.

Muraven, M., & Baumeister, R. F. (2000). Self-regulation and depletion of limited resources: Does self-control resemble a muscle? *Psychological Bulletin, 126*, 247–259.

Myers, D. (2000). The funds, friends, and faith of happy people. *American Psychologist, 55*, 56–67.

Nedeljkovic, M., Wirtz, P. H., & Ausfeld-Hafter, B. (2012). Effects of Taiji practice on mindfulness and self-compassion in healthy participants: A randomized controlled trial. *Mindfulness, 3*(3), 200–208.

Neely, M., Schallert, D., Mohammed, S., Roberts, R., & Chen, Y. (2009). Self-kindness when facing stress: The role of self-compassion, goal regulation, and support in college students' well-being. *Motivation and Emotion, 33*, 88–97.

Neff, K. D. (2003a). Self-compassion: An alternative conceptualization of a healthy attitude toward oneself. *Self and Identity, 2*, 85–101.

Neff, K. D. (2003b). Development and validation of a scale to measure self-compassion. *Self and Identity, 2*, 223–250.

Neff, K. D. (2011). *Self-compassion: Stop beating yourself up and leave insecurity behind.* New York, NY: William Morrow.

Neff, K. D., & Rude, S. S., & Kirkpatrick, K. (2007). An examination of self-compassion in relation to positive psychological functioning and personality traits. *Journal of Research in Personality, 41*, 908–916.

Neff, K. D., & Vonk, R. (2009). Self-compassion versus global self-esteem: Two different ways of relating to oneself. *Journal of Personality, 77*, 23–50.

Nhat Hanh, T. (1979). *The miracle of mindfulness: An introduction to the practice of meditation.* Boston, MA: Beacon.

Nhat Hanh, T. (1991). *Peace is every step.* New York, NY: Bantam Books.

Nhat Hanh, T. (1992). *Touching peace.* Berkeley, CA: Parallax Press.

Nhat Hanh, T. (1993). *For a future to be possible: Commentaries on the five mindfulness trainings.* Berkeley, CA: Parallax Press.

Nhat Hanh, T. (1998). *The heart of the Buddha's teaching.* New York, NY: Broadway.

Nhat Hanh, T. (2001). *Anger: Wisdom for cooling the flames.* New York, NY: Riverhead Books.

Nhat Hanh, T. (2006). *True love: A practice for awakening the heart.* Boston, MA: Shambhala.

Nhat Hanh, T. (2009). *Happiness.* Berkeley, CA: Parallax Press.

Nhat Hanh, T., & Cheung, L. (2010). *Savor: Mindful eating, mindful life.* New York, NY: HarperCollins.

Nidich, S. I., Ryncarz, R. A., Abrams, A. I., Orme-Johnson, D. W., & Wallace, R. K. (1983). Kohlbergian cosmic perspective responses, EEG coherence, and the TM and TM-Sidhi program. *Journal of Moral Education, 12*, 166–173.

Niemiec, R. M. (2005). The expansion of mindfulness meditation [Review of the video *Mindfulness-based cognitive therapy for depression*] *PsycCRITIQUES, 50*(23), Article 13.

Niemiec, R. M. (2012). Mindful living: Character strengths interventions as pathways for the five mindfulness trainings. *International Journal of Wellbeing, 2*(1), 22–33.

Niemiec, R. M. (2013). VIA character strengths: Research and practice (The first 10 years). In H. H. Knoop & A. Delle Fave (Eds.), *Well-being and cultures: Perspectives on positive psychology* (pp. 11–30). New York, NY: Springer.

Niemiec, R. M., Rashid, T., & Spinella, M. (2012). Strong mindfulness: Integrating mindfulness and character strengths. *Journal of Mental Health Counseling, 34*(3), 240–253.

Niemiec, R. M., & Wedding, D. (2014). *Positive psychology at the movies 2: Using films to build character strengths and well-being.* Boston, MA: Hogrefe Publishing.

Norris, K. (2008). *Acedia and me: A marriage, monks, and a writer's life.* New York, NY: Riverhead.

Nyklicek, I., Vingerhoets, A., & Zeelenberg, M., (2010). *Emotion regulation and well-being.* New York, NY: Springer.

Oman, D., Shapiro, S. L., Thoresen, C. E., Flinders, T., Driskill, J. D., & Plante, T. G. (2007). Learning from spiritual models and meditation: A randomized evaluation of a college course. *Pastoral Psychology, 55*(4), 473–493.

Oman, D., Shapiro, S. L., Thoresen, C. E., Plante, T. G., & Flinders, T. (2008). Meditation lowers stress and supports forgiveness among college students: A randomized controlled trial. *Journal of American College Health, 56,* 569–578.

Pace, T. W., Negi, L. T., Adame, D. D., Cole, S. P., Sivilli, T. I., Brown, T. D., ... Raison, C. L. (2009). Effect of compassion meditation on neuroendocrine, innate immune and behavioral responses to psychosocial stress. *Psychoneuroendocrinology, 34,* 87–98.

Papies, E. K. (2012). Mindful attention prevents mindless impulses. *Social Psychological and Personality Science, 3*(3), 291–299. doi: 10.1177/19485506 11419031

Park, N., & Peterson, C. (2006a). Character strengths and happiness among young children: Content analysis of parental descriptions. *Journal of Happiness Studies, 7,* 323–341.

Park, N., & Peterson, C. (2006b). Moral competence and character strengths among adolescents: The development and validation of the Values in Action Inventory of Strengths for Youth. *Journal of Adolescence, 29,* 891–905.

Park, N., & Peterson, C. (2006c). Methodological issues in positive psychology and the assessment of character strengths. In A. D. Ong & M. van Dulmen (Eds.), *Handbook of methods in positive psychology* (pp. 292–305). New York, NY: Oxford University Press.

Park, N., & Peterson, C. (2009). Character strengths: Research and practice. *Journal of College and Character, 10*(4). Retrieved from http://www.degruyter.com/view/j/jcc.2009.10.4/jcc.2009.10.4.1042/jcc.2009.10.4.1042.xml?format=INT

Park, N., Peterson, C., & Seligman, M. E. P. (2004). Strengths of character and well-being. *Journal of Social & Clinical Psychology, 23,* 603–619.

Park, N., Peterson, C., & Seligman, M. E. P. (2006). Character strengths in fifty-four nations and the fifty US states. *Journal of Positive Psychology, 1* (3), 118–129.

Passmore, J., & Marianetti, O. (2007). The role of mindfulness in coaching. *The Coaching Psychologist, 3*(3), 130–136.

Petchsawang, P., & Duchon, D. (2012). Workplace spirituality, meditation, and work performance. *Journal of Management, Spirituality & Religion, 9*(2), 189–208.

Peters, M. L., Flink, I. K., Boersma, K., & Linton, S. J. (2010). Manipulating optimism: Can imagining a best possible self be used to increase positive future expectancies? *Journal of Positive Psychology, 5*(3), 204–211.

Peterson, C. (2000). The future of optimism. *American Psychologist, 55*(1), 44–55.

Peterson, C. (2006). *A primer in positive psychology.* New York, NY: Oxford University Press.

Peterson, C., Ruch, W., Beermann, U., Park, N., & Seligman, M. E. P. (2007). Strengths of character, orientations to happiness, and life satisfaction. *The Journal of Positive Psychology, 2,* 149–156.

Peterson, C., & Seligman, M. E. P. (2004). *Character strengths and virtues: A handbook and classification.* New York, NY: Oxford University Press.

Peterson, C., Stephens, J. P., Park, N., Lee, F., & Seligman, M. E. P. (2010). Strengths of character and work. Oxford handbook of positive psychology and work. In Linley, P. A., Harrington, S., & Garcea, N. (Eds.). *Oxford handbook of positive psychology and work* (pp. 221–231). New York, NY: Oxford University Press.

Peterson, T. D., & Peterson, E. W. (2008). Stemming the tide of law student depression: What law schools need to learn from the science of positive psychology. *Yale Journal of Health Policy, Law, and Ethics, 9*(2), 357–434.

Plante, T. G. (2008). *Using spiritual and religious tools in psychotherapy.* Washington, DC: American Psychological Association.

Post, S. G. (2005). Altruism, happiness, and health: It's good to be good. *International Journal of Behavioral Medicine, 12,* 66–77.

Proctor, C., & Fox Eades, J. (2011). *Strengths gym: Build and exercise your strengths!* St. Peter Port, UK: Positive Psychology Research Centre.

Proctor, C., Maltby, J., & Linley, P. A. (2009) Strengths use as a predictor of well-being and health-related quality of life. *Journal of Happiness Studies, 10,* 583–630.

Proctor, C., Tsukayama, E., Wood, A., M., Maltby, J., Fox Eades, J., & Linley, P. A. (2011). Strengths gym: The impact of a character strengths-based intervention on the life satisfaction and well-being of adolescents. *Journal of Positive Psychology, 6* (5), 377–388.

Proulx, K. (2008). Experiences of women with bulimia nervosa in a mindfulness-based eating disorder treatment group. *Eating Disorders: The Journal of Treatment & Prevention, 16,* 52–72.

Proyer, R. T., Ruch, W., & Buschor, C. (2012). Testing strengths-based interventions: A preliminary study on the effectiveness of a program targeting curiosity, gratitude, hope, humor, and zest for enhancing life satisfaction. *Journal of Happiness Studies.* Advance online publication. doi: 10.1007/s10902-012-9331-9

Proyer, R. T., Sidler, N., Weber, M., & Ruch, W. (2012). A multi-method approach to studying the relationship between character strengths and vocational interests in adolescents. *International Journal for Educational and Vocational Guidance, 12*(2), 141–157.

Pury, C. (2008). Can courage be learned? In S. J. Lopez (Ed.), *Positive psychology: Exploring human strengths* (pp. 109–130). Westport, CT: Praeger.

Pury, C. L. S., & Kowalski, R. M. (2007). Human strengths, courageous actions, and general and personal courage. *Journal of Positive Psychology, 2*(2), 120–128.

Putman, D. (1997). Psychological courage. *Philosophy, Psychiatry, and Psychology, 4,* 1–11.

Rashid, T. (2008). Positive psychotherapy. In S. J. Lopez (Ed.), *Positive psychology: Exploring the best in people, vol. 4* (pp. 187–217). Westport, CT: Praeger.

Rashid, T. (2009). Positive interventions in clinical practice. *Journal of Clinical Psychology: In Session, 65*(5), 461–466.

Reb, J., Narayanan, J., & Chaturvedi, S. (2012). Leading mindfully: Two studies on the influence of supervisor trait mindfulness on employee well-being and performance. *Mindfulness.* Advance online publication. doi: 10.1007/s12671-012-0144-z

Rehg, W. (2002). Christian mindfulness: A path to finding God in all things. *Studies in the Spirituality of Jesuits, 34*(3), 1–32.

Reibel, D. K., Greeson, J. M., Brainard, G. C., & Rosenzweig, S. (2001). Mindfulness-based stress reduction and health-related quality of life in a heterogeneous patient population. *General Hospital Psychiatry, 23*(4), 183–192.

Reis, H. T., Smith, S. M., Carmichael, C. L., Caprariello, P. A., Tsai, F.-F., Rodrigues, A., & Maniaci, M. R. (2010). Are you happy for me? How sharing positive events with others provides personal and interpersonal benefits. *Journal of Personality and Social Psychology, 99*(2), 311–329.

Ritchie, T. D., & Bryant, F. B. (2012). Positive state mindfulness: A multidimensional model of mindfulness in relation to positive experience. *International Journal of Wellbeing, 2*(3), 150–181. doi: 10.5502/ijw.v2.i3.1

Roemer, L., & Orsillo, S. M. (2002). Expanding our conceptualization of and treatment for generalized anxiety disorder: Integrating mindfulness/acceptance-based approaches with existing cognitive-behavioral models. *Clinical Psychology: Science and Practice, 9,* 54–68.

Roemer, L., & Orsillo, S. M. (2009). *Mindfulness- and acceptance-based behavioral therapies in practice.* New York, NY: Guilford.

Rollnick, S., & Miller, W. R. (1995). What is motivational interviewing? *Behavioural and Cognitive Psychotherapy, 23,* 325–334.

Rothaupt, J. W., & Morgan, M. M. (2007). Counselors' and counselor educators' practice of mindfulness: A qualitative inquiry. *Counseling and Values, 52,* 40–54.

Rust, T., Diessner, R., & Reade, L. (2009). Strengths only or strengths and relative weaknesses? A preliminary study. *Journal of Psychology, 143*(5), 465–476.

Ryan, R. M., & Frederick, C. (1997). On energy, personality, and health: Subjective vitality as a dynamic reflection of well-being. *Journal of Personality, 65*(3), 529–565.

Saleebey, D. (1996). The strengths perspective in social work practice: Extensions and cautions. *Social Work, 41*(3), 296–306.

Salzberg, S. (1995). *Lovingkindness: The revolutionary art of happiness.* Boston, MA: Shambhala.

Salzberg, S. (2011). Mindfulness and loving-kindness. *Contemporary Buddhism, 12*(1), 177–182.

Sauer-Zavala, S., Walsh, E., Eisenlohr-Moul, T., & Lykins, E. (2012). Comparing mindfulness-based intervention strategies: Differential effects of sitting meditation, body scan, and mindful yoga. *Mindfulness.* Advance online publication. doi: 10.1007/s12671-012-0139-9

Schutte, N. S., & Malouff, J. M. (2011). Emotional intelligence mediates the relationship between mindfulness and subjective well-being. *Personality and Individual Differences, 50*(7), 1116–1119.

Schwartz, B., & Sharpe, K. E. (2006). Practical wisdom: Aristotle meets positive psychology. *Journal of Happiness Studies, 7,* 377–395.

Scott, G., Leritz, L. E., & Mumford, M. D. (2004). The effectiveness of creativity training: A quantitative review. *Creativity Research Journal, 16*(4), 361–388.

Sears, R. W., Tirch, D. D., & Denton, R. B. (2011). *Mindfulness in clinical practice.* Sarasota, FL: Professional Resource Press.

Sears, S., & Kraus, S. (2009). I think therefore I Om: Cognitive distortions and coping style as mediators for the effects of mindfulness meditation on anxiety, positive and negative affect, and hope. *Journal of Clinical Psychology, 65,* 1–13.

Sedlmeier, P., Eberth, J., Schwarz, M., Zimmermann, D., Haarig, F., Jaeger, S., & Kunze, S. (2012). The psychological effects of meditation:

A meta-analysis. *Psychological Bulletin, 138* (6),1139–1171.

Seear, K. H., & Vella-Brodrick, D. A. (2012). Efficacy of positive psychology interventions to increase well-being: Examining the role of dispositional mindfulness. *Social Indicators Research.* Advance online publication. doi: 10.1007/s11205-012-0193-7

Segal, Z. V., Williams, J. M. G., & Teasdale, J. D. (2002). *Mindfulness-based cognitive therapy for depression: A new approach to preventing relapse.* New York, NY: Guilford.

Segal, Z. V., Williams, J. M. G., & Teasdale, J. D. (2013). *Mindfulness-based cognitive therapy for depression: A new approach to preventing relapse* (2nd ed.). New York, NY: Guilford.

Seligman, M. E. P. (1999). The president's address. *American Psychologist, 54*, 559–562.

Seligman, M. E. P. (2002). *Authentic happiness: Using the new positive psychology to realize your potential for lasting fulfillment.* New York, NY: Free Press.

Seligman, M. E. P., & Csikszentmihalyi, M. (2000). Positive psychology: An introduction. *American Psychologist, 55*, 5–14.

Seligman, M. E. P, Ernst, M. E., Gillham, J., Reivich, K., & Linkins, M. (2009). Positive education: positive psychology and classroom interventions. *Oxford Review of Education, 35*(3), 293–311.

Seligman, M. E. P., Steen, T. A., Park, N., & Peterson, C. (2005). Positive psychology progress: Empirical validation of interventions. *American Psychologist, 60*, 410–421.

Selvam, S. G. (2012). Character strengths as mediators in a mindfulness based intervention for recovery from addictive behaviour: A study in psychology of religion and positive psychology. Unpublished doctoral dissertation, Heythrop College, University of London, UK. Available at: http://www.sahayaselvam.org/wp-content/uploads/2012/08/Sel_Phd_Public_Aug12.pdf

Semple, R. J., Lee, J., & Miller, L. F. (2006). Mindfulness-based cognitive therapy for children. In R. A. Baer (Ed.), *Mindfulness-based treatment approaches: Clinician's guide to evidence base and applications* (pp. 143–166). Burlington, MA: Academic Press.

Shapira, L. B., & Mongrain, M. (2010). The benefits of self-compassion and optimism exercises for individuals vulnerable to depression. *Journal of Positive Psychology, 5*(5), 377–389.

Shapiro, S. L., Astin, J. A., Bishop, S. R., & Cordova, M. (2005). Mindfulness-based stress reduction for health care professionals: Results from a randomized trial. *International Journal of Stress Management, 12*, 164–176.

Shapiro, S. L., & Carlson, L. E. (2009). *The art and science of mindfulness: Integrating mindfulness into psychology and the helping professions.* Washington, DC: American Psychological Association.

Shapiro, S. L., Jazaieri, H., & Goldin, P. R. (2012). Mindfulness-based stress reduction effects on moral reasoning and decision making. *Journal of Positive Psychology, 7*(6), 504–515.

Shapiro, S. L., & Schwartz, G. E. (2000). The role of intention in self-regulation: Toward intentional systemic mindfulness. In M. Boekaerts, P. R. Pintrich, & M. Zeidner (Eds.), *Handbook of self-regulation* (pp. 253–273). New York, NY: Academic Press.

Shapiro, S. L., Schwartz, G. E. R., & Santerre, C. (2002). Meditation and positive psychology. In C. R. Snyder & S. J. Lopez (Eds.), *Handbook of positive psychology* (pp. 632–645). New York, NY: Oxford University Press.

Shapiro, S. L., Schwartz, G. E. R., & Bonner, G. (1998). The effects of mindfulness-based stress reduction on medical and pre-medical students. *Journal of Behavioral Medicine, 21*, 581–599.

Sheethal, D., Reddy, S. D., Negi, L. T., Dodson-Lavelle, B., Ozawa-de Silva, B., Pace, T. W. W., ... Craighead, L. W. (2013). Cognitive-based compassion training: A promising prevention strategy for at-risk adolescents. *Journal of Child and Family Studies, 22*(2), 219–230.

Sheldon, K. M., & Kasser, T. (1998). Pursuing personal goals: Skills enable progress but not all progress is beneficial. *Personality and Social Psychology Bulletin, 24*, 546–557.

Sheldon, K., & King, L. (2001). Why positive psychology is necessary. *American Psychologist, 56* (3), 216–217.

Sheldon, K. M., & Lyubomirsky, S. (2006). How to increase and sustain positive emotion: the effects of expressing gratitude and visualizing best possible selves. *Journal of Positive Psychology, 1*, 73–82.

Shoshani, A., & Ilanit Aviv, I. (2012). The pillars of strength for first-grade adjustment – Parental and children's character strengths and the transition to elementary school. *Journal of Positive Psychology, 7*(4), 315–326.

Shoshani, A., & Slone, M. (2012). Middle school transition from the strengths perspective: Young adolescents' character strengths, subjective well-being, and school adjustment. *Journal of Happiness Studies.* Advance online publication. doi: 10.1007/s10902-012-9374-y

Siegel, D. J. (2007). *The mindful brain: Reflection and attunement in the cultivation of wellbeing*. New York, NY: Norton.

Siegel, D. J. (2010). *The mindful therapist*. New York, NY: W. W. Norton & Company.

Silberman, J. (2007, March 27). Mindfulness and VIA signature strengths. *Positive Psychology News Daily*. Available at: http://positivepsychologynews.com/news/jordan-silberman/20070327179

Simonton, D. K. (2000). Creativity: Cognitive, developmental, personal, and social aspects. *American Psychologist, 55*, 151–158.

Sirgy, M. J. (1998). Materialism and quality of life. *Social Indicators Research, 43*, 227–260.

Slagter, H. A., Lutz, A., Greishar, L. L., Francis, A. D., Nieuwenhuis, S., Davis, J. M., & Davidson, R. J. (2007). Mental training affects distribution of limited brain resources. *PLoS Biology, 5*(6), e138.

Smallwood, J., Mrazek, M. D., & Schooler, J. W. (2011). Medicine for the wandering mind: Mind wandering in medical practice. *Medical Education, 45* (11), 1072–80.

Smith, E. J. (2006). The strength-based counseling model. *The Counseling Psychologist, 34*(1), 13–79.

So, K., & Orme-Johnson, D. (2001). Three randomized experiments on the longitudinal effects of the transcendental meditation technique on cognition. *Intelligence, 29*(5), 419–440.

Son, V., Jackson, B., Grove, J. R., & Feltz, D. L. (2011). "I am" versus "we are": Effects of distinctive variants of self-talk on efficacy beliefs and motor performance. *Journal of Sports Sciences, 29*, 1417–24. doi: 10.1080/02640414.2011.593186

Sosik, J. J., Gentry, W. A., & Chun, J. A. (2012). The value of virtue in the upper echelons: A multisource examination of executive character strengths and performance. *Leadership Quarterly, 23*, 367–382.

Staats, S., Hupp, J. M., & Hagley, A. M. (2008). Honesty and heroes: A positive psychology view of heroism and academic honesty. *The Journal of Psychology, 142*(4), 357–372.

Steen, T. A., Kachorek, L. V., & Peterson, C. (2003). Character strength among youth. *Journal of Youth & Adolescence, 32*(1), 5–16.

Steindl-Rast, D. (1984). *Gratefulness, the heart of prayer: An approach to life in the fullest*. Ramsey, NJ: Paulist Press.

Stern, D. N. (2004). *The present moment: In psychotherapy and everyday life*. New York, NY: W. W. Norton & Company.

Sugiura, Y. (2004). Detached mindfulness and worry: A meta-cognitive analysis. *Personality and Individual Differences, 37*(1), 169–179.

Surawy, C., Roberts, J., & Silver, A. (2005). The effect of mindfulness training on mood and measures of fatigue, activity, and quality of life in patients with chronic fatigue syndrome on a hospital waiting list: A series of exploratory studies. *Behavioural and Cognitive Psychotherapy, 33*(1), 103–109.

Surya Das, L. (1999). *Awakening to the sacred*. New York, NY: Broadway Books.

Sweet, M. J., & Johnson, C. G. (1990). Enhancing empathy: The interpersonal implications of a Buddhist meditation technique. *Psychotherapy: Theory, Research, Practice, Training, 27*(1), 19–29.

Teasdale, J. D. (1999). Metacognition, mindfulness and the modification of mood disorders. *Clinical Psychology and Psychotherapy, 6*, 146–155.

Teasdale, J. D., Segal, Z. V., Williams, J. M. G., Ridgeway, V. A., Soulsby, J. M., & Lau, M. A. (2000). Prevention of relapse/recurrence in major depression by mindfulness-based cognitive therapy. *Journal of Consulting and Clinical Psychology, 68*(4), 615–623.

Tetlock, P. E. (1986). A value pluralism model of ideological reasoning. *Journal of Personality and Social Psychology, 50*, 819–827.

Tloczynski, J., & Tantriella, M. (1998). A comparison of the effects of Zen breath meditation or relaxation on college adjustment. *Psychologia: An International Journal of Psychology in the Orient, 41*(1), 32–43.

Toner, E., Haslam, N., Robinson, J., & Williams, P. (2012). Character strengths and wellbeing in adolescence: Structure and correlates of the Values in Action Inventory of Strengths for Children. *Personality and Individual Differences, 52*(5), 637–642.

Twohig, M. P., Field, C., Armstrong, A., & Dahl, A. (2010). Acceptance and mindfulness as mechanisms of change in mindfulness-based interventions for children and adolescents. In R. Baer (Ed.), *Assessing mindfulness and acceptance: Illuminating the process of change* (pp. 225–250). Oakland, CA: New Harbinger.

Vaillant, G. E. (2008). *Spiritual evolution*. New York, NY: Broadway.

Vettese, L. C., Toneatto, T., Stea, J. N., Nguyen, L., & Wang, J. J. (2009). Do mindfulness meditation participants do their homework and does it make a difference? A review of the empirical evidence. *Journal of Cognitive Psychotherapy: An International Quarterly, 23*(3), 198–225.

Wallace, B. A., & Hodel, B. (2008). *Embracing mind: The common ground of science & spirituality*. Boston, MA: Shambhala Publications.

Wallace, B. A., & Shapiro, S. L. (2006). Mental balance and well-being: Building bridges between Buddhism and Western psychology. *American Psychologist, 61*(7), 690–701.

Walsh, R. (1999). *Essential spirituality: The 7 central practices to awaken heart and mind.* New York, NY: John Wiley & Sons.

Wansink, B. (2006). *Mindless eating: Why we eat more than we think.* New York, NY: Bantam-Dell.

Wayment, H. A., & Bauer, J. J. (Eds.). (2008). *Transcending self-interest: Psychological explorations of the quiet ego.* Washington, DC: American Psychological Association.

Wayment, H. A., Wiist, B., Sullivan, B. M., & Warren, M. A. (2011). Doing and being: Mindfulness, health, and quiet ego characteristics among Buddhist practitioners. *Journal of Happiness Studies, 12*, 575–589.

Webb, J. R., Phillips, T. D., Bumgarner, D., & Conway-Williams, E. (2012). Forgiveness, mindfulness, and health. *Mindfulness.* Advance online publication. doi: 10.1007/s12671-012-0119-0

Weber, M., & Ruch, W. (2012a). The role of character strengths in adolescent romantic relationships: An initial study on partner selection and mates' life satisfaction. *Journal of Adolescence, 35*(6), 1537–1546.

Weber, M., & Ruch, W. (2012b). The role of a good character in 12-year-old school children: Do character strengths matter in the classroom? *Child Indicators Research, 5*(2), 317–334.

Whelton, W. J. (2004). Emotional processes in psychotherapy: Evidence across therapeutic modalities. *Clinical Psychology and Psychotherapy, 11*, 58–67.

Whitmore, J. (2002). *Coaching for performance: GROWing people, performance and purpose.* London, UK: Nicholas Brealey.

Williams, J. C., & Lynn, S. J. (2010–2011). Acceptance: An historical and conceptual review. *Imagination, Cognition, and Personality, 30*(1), 5–56.

Williams, J. M. G., Teasdale, J. D., Segal, Z. V., & Kabat-Zinn, J. (2007) *The mindful way through depression: Freeing yourself from chronic unhappiness.* New York, NY: Guilford.

Wilson, K., Sandoz, E. K., Flynn, M. K., Slater, R. M., & DuFrene, T. (2010). Understanding, assessing, and treating values processes in mindfulness- and acceptance-based therapies. In R. A. Baer (Ed.), *Assessing mindfulness & acceptance processes in clients: Illuminating the theory and practice of change* (pp. 77–106). Oakland, CA: New Harbinger.

Winbush, N. Y., Gross, C. R., & Kreitzer, M. J. (2007). The effects of mindfulness-based stress reduction on sleep disturbance: A systematic review. *Explore, 3*(6), 585.

Wisniewski, L., & Kelly, E. (2003). Can DBT be used to effectively treat eating disorders? *Cognitive and Behavioral Practice, 10*, 131–138.

Witvliet, C. V. O., DeYoung, N. J., Hofelich, A. J., & DeYoung, P. A. (2011). Compassionate reappraisal and emotional suppression as alternatives to offense-focused rumination: Implications for forgiveness and psychophysiological well-being. *Journal of Positive Psychology, 6*(4), 286–299.

Witvliet, C. V. O., Knoll, R. W., Hinman, N. G., & DeYoung, P. A. (2010). Compassion-focused reappraisal, benefit-focused reappraisal, and rumination after an interpersonal offense: Emotion-regulation implications for subjective emotion, linguistic responses, and physiology. *Journal of Positive Psychology, 5*(3), 226–242.

Wolever, R. Q., Bobinet, K. J., McCabe, K., Mackenzie, E. R., Fekete, E., Kusnick, C. A., & Baime, M. (2012). Effective and viable mind-body stress reduction in the workplace: A randomized controlled trial. *Journal of Occupational Health Psychology, 17*, 246–258.

Wong, Y. J. (2006). A strength-centered therapy: A social constructionist, virtues-based psychotherapy. *Psychotherapy: Theory, Research, Practice, Training, 43*, 133–146.

Wood, A. M., Linley, P. A., Maltby, J., Kashdan, T. B., & Hurling, R. (2011). Using personal and psychological strengths leads to increases in well-being over time: A longitudinal study and the development of the strengths use questionnaire. *Personality and Individual Differences, 50*, 15–19.

World Health Organization. (1990). *International classification of diseases and related health problems* (10th rev. ed.). Geneva, Switzerland: Author.

Worthington, E. L. (2007). *Humility: The quiet virtue.* Philadelphia, PA: Templeton Foundation Press.

Yamada, K., & Victor, T. L. (2012). The impact of mindful awareness practices on college student health, well-being, and capacity for learning: A pilot study. *Psychology Learning & Teaching, 11*(2), 139–145.

Yapko, M. D. (2011). *Mindfulness and hypnosis: The power of suggestion to transform experience.* New York, NY: W. W. Norton & Company.

Yeager, J. M., Fisher, S. W., & Shearon, D. N. (2011). *Smart strengths: Building character, resilience and relationships in youth.* New York, NY: Kravis Publishing.

Yearley, L. H. (1990). *Mencius and Aquinas: Theories of virtue and conceptions of courage.* Albany, NY: State University of New York Press.

Young-Eisendrath, P. (1996). *The resilient spirit: Transforming suffering into insight and renewal.* Reading, MA: Addison-Wesley Publishing.

Zeidan, F., Gordon, N. S., Merchant, J., & Goolkasian, P. (2010). The effects of brief mindfulness meditation training on experimentally induced pain. *Journal of Pain, 11*(3), 199–209.

Zgierska, A., Rabago, D., Chawla, N., Kushner, K., Koehler, R., & Marlatt, A. (2009). Mindfulness meditation for substance use disorders: A systematic review. *Substance Abuse, 30*(4), 266–294.

Zhang, L., Layne, C., Lowder, T., & Liu, J. (2012). A review focused on the psychological effectiveness of tai chi on different populations. *Evidenced-Based Complementary and Alternative Medicine.* doi:10.1155/2012/678107.

Index

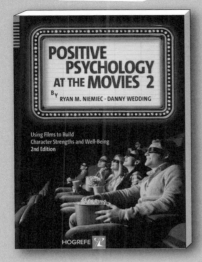
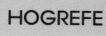